Ovarian Cancer: Translational Research

Ovarian Cancer: Translational Research

Editor: Susan Conway

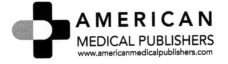

AMERICAN
MEDICAL PUBLISHERS
www.americanmedicalpublishers.com

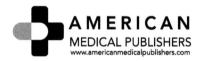

AMERICAN
MEDICAL PUBLISHERS
www.americanmedicalpublishers.com

Cataloging-in-Publication Data

Ovarian cancer : translational research / edited by Susan Conway.
    p. cm.
Includes bibliographical references and index.
ISBN 978-1-63927-777-3
1. Ovaries--Cancer. 2. Ovaries--Cancer--Research. 3. Ovaries--Cancer--Diagnosis.
4. Ovaries--Cancer--Treatment. 5. Ovaries--Diseases. I. Conway, Susan.
RC280.O8 O933 2023
616.994 65--dc23

American Medical Publishers,
41 Flatbush Avenue,
1st Floor, New York,
NY 11217, USA

ISBN 978-1-63927-777-3 (Hardback)

Contents

Preface..VII

Chapter 1   **The Communication between the PI3K/AKT/mTOR Pathway and Y-Box Binding Protein-1 in Gynecological Cancer**..1
Monika Sobočan, Suzana Bračič, Jure Knez, Iztok Takač and Johannes Haybaeck

Chapter 2   **Zoledronic Acid Abrogates Restraint Stress-Induced Macrophage Infiltration, PDGF-AA Expression and Ovarian Cancer Growth**..19
Claudia B. Colon-Echevarria, Tatiana Ortiz, Lizette Maldonado, Melanie J. Hidalgo-Vargas, Jaileene Pérez-Morales, Alexandra N. Aquino-Acevedo, Roberto Herrera-Noriega, Margarita Bonilla-Claudio, Eida M. Castro and Guillermo N. Armaiz-Pena

Chapter 3   **The Tumor Microenvironment of Epithelial Ovarian Cancer and its Influence on Response to Immunotherapy**..35
Galaxia M. Rodriguez, Kristianne J. C. Galpin, Curtis W. McCloskey and Barbara C. Vanderhyden

Chapter 4   **The Role of Inflammation and Inflammatory Mediators in the Development, Progression, Metastasis and Chemoresistance of Epithelial Ovarian Cancer**..64
Sudha S. Savant, Shruthi Sriramkumar and Heather M. O'Hagan

Chapter 5   **Ovarian Tumor Microenvironment Signaling: Convergence on the Rac1 GTPase**..94
Laurie G. Hudson, Jennifer M. Gillette, Huining Kang, Melanie R. Rivera and Angela Wandinger-Ness

Chapter 6   **The Endometriotic Tumor Microenvironment in Ovarian Cancer**..120
Jillian R. Hufgard Wendel, Xiyin Wang and Shannon M. Hawkins

Chapter 7   **The Impact of Mesothelin in the Ovarian Cancer Tumor Microenvironment**..149
Tyvette S. Hilliard

Chapter 8   **Can Stemness and Chemoresistance be Therapeutically Targeted via Signaling Pathways in Ovarian Cancer?**..162
Lynn Roy and Karen D. Cowden Dahl

Chapter 9   **Cancer Associated Fibroblasts: Naughty Neighbors that Drive Ovarian Cancer Progression**..185
Subramanyam Dasari, Yiming Fang and Anirban K. Mitra

Chapter 10   **Targeting the Microenvironment in High Grade Serous Ovarian Cancer**..203
Nkechiyere G. Nwani, Livia E. Sima, Wilberto Nieves-Neira and Daniela Matei

Permissions

List of Contributors

Index

Preface

It is often said that books are a boon to mankind. They document every progress and pass on the knowledge from one generation to the other. They play a crucial role in our lives. Thus I was both excited and nervous while editing this book. I was pleased by the thought of being able to make a mark but I was also nervous to do it right because the future of students depends upon it. Hence, I took a few months to research further into the discipline, revise my knowledge and also explore some more aspects. Post this process, I begun with the editing of this book.

Ovarian cancer is a gynecologic malignancy in which the development of cancer cells occurs in the ovaries. The cells reproduce rapidly and have the ability to infiltrate and impair healthy body tissue. Majority of the times ovarian cancers are diagnosed at an advanced stage and traditional treatments provide minimal improvements in overall survival. Tumor heterogeneity and clonal evolution in ovarian cancer can be critical with respect to drug resistance. Hence, liquid biopsies become necessary for monitoring cancer development. The complexity of ovarian cancer, as compared to other solid cancers, makes the development of alternative targeted therapies a difficult and time consuming process. Antiangiogenic medications have been proven to be effective in the treatment of ovarian cancer with modest patient outcomes. This book unfolds the translational researches on ovarian cancer, which will be crucial for the progress of the study of this medical condition in the future. It consists of contributions made by international experts. The readers would gain knowledge that would broaden their perspective on this medical condition as well as its treatment.

I thank my publisher with all my heart for considering me worthy of this unparalleled opportunity and for showing unwavering faith in my skills. I would also like to thank the editorial team who worked closely with me at every step and contributed immensely towards the successful completion of this book. Last but not the least, I wish to thank my friends and colleagues for their support.

Editor

The Communication between the PI3K/AKT/mTOR Pathway and Y-Box Binding Protein-1 in Gynecological Cancer

Monika Sobočan [1,2,3,*] ⓘ, Suzana Bračič [4,5], Jure Knez [2,3] ⓘ, Iztok Takač [2,3] and Johannes Haybaeck [6,7,8]

1. Department of Pharmacology, Faculty of Medicine, University of Maribor, 2000 Maribor, Slovenia
2. Divison of Gynecology and Perinatology, University Medical Centre Maribor, 2000 Maribor, Slovenia; knez.jure@gmail.com (J.K.); iztok.takac@ukc-mb.si (I.T.)
3. Department of Obstetrics and Gynecology, Faculty of Medicine, University of Maribor, 2000 Maribor, Slovenia
4. Department of Pathology, Hospital Graz II, West, 8020 Graz, Austria; suzy.bracic@gmail.com
5. Department of Pathology, Faculty of Medicine, University of Maribor, 2000 Maribor, Slovenia
6. Department of Pathology, Medical Faculty Otto-von-Guericke University Magdeburg, 39120 Magdeburg, Germany; johannes.haybaeck@med.ovgu.de
7. Department of Pathology, Neuropathology and Molecular Pathology, Medical University of Innsbruck, 6020 Innsbruck, Austria
8. Diagnostic and Research Institute of Pathology, Medical University of Graz, 8036 Graz, Austria
* Correspondence: monika.sobocan@gmail.com

Abstract: Studies of the mechanistic (mammalian) target of rapamycin inhibitors (mTOR) represent a step towards the targeted treatment of gynecological cancers. It has been shown that women with increased levels of mTOR signaling pathway targets have worse prognosis compared to women with normal mTOR levels. Yet, targeting mTOR alone has led to unsatisfactory outcomes in gynecological cancer. The aim of our review was therefore to provide an overview of the most recent clinical results and basic findings on the interplay of mTOR signaling and cold shock proteins in gynecological malignancies. Due to their oncogenic activity, there are promising data showing that mTOR and Y-box-protein 1 (YB-1) dual targeting improves the inhibition of carcinogenic activity. Although several components differentially expressed in patients with ovarian, endometrial, and cervical cancer of the mTOR were identified, there are only a few investigated downstream actors in gynecological cancer connecting them with YB-1. Our analysis shows that YB-1 is an important player impacting AKT as well as the downstream actors interacting with mTOR such as epidermal growth factor receptor (EGFR), Snail or E-cadherin.

Keywords: mTOR signaling; YB-1; endometrial cancer; ovarian cancer; cervical cancer

1. Introduction

Malignancies of the endometrium, cervix, and ovaries represent the most common gynecological malignancies. It is a particular challenge to treat these cancers at advanced disease stages or at the time of recurrence. Several attempts have already been made to target signaling pathways in order to improve the overall survival (OS) and progress-free survival (PFS) of women with gynecological malignancies. One approach towards targeted treatment is the use of a mechanistic (mammalian) target of rapamycin (mTOR) inhibitors [1]. The current level of knowledge is that the outcomes for women with gynecological cancer and elevated levels of mTOR signaling pathway targets seem to be significantly worse than those for women with normal mTOR levels [2]. Significantly increased levels of mTOR resulted in poorly differentiated tumors and correlated positively with lymph node involvement. If nuclear mTOR expression was increased, the PFS rate was also lower. However, the overexpression of mTOR or protein kinase B (more commonly referred to as Akt) was not associated with specific histological subtype features of the tumor [3]. This led to the development and clinical testing of mTOR inhibitors in gynecological cancers. However, in gynecological cancers, the success of the clinical trials was limited [1]. Therefore, an investigation of different processes involved in tumor development and progression interacting with the mTOR pathway is warranted. One possibility of such an interaction is the interplay between cold shock proteins, one of the most evolutionary conserved proteins [4], and the mTOR pathway. This review addresses recent advances made in the study of aberrations and triggers of the mTOR signaling pathway in gynecological malignancies in the context of their interaction with cold shock proteins, thus allowing us to better understand the stratification of patients undergoing mTOR therapy and future disease prediction.

Cold shock proteins (CSP) are a family of proteins where Y-box binding protein-1 (YB-1) is one of the best characterized proteins [5]. An important feature of CSP is their presence in one or more cold shock domains (CSD). The domains possess nucleic acid binding properties and thus function pleiotropically in processes such as transcription, translation, and cell proliferation [4,6]. In humans, YB-1 represents the predominant form of CSP. It functions in the nucleus as a transcription factor as well as in the cytoplasm where it directly interacts with mRNA splicing and the storage of mRNA. By binding to internal ribosomal entry sites (IRES), YB-1 impacts the translation in Snail, Twist, and HIF1alpha and effects the epithelial mesenchymal transition (EMT) [6]. Recent studies in colorectal cancer showed that combining strategies of silencing a dual target, YB-1 through the inhibition of p90 ribosomal S6 kinase (RSK) and Akt, lead to improved sensitivity to standard systemic therapy [7]. This warrants the attempt to connect and understand the impactful molecular mechanisms behind the signaling.

2. Clinical Investigation into mTOR Signaling and Inhibition in Women with Gynecological Cancers

2.1. Endometrial Cancer

Endometrial cancer (EC) is the most frequently diagnosed gynecological malignancy [8]. It mostly consists of type I tumors, characterized as endometrioid adenocarcinomas or, in rare occasions, as mucinous carcinomas. These tumors are low-grade and estrogen-related tumors. This is in contrast to type II non-endometrioid carcinomas, which are histologically serous or clear cell carcinomas, and are unrelated to estrogen. Type II EC also behaves more aggressively [8,9]. To stratify patients, one of the emerging markers connecting a personalized prognosis for women with endometrial EC is the presence of the nuclear p-Ser167-Era, an estrogen receptor that interacts with the mitogen-activated protein kinase (MAPK) and mTOR pathway. Patients with positively stained p-Ser167-Era had a shorter recurrence-free survival (RFS), and p-Ser167-Era was positively correlated with pS6K1 and pMAPK staining [10]. Against the background of a growing understanding of mTOR signaling, trials investigating mTOR inhibitors in EC have been conducted in recent years. The inhibition of mTOR was used as monotherapy or as a combination therapy with other substances, whose focus is the determination of different targets in the mTOR signaling pathway. The most common therapy trials in EC are carried out using mammalian target of rapamycin complex 1 (mTORC1) inhibitors (temsirolimus, everolimus) as well as mTORC1/2 inhibitors (AZD2014), AKT inhibitors (AZD5363, MIK2206, GSK2141795), and dual mTOR/AKT inhibitors (MKC1) [11]. Interestingly very scarce literature is available on the expression of YB-1 in endometrial tissue or EC. Silvera et al. [12] found, that, in patients with endometriosis, in comparison to patients without endometriosis, there are high levels of YB-1 expression present. A knockdown of YB-1 resulted in cell growth inhibition, a cessation of YB-1 proliferation and an increase in apoptosis [12]. To the best of our knowledge, there is currently no published research investigating the role ob YB-1 and mTOR signaling in EC.

2.2. Cervical Cancer

Cervical cancer (CC) is the fourth leading cause of cancer-related deaths in women. Although the number of deaths caused by CC has decreased, especially in countries implementing screening programs, the prognosis for patients affected by this disease is still poor [13]. The different CC subtypes show significant differences as regards the clinical aspects and biology. Clinically, squamous cell carcinomas (SCC) account for the majority of cervical tumors. As far as their incidence is concerned, adenocarcinomas in CC follow in second place. They account for approximately 10–20% of all CC cases, and their incidence is increasing [9]. Considering its development, CC is a multifactorial disease related to HPV (human papilloma virus), tumor suppressor genes, oncogenes, and others [14]. It is driven by different molecular mechanisms that are not yet fully understood. The mTOR signaling pathway is assumed to be one of those mechanisms. A study investigating mTOR signaling of cervical cancer cell lines revealed high mTOR activity in CC [15]. Immunohistochemical analysis of the mTOR pathway markers phosphorylated-mTOR (p-mTOR), p-p70S6K, and EGFR revealed a highly positive expression in high grade squamous intraepithelial lesions (HSIL) and all SCC stains. Especially SCCs showed increased nuclear translocation of p-mTOR and p-p70S6K in all cases and in most HSIL cases [16]. A few trials have evaluated the value of mTOR inhibitors in CC. These trials used mTORC1 inhibitors (everolimus or trials including temsirolimus) [17]. Nishio et al [5] explored YB-1 overexpression in cervical cancer. It was shown, that YB-1 expression correlated with epidermal growth factor receptor (EGFR) overexpression, human epidermal growth factor receptor 2 (HER2) overexpression, and worse OS [5]. Research on the clinical impact of YB-1 showed that, in patients with overexpressed YB-1, chemoradiosensitivity was decreased [18]. This might be due to the interaction of YB-1 with HPV18 E6 mRNA regulation [19].

2.3. Ovarian Cancer

Different subtypes and clinicopathological features are even more evident in ovarian cancer (OC) [9,20]. The classification of ovarian carcinomas is based on the histological differentiation of the tumors according to the World Health Organization (WHO). Tumors are divided into epithelial, sex cord-stromal, and germ cell neoplasms. The tumors with the highest incidence of ovarian carcinoma are epithelial ovarian tumors. They are subdivided into serous, mucinous, endometrioid, clear cell and transitional cell tumors (inclusive of Brenner tumors) [20]. The understanding of carcinogenesis in OC is currently based on a model that divides OC in two groups: (i) Type I: low-grade serous, endometrioid, clear cell, mucinous carcinoma, and Brenner tumors and (ii) Type II: high grade serous, high-grade endometrioid, undifferentiated carcinomas, and mixed mesodermal tumors. The slow-growing type I tumors can turn into Type II tumors over time [20]. As in endometrial cancer, targets of mTOR inhibitors in ovarian carcinoma are in most cases the mTORC1 complex, as well as the mTORC1/2 complex inhibitor in combination with AKT inhibition [11]. Molecular studies found no specific mTOR target that pointed to statistically significant clinical outcomes for patients treated with common mTOR inhibitors IND160A and IND160B (temsirolimus) as well as IND192 (ridaforolimus) [21]. YB-1 has been proposed to be an oncogene for OC for more than a decade. It has been connected to promote tumor growth and multi drug resistance through interaction with genes and growth factors [12]. In exploring the possibility of determining YB-1 in serum samples, it was further shown that a decreased level of YB-1/p18 correlated with ovarian cancer compared to the control group of healthy volunteers. This initially contradictory data can be understood as the formation of homodimers and multimer-formation in the extracellular space, and as such leads to lower levels of YB-1/p18 in OC patients [22].

2.4. Ongoing Clinical Trials

Current ongoing trials investigating the role of different mTOR pathway inhibitors are depicted in Table 1. The current clinical trials use the knowledge on signaling pathways in gynecological cancer and combine inhibition in most cases of at least two pathways. This is particularly illustrated in NCT01596140 where the trial is investigating the inhibition of the B-Raf/MEK step on the mitogen activated protein kinase/extracellular signal-related kinase (B-Raf/MEK/ERK) pathway through vemurafenib and the mTOR pathway through everolimus or temsirolimus. Some clinical trials have moved to the investigation of molecular targeted therapy for mTOR using the alterations in the mTOR signaling pathway as landmarks for patient selection (e.g., NCT02029001 or NCT02465060). However, to our current knowledge there are no clinical trials investigating YB-1 as a marker in gynecological cancer. However, knowledge is emerging that momelotinib (CYT387), a pharmacological inhibitor of noncanonical IkB kinase/TANK-binding kinase 1 (IKBKE/TBK1) which is used in acute myeloid leukemia, might be able to regulate tumor MYC-dependent survival through YB-1 [9,23]. This opens new pathways of investigation for the enhancement of current mTOR inhibition or YB-1 regulation.

Table 1. Ongoing clinical trials * involving mTOR in gynecological cancer.

Target	Therapeutic Agent	Carcinoma	Trial Drug Design	Reg. Nr.
mTORC1	everolimus	EC	Everolimus (RAD001) and Letrozole or Hormonal Therapy	NCT02228681
		Atypical hyperplasia or FIGO stage IA EC	Levonorgestrel-Releasing Intrauterine System with or without Everolimus	NCT02397083
		OC, EC, CC	Patients with alterations in PIK3CA, PIK3R1, AKT1, AKT2, mTOR, RICTOR, RAPTOR genes, or with TSC1, TSC2 or PTEN loss for maintenance therapy	NCT02029001
	everolimus temsirolimus	Advanced OC	Vemurafenib in Combination with Everolimus or Temsirolimus	NCT01596140
	sirolimus	Stage II-IV OC	The effects of TRICOM vaccine with sirolimus	NCT01536054
mTORC1/2	Vistusertib (AZD2014)	HR positive EC	AZD2014 and anastrozole vs. anastrozole alone	NCT02730923
	Sapanisertib MLN0128	EC and other solid tumors	Single experimental arm: bevacizumab and MLN0128	NCT02142803
	Sapanisertib MLN0128	EC, OC	Patients with mTOR mutation receive sapanisertib as a single experimental arm	NCT02465060
AKT inhibitors	miransertib ARQ 092	OC, CC, EC	ARQ 092 + paclitaxel or ARQ 092 + anastrozole	NCT02476955
PI3K inhibition	Copanlisib Hydrochloride	CC, OC, EC	Patients with a PI3K or a PTEN mutation receive copanlisib	NCT02465060
	GSK2636771	CC, OC, EC	Patients with a PTEN mutation/expression/loss	NCT02465060
Dual PI3K/mTOR inhibition	Gedatolisib PF-05212384	EC and other solid tumors	Single experimental arm: palbociclib and gedatolisib	NCT03065062
mTORC1/2 vs. AKT inhibition	vistusertib AZD2014 vs. capivasertib AZD5363	Recurrent EC or OC	(olaparib, vistusertib) vs. (olaparib, capivasertib)	NCT02208375
Dual Akt/ERK inhibition	ONC201	Recurrent or metastatic EC	Single experimental arm: ONC201 treatment	NCT03099499

* accurate data as of 3rd January 2020. Abbreviations: EC: endometrial cancer, OC: ovarian cancer, CC: cervical cancer, HR: hormone receptor; mTORC1: mammalian target of rapamycin complex 1, AKT: protein kinase B, PI3K: Phosphoinositide 3-kinase, mTOR: mammalian target of rapamycin.

3. The PI3K/AKT/mTOR Impact on Molecular Pathophysiology of Gynecological Cancer

3.1. PI3K/AKT/mTOR Pathway

The phosphoinositide 3-kinases/protein kinase B/mammalian target of rapamycin (PI3K/AKT/mTOR) pathway is a signaling pathway long known to be present in the normal cell physiology and oncogenesis [2]. It regulates cell growth and cell cycle progression through growth stimuli and signal integration [9]. The cascade is frequently hyperactivated in several cancer subtypes [24]. Factors dysregulating the pathway, such as increased growth factor stimuli, mutation activation, loss of gene function, or kinase gene activation, contribute to aberrant signaling, leading to carcinogenic events [9]. Studies have shown that the dysregulation of mTOR pathway influences the process of carcinogenesis in many cancers, such as ovarian cancer, lung cancer, prostate cancer, and mantle cell lymphoma [15].

The PI3K/AKT/mTOR pathway consists of three driving molecules: (i) PI3K, a member of the lipid kinase family that phosphorylates the 3-hydroxyl group of phosphoinositide; (ii) AKT, a serine/threonine kinase; and (iii) the mTOR [2]. The mechanism of action starts with the stimulation of the PI3K through growth factors, which leads to activation of the cascade by the phosphorylation of phosphatidylinositol-4,5-bis-phosphate (PIP2) to develop phosphatidylinositol-3,4,5-triphosphate (PIP3). Once PIP3 is accumulated, the cascade events start to unfold. Activation starts by the phosphorylation of AKT through phosphoinositide-dependent kinase-1 (PDK1) [9]. AKT then phosphorylates and inhibits the tuberous sclerosis complex (TSC), influencing the inhibition effect of Ras-related small GTPase Rheb (Ras-homolog-enriched-in-brain). This leads to the positive up-stream regulation of mTOR, which is an atypical serine/threonine kinase that belongs to the PIKK (phosphoinositide 3-kinase related protein kinase) family [9,25]. Only one mTOR gene has been identified in mammalian cells. mTOR is activated in coordination with other protein complexes [6,7]. It functions as a catalytic subunit of two protein kinase complexes, referred to as mTORC1 and mTORC2 [26]. mTORC1 activation is associated with the Regulatory-associated protein of mTOR (RAPTOR), the regulatory-associated protein of mTOR. This leads to the phosphorylation of the eukaryotic translation initiation factor (4E-BP1) and the ribosomal protein kinase 1 (S6K1). Downstream, the mechanism of action therefore initiates protein synthesis, such as cell cycle proteins, vascular endothelial growth factor (VEGF), or c-Myc [9]. The complex mTORC2 is different from mTORC1 since it is not sensitive to rapamycin. It participates in cell survival and proliferation by its ability to control AKT activity through the phosphorylation of AKT at serine-473 [2].

3.2. mTORC1 and mTORC2 Complexes in Gynecological Malignancies

Montero et al. [27] investigated the function of mTORC1 and mTORC2 in ovarian cancer cell proliferation. Through the knockdown of RAPTOR or rapamycin-insensitive companion of mammalian target of rapamycin (RICTOR), they found that, compared to mTORC2, mTORC1 played a predominant role in ovarian cancer. The inhibition was visible on the level of S6 phosphorylation, a marker of mTORC1 function [27]. Interestingly, rapamycin had a small effect on 4E-BP1, another substrate of mTORC1 [27]. Noske et al. then further investigated [28] the overexpression of p-eIF-4E (56%) in primary ovarian carcinomas in a comparison to borderline tumors. They found that p-mTOR expression correlated with p-eIF-4E and the serous histological type. The increased p-mTOR and p-eIF-4E values were correlated with a higher mitotic rate ($p = 0.004$) and with poor differentiation ($p = 0.04$). Recent studies have tried to gain a deeper understanding of the role of mTORC2 in carcinogenesis. Liu et al. therefore explored the role of Sin1 in mTORC2 complex and found that phosphorylation of AKT or S6K was a prerequisite for the Sin1 activation of mTORC2 [29]. Especially 4E-BP seemed promising as a marker for mTOR signaling inhibition as it was previously implied, that 4EBP and p70S6 kinase communicate and inhibit the oncogene YB-1. However, studies by Lyabin and Ovchinnikov [30] on the inhibition of YB-1 synthesis through rapamycin showed, that inhibition produced no effect on YB-1 synthesis in CC cell lines as well as no effect on translation. It was suggested that previously visible inhibition of YB-1 mRNA was not specifically due to targeted interaction on 4E-BP, but to a dependence of YB-1 mRNA on the eIF4F-group factors. Thus, once inhibition targeted eIF4F and impacted mRNA availability, this also downregulated YB-1 mRNA [30].

3.3. Metabolic Impact on Carcinogenesis by mTOR

Using a well-established phosphatase and tensin homologue (PTEN) knockout model, Iglesias and colleagues found that in endometrial hyperplasia (EH), obesity or lean body weight in mouse models did not affect the development of EH. There was no significant difference between lean and obese mice in the progression of normal endometrium to EH, nor were there any significant differences in the alteration of the mTOR pathway [31]. Studies have associated higher body mass index (BMI) with EC for a long time. To understand this mechanism on a molecular level, Sahoo and colleagues examined the effects of adipocyte-conditioned medium (ACM) on EC cell lines in a comparison with pre-adipocyte-conditioned medium (PACM). They found that in ACM, the vascular endothelial growth factor (VEGF), a downstream signaling pathway connected to the mTOR pathway, was upregulated. This correlates with the finding that mTOR pathway upregulation leads to larger EC tumors [32]. Zhu et al. report that the clinical outcome of EC is influenced by the expression of fat mass and the obesity-associated gene (FTO). Using immunohistochemistry and Western blotting, they observed that obese women with endometrial cancer showed estrogen (ERα-dependent)-induced FTO nuclear accumulation in the mTOR signaling pathway, which contributed to worse clinical outcomes [33]. In vitro tests carried out to determine the cell response to glucose in terms of cytotoxicity, apoptosis, cell cycle and adhesion/invasion revealed increased cell growth in the presence of high glucose levels. The behavior of EC cells was dependent on the level of glucose and influenced adhesion and invasion. E-Cadherin expression was decreased, while Snail expression was increased. The adenosine monophosphate-activated protein kinase/(AMPK)/mTOR/S6 and mitogen-activated protein kinase (MAPK) pathway was affected by upregulation of glucose metabolism [34]. A downregulation of E-cad with a Snail upregulation is considered to be a hallmark of EMT [19].

3.4. Carcinogenesis in Presence and Absence of HPV

It is increasingly recognized that HPV oncoproteins E6 and E7 induce the process of carcinogenesis not only by affecting p53 and pRb, but also by molecular events in mTOR signaling [35]. In Figure 1, the cascade of mTOR signaling in coordination with the human papilloma virus (HPV) E6 is shown. This protein expression was shown by Pang et al [19] to regulate the levels of mRNA expression of YB-1 and by this promoting the progression of CC: The mechanism is based on the observations that E6 promoted enhanced expression of Snail [19]. Further on, studies investigating oncogenic protein RAS show that by the background expression of E6 E7, transformation of human cervical keratinocytes (HCK) is initiated, and that MYC and HRAS-oncogene are critical stakeholders in tumorigenic transformation. Increased levels of MYC lead to an increase in survivin and p-4EBP1 levels, as well as in p70S6K levels, but to decreased Tuberous Sclerosis Complex 2 (TSC2) levels [36]. Molinolo et al. compared the expression of pS6 and Akt^{S473} in HPV-positive and HPV-negative oral and cervical squamous cancers. They found that while stable HPV infections had no particular impact on proliferation, the presence of p16, a staining marker for the E6 HPV oncoprotein, triggered the degradation of TSC2, a downstream target of mTORC1. Further investigations then showed that mTOR inhibitors had a particular effect on mTORC1 signaling pathway in SCC, but access to the mTORC2 pathway was limited.

Studies using a model of LKB1 deficiency have shown that carcinogenesis is influenced not only by HPV oncogene initiation of mTOR pathway overexpression, but also plays an important role in the initiation of the pathway [37]. Furthermore, phosphoacidic acid (PA), a product of phospholipase D (PLD), has been shown to be required for the activation of mTORC1 through mitogen and amino acid signaling, and to be able to intervene independently with DEP Domain Containing MTOR Interacting Protein (DEPTOR), the mTOR protein for mTORC1 and mTORC2 inhibition. This cascade of E7-based initiation of carcinogenesis is known to contribute to AKT activation in in vivo experiments [38].

A smaller proportion of CC pathologies are unrelated to the presence of high-risk HPV. A histological subtype unrelated to the HPV carcinogenesis initiation is the clear cell cervical carcinoma (CCCC). A small study investigated the impact of autophosphorylation of EGFR, HER2, p-mTOR, and pAKT and its contribution to downstream pathways of the four core protein kinases (RAS/RAF/MEK/ERK) and to the PI3K/AKT/mTOR pathway. All cases of CCCC showed increased expression of EGFR, HER2, AKT or mTOR [39]. This is especially interesting as the overexpression of EGFR and HER2 was associated with YB-1 overexpression enabling us to further hypothesize the underlying linkage between HPV and YB-1. However, mTOR signaling activation was also shown to be activated in the absence of E6 or p53 under the influence of the transcriptional factor PPARbeta. It was shown that PPARbeta acts as an agonist for VEGF in CC cell lines and did not require target nuclear receptors for higher levels of VEGF mRNA [40].

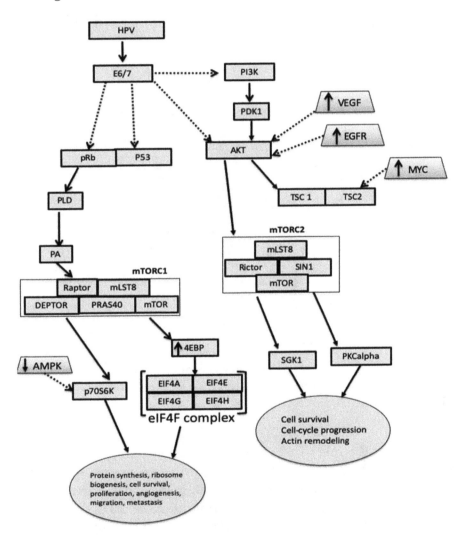

Figure 1. A simplistic model of the mTOR signaling pathway in cervical cancer. Abbreviations: EIF: eukaryotic initiation factor, AMPK: adenosine monophosphate-activated protein kinase, PKCalpha: Protein kinase C-alpha, SGK1: serum and glucocorticoid-regulated kinase 1, 4EBP: Eukaryotic translation initiation factor 4E-binding protein 1, mTOR: mammalian target of rapamycin, SIN1: mammalian stress-activated protein kinase interacting protein 1, Rictor: Rapamycin-insensitive companion of mammalian target of rapamycin, mTORC1: rapamycin-sensitive mTOR-Raptor, mTORC2: rapamycin-insensitive mTOR-Rictor, mLST8: target of rapamycin complex subunit LST8, Raptor: regulatory-associated protein of mTOR, PRAS40: roline-rich Akt substrate of 40 kDa, PA: phosphatidic acid, PLD: phospholipase D, pRb: retinoblastoma protein, HPV: Human Papilloma Virus, PI3K: phosphoinositide 3-kinase, PDK1: Pyruvate Dehydrogenase Kinase 1, Akt: Protein kinase B, VEGF: Vascular endothelial growth factor, EGFR: epidermal growth factor receptor, TSC: Tuberous sclerosis 1.

3.5. Growth Factors in mTOR Dysregulation

A group of effectors triggering gynecological cancer development through the mTOR pathway can be identified as growth factors. Especially the epidermal growth factor receptor (EGFR) overexpression has been connected to a more aggressive tumor behavior [41]. Nishio et al [5] reported especially an important correlation of the EGFR overexpression with YB-1 expression in cervical cancer. As depicted in Figure 2, the overexpression of EGFR was connected with worse OS in patients. Additionally, VEGF (vascular endothelial growth factor) [42], IGF (insulin like growth factor) [43], GDF-15 (growth differentiation factor 15) [44] and CYR61 (cysteine rich protein 61) were involved in influencing the mTOR signaling pathway [45].

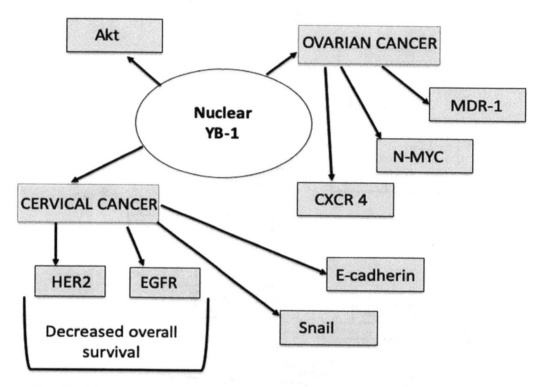

Figure 2. Identified downstream targets of YB-1 in gynecological cancer. Abbreviations: YB-1: Y box binding protein 1, HER2: human epidermal growth factor receptor 2, EGFR: epidermal growth factor receptor, CXCR4: chemokine receptor type 4, MDR-1: multidrug resistance mutation 1, AKT: Protein kinase B.

Early investigations on the role of VEGF in epithelial OC showed that the VEGF-A receptor (VEGFR2) upregulation especially was connected with the overexpression of pS6. The interplay between VEGFR2 activation and pS6 activation led to an increased incidence of ascites, and reduced the response to the standard chemotherapy [42]. By inhibiting the mTOR pathway, Chen et al. found that, in CC, VEGF-A overexpression correlated with cell growth through cyclinD1, CDK4 activation, and invasion through Matrix Metallopeptidase 2 (MMP2) and MMP3 [46].

An investigation on Insulin-like growth factor 1 (IGF 1) revealed elevated levels in women with OC. Lau and Leung [43] then further investigated the mechanism of action to answer the question of how tumor progression is possible through the involvement of IGF1. They found that the mTOR signaling pathway is necessary for IGF-1-affected E-cadherin down-regulation [43], revealing a novel mechanism of action of IGF-1 in OC carcinogenesis. Conducting carboplatin-induced apoptosis studies, Lee et al. [45] reported overexpression of CYR61 growth factor, a member of the CCN protein family, in OC. Using that model, CYR61 was found to promote cell proliferation and to inhibit apoptosis. Carboplatin-induced apoptosis cells showed increased AKT phosphorylation, which was not the case in the rapamycin-treated group [45].

Studies on the impact of EGF on EMT in a model of endometrioid ovarian carcinoma revealed that EGF induction activated AKT and reduced levels of expressed PTEN, but did not increase cell proliferation. This was assumed to be due to the persistently low levels of mTOR, which were sufficient to maintain low cell proliferation or impact autophagy [41].

Focal adhesion kinase (FAK) also makes an important contribution to growth factor receptor and integrin signaling [47]. Studies focusing on esophagus squamous carcinoma linked pFAK to high mTOR S6K1 expression and consequently to the mTOR pathway. Investigations on FAK autophosphorylation in epithelial OC showed that while elevated levels of FAK were associated with distant and lymph-node metastasis, high levels of FAK were concurrently linked to improved OS [48], thus presenting an intriguing entity in gynecological cancer. Investigating ovarian clear cell carcinoma, Sato and colleagues found that phosphorylation of FAK was increased in spheroids, but not in adherent cells. This, in turn, provides a rationale for considering FAK inhibition as a supplement to current inhibition routes [49].

GDF-15 has already been associated with oncogenesis and worse outcomes in breast cancer and brain tumor models. Due to the unknown mechanism of action in tumor progression, subsequent investigations were also performed in ovarian cancer. It was shown that overexpression of GDF-15 contributed to the upregulation of MMP2, MMP9 and VEGF. This effect, however, could be inhibited by the use of inhibitors p38, MEK, and PI3K [44].

In the light of the impact of growth factors on endometrial cells, Subramaniam and colleagues [50] investigated cancer-associated fibroblasts (CAFs) in the vicinity of the EC cells. They reported that, compared to normal fibroblasts, CAFs secreted higher levels of macrophage chemoattractant protein (MCP)-1, interleukin (IL)-6, IL-8, RANTES, and vascular endothelial growth factor (VEGF). This suggests that fibroblasts can have a pro-tumorigenic effect on the progression of endometrial cancer, and PI3K/AKT and MAPK/ERK signaling may be critical regarding their maintenance [50]. Cell line studies have shown that inhibition of fibroblast growth factor receptor 2 (FGFR2), together with inhibition of mTOR, leads to a synergistic positive effect in EC.

The FGFR2 mutations are present in approximately 10% of EC and are mutually exclusive with KRAS mutations. FGFR2 is highly associated with PTEN loss, and a majority of tumors with FGFR2 mutations also carry PTEN mutations [51].

3.6. Genomic Aberrations Interacting with mTOR Signaling Pathway Activation

A recent analysis of genomic data on endometrial cancer has identified the IGF-1/mTOR pathway in genome-wide association study (GWAS) and exome-Seq data as a relevant pathway, following the p53 pathway, which is the most relevant one [52]. The downstream targets of the IGF1 signaling, i.e., EIF2S1 and EIF2B5, have been associated with EC. In addition, according to findings based on the Human cancer genome atlas (HCGA), single nucleotide polymorphisms (SNPs) connected to PIK3CA, PIK3R1, and IGF1R are commonly found in EC [52]. In order to understand functional SNPs and target genes, Painter and colleagues carried out in silico fine mapping of patients with EC. They found that SNP rs2494737, a member of the PI3K/AKT/mTOR pathway located within AKT1, is activated in EC. The SNPs, however, also influence the silencer activity and affect YY1 siRNA, a positive regulator of AKT1. The expression of this SNP is therefore also related to the risk of EC development [53]. In a Taiwanese population, 50% of endometrial cancers displayed mutations in the PTEN gene. A smaller number of cases, however, showed aberrations in PIK3R1, AKT2, FOXO1, which contributed to the activation of the IL-7 signaling pathway [54].

Genetic analysis carried out in serous high-grade ovarian cancer shows that PI3KCA mutations are present in 18% of the cases and PTEN mutations in 7% of the cases. This is also true for mutations (PIK3CA) in endometrioid and mucinous carcinomas (20% of cases had mutations) as well as in clear cell tumors (46% of the case series had carcinomas). Activation of the AKT2 kinase was also observed in 40% of mostly high grade serous ovarian tumors. A simultaneous activation of AKT and mTOR occurred in 87% of ovarian tumors [55].

PI3K is at the modification level of the mTOR initiation cascade. Of importance are changes in Gab2 expression, which impact the EMT through the PI3K-Zeb1 pathway in OC. This mechanism is activated by the inhibition of E-cadherin expression [56]. Duckworth et al. then investigated the role of Gab2 expression in chemokine expression. They found that overexpression of Gab2 upregulated chemokine ligand 1 (CXCL1), CXCL2, and CXCL8. Interestingly, however, only pharmacological inhibition of IKKbeta, a target in NF kappa-B signaling, leads to the suppression of Gab2-induced chemokine expression. Other targets, among them PI3K, did not lead to the suppression of chemokine activity, thus showing that co-regulating the nuclear factor kappa B (NF-KB) and the mTOR pathways could be beneficial in OC [57]. Wang and colleagues [56] then further investigated the role of Zeb1 in the transcription process in ovarian cancer. Through the expression of the Gab2 protein, they found that if mutant Gab2 variants were present, the activation of PI3K and Shp2-ERK pathways was defective. Gab2 presence enhanced the expression of Zeb1, a factor involved in the epithelial-to-mesenchymal transition, cell migration and invasion, thus worsening the prognosis of the malignancy.

3.7. Epithelial-Mesenchymal Transition and mTOR Signaling

Understanding the induction of EMT in gynecological cancers is important in terms of understanding metastasis mechanisms. Regardless of our knowledge that EMT changes lead to cell migration and invasion ability, the mechanism how mTOR interacts with EMT is unclear. A proposed trigger of EMT transformation is the Transforming Growth Factor beta (TGF-b). TGF-b activates AKT through PI3K and subsequently activates the mTORC1 cascade and its downstream targets of p70S6 and eukaryotic initiation factors. Studying the role of TGF-b, Chen and colleagues found that inhibiting the mTOR signaling leads to downregulation of pyruvate kinase M2 (PKM2), which is needed to induce EMT in cervical cancer cells [58]. EMT was studied in histologically high-grade OC. An analysis of cell lines and Western Blot revealed that the expression of PI3K, pAKT, and p-mTOR was decreased after γ-Glutamyl cyclotransferase (GGCT) knockdown. This resulted in decreased proliferation, clone formation, and migration, which led some authors to conclude that GGCT could be used as a biomarker or potential therapeutic target [59]. Forkhead Box P3 (Foxp3) was also examined for its function in carcinogenesis. The upregulation of Foxp3 showed a decrease of Ki-67 and cyclin-dependent kinases (CDKs), as well as downregulation of matrix metalloproteinase-2 (MMP-2) and urokinase-type plasminogen activator (uPA). In malignancies, MMPs and uPA are involved in the development of metastasis. Their role is defined by the inhibition of cell migration and invasion, and they inhibited mTOR signaling and NF-kB signaling [60]. These molecules can be involved as downstream actors (Figure 2) in connection with the enhanced Snail expression, which is associated with YB-1 mRNA expression [19].

3.8. RNA-Based Alterations Interacting with mTOR

RNA-based alterations can be evaluated through long non-coding RNA (lncRNA) and microRNA (miRNA) changes. miRNA consists of short RNAs of 18–22 nucleotides with non-coding characteristics and regulates the expression of a variety of genes. miRNA regulates the gene expression by binding to the 3'-untranslated regions (3'-UTRs) of messenger RNA (mRNA) [61,62]. It is assumed that more than half of the mRNAs are regulated by miRNA, which was found to enhance degradation or inhibit post-transcriptional translation of mRNA. As approximately half of the miRNA genes are located in cancer-associated regions of the genome or at sites vulnerable to cancer-based aberrations, miRNAs are suggested to play an important role in carcinogenesis [61]. Investigating cervical cancer transfected with HPV 16, Nair and colleagues described a specific miRNA profile correlating with HPV16-transfected cervical cancer (downregulation of miR-1184, miR-377-3p, miR-136-5p, miR-218-5p, miR-4687-3p, miR-497-5p, and miR-5572 and upregulation of miR-21-5p, miR-429, miR-135b-5p, and miR-363-3p [63]). Analysis of the cancer genome atlas (TCGA) miRNA data further on identified a signature of miRNA for cervical cancer. Their risk scoring showed that an interplay of miR-3154 and miR-7-3 was correlated with shortened OS, and the miR-600 was significantly associated with improved OS [64]. Table 2 depicts the miRNAs identified for different gynecological cancer subtypes. In gynecological cancers, only a few miRNAs overlap due to the regulation of the mTOR pathway. These consist of the miR99 family (consisting of miR-99a and miR-100), which is present in all gynecological malignancies, and the miR-199 family, detected in endometrial and ovarian carcinoma. According to Torres et al., the three mTOR signature of miR-99a, miR-100 and miR199b is an miRNA signature that needs to be down-regulated in order to enable mTOR kinase upregulation [65].

Table 2. Overview of miRNA molecules identified interacting with gynecological cancers through the PI3K/Akt/mTOR pathway.

Type of Investigated Cancer	miRNA	Component	Impact of Aberration on Signaling
Endometrial cancer	miR-101 [66]	mTORC1/mTORC2	Downregulation leads to mTOR upregulation
	miR-205 [67]	PTEN expression regulation	Low levels of miR-205 lead to reduced pmTOR and pAKT expression
	miR99 family [65,68]	PI3K through direct target IGF/IGFR	Low levels of expression correlated with better tumor differentiation
	miR-199a-3p [69]	mTORC1/mTORC2	Upregulation inhibits tumor cell proliferation through negative regulation of mTOR expression
	miR-199b [65]	mTOR kinase	High expression in better differentiated EC
	miR-152 [70]	Impacts RICTOR and the mTORC2-AKT cascade	Downregulation enables CpG island hypermethylation
Cervical cancer	miR-155 family [71,72]	3'UTR of PDK1	Enables PDK1 the activation of the mTOR pathway when under expression
	miR-99 family [73]	PI3K through the direct target IGF/IGFR	Upregulation directly negatively regulates mTOR expression
	miR-634 [74]	Direct binding to 3ÚTR of mTOR	Upregulation represses mTOR expression
	miR-338 [13]	No direct information—downregulation of PI3K and AKT, upregulation of pmTOR and p70S6	Downregulation inhibits autophagy by targeting ATF2
Ovarian cancer	miR-206 [75]	c-Met	Downregulation impacts estrogen receptor as a direct target, enables growth and invasion in EOC
	miR-130a [76]	TSC1	Downregulation enables enhanced mTOR activity
	miR-199a [77]	mTOR	Upregulation blocks mTOR expression
	miR-100 [78]	FRAP1/mTOR	Down regulation leads to enhanced mTOR pathway activity
	MiR-206 [75]	c-Met	Direct activation of downstream AKT/mTOR signaling pathway

mTORC1- mammalian target of rapamycin complex 1; PTEN - Phosphatase and tensin homolog; PI3K- Phosphoinositide 3-kinases; IGF/IGFR: Insulin growth factor/receptor, RICTOR: rapamycin-insensitive companion of mammalian target of rapamycin, UTR: untranslated region, PDK1: Pyruvate Dehydrogenase Kinase 1, TSC1: Tuberous sclerosis protein, FRAP1/mTOR: FK506-binding protein 12-rapamycin-associated protein 1/ mammalian target of rapamycin.

Discoveries made over the last few years have identified long non-coding RNA (lncRNA), an important stakeholder in carcinogenesis signaling. Previously, lncRNAs were considered a transcriptional noise. This class of RNA, containing more than 200 nucleotides, is involved in the processes of translation, RNAsplicing and gene regulation [79,80]. In the understanding of pathological processes, lncRNA was given the role of a co-player influencing proliferation, apoptosis, cell cycle inference, migration, invasion, metastasis, and drug resistance [79]. A few lncRNAs have been identified in gynecological cancers. A systematic analysis of the literature showed that among currently identified lncRNAs, there are two overlapping lncRNAs in gynecological malignancies. These are MEG3 (maternally expressed gene 3) [81–83] and DLEU1 (deleted in lymphocytic leukemia 1) [84–86], which have been identified in all three gynecological cancers. MEG3 is a maternally imprinted gene functioning as a tumor suppressor. It is often found in normal tissue and is expressed only in some cancer tissue types. In EC, it was demonstrated that lncRNA MEG3 can be directly combined with PI3K, thus impacting tumor growth. Compared to normal tissue, endometrial and ovarian carcinomas showed high expression of lncRNA DLEU1 [84,86]. This overexpression has been reported to increase cell viability, proliferation, migration, and invasion. Subsequent studies have shown that changes in the expression of AKT1, p70S6K, rpS6, GSK3beta, signal transducer and activator of transcription 3 (STAT3), and B-cell lymphoma-extra large (Bcl-xl) were correlated with changes of lncRNA, DLEU1, and mTOR in endometrial carcinoma [84]. A significantly low expression of lncRNA Cancer Susceptibility 2 (CASC2) was identified in ovarian carcinoma. The initiation factor eIF4A3 acted as a CASC2-binding protein [87].

3.9. Hypoxic Modulation of Carcinogenesis via mTOR Signaling

Rapidly expanding tumors outgrow their vascular supply and as such become hypoxic. Hypoxic conditions enable the enhancement of tumor invasiveness. The process is mostly regulated by the expression of hypoxia inducible factors (HIFs) [88]. Investigating OC, Gomez-Roman et al. have found that HIFs, in order to become invasive, need to be induced by Rab25, a small GTPase. Rab25 functions as a downstream target of p70S6K. The protein p70S6K was overexpressed in cells with levels of Rab25, which were overexpressed as well. This indicates that the activation of the mTOR signaling, specifically the downstream targets of p70S6K, is needed to induce HIF [88]. Research on CC showed that the induction of HIF-1alpha is controlled by Pak4, another p21-activated kinase of the serine/threonine kinase family affecting the Rho-related GTPases, such as Rac and Cdc42, in hypoxic conditions. In vitro experiments showed that the knockdown of Rac4 attenuated the expression of HIF-1alpha. The process of Pak4 control was modulated by AKT and the downstream modulation of the translation inihibitor 4E-BP1 [89]. The regulation of HIF, however, is not yet fully understood, and is most likely dependent not only on the regulation through GTPases. Investigation into the protein kinase C (PKC) family showed that, in cancer cells, PKC accumulation is dependent on HIF-1a. Tests conducted in three different cell lines (cervical and prostate cancer as well as fibrosarcoma) led to the hypothesis that tumor-caused hypoxia most likely induces PKC isoform-dependent HIF-1a accumulations. Cell line studies have shown that the HIF1alpha activation was initiated by the AKT-mTOR and NF-kB cascade [90,91].

Hypoxia has been interconnected with autophagy [71]. Autophagy, as a cytoprotective process, represents an important step in carcinogenesis as it facilitates cell survival and accompanies a multistep process to degrade cell components. Dysregulation of this process contributes to tumor progression [13]. Autophagy, which is lower in cancerous than in normal cells, has been observed in malignant cells and cells with malignant potential [72]. An evaluation of the levels of miR155 in cervical and nasopharyngeal cancer shows that if members of the mTOR pathway (RHEB, RICTOR and RPS6KB2) are activated, the levels of miR155 are lowered and autophagy is decreased. This is most likely a consequence of miR-155 impacting PDK1, which is an upstream kinase of AKT that can activate AKT. An attenuation of the pathway leads to an increase in autophagy in the in vitro models. This had an impact on cell proliferation and G1/S cell cycle progression [71]. Furthermore, due to the impact of PTEN, miR-205 induced autophagy was attenuated. [67]. Processes interconnecting authophagy dysregulation linked to the mTOR pathway have been observed on different levels. In OC, the expression of DIRAS 1 and 2, GTP-ases, leads to the inhibition of S473 AKT1 and S448 mTOR phosphorylation. DIRAS 1 and 2 expression was downregulated and correlated with lower DFS and OS [92]. Further studies investigating ARHI (also known as DIRAS3) in OC found that it induces autophagy by blocking mTOR and PI3K signaling. Further, 60% of OC samples in that study showed downregulated expression of DIRAS3. However, this study also showed that ARHI overexpression leads to autophagic cell death, but enabled dormant carcinoma cell survival [93].

4. Conclusions

YB-1 interacts with mTOR mostly through the nuclear YB-1. The data demonstarte that dual inhibition of mTOR and YB-1 shows promising decreases in carcinogenic activity. The downstream effects in gynecological cancer (Figure 2) show an important interconnection of mTOR with YB-1 activity. However, in gynecological cancers, there have only been a few identified targets of YB-1 action until now.

Our imperfect understanding of the interplay of YB-1 and mTOR is even more pronounced in endometrial cancer. While we have observed that YB-1 influences VEGF, our observation of the communication of cancer-associated fibroblasts (CAFs) with the overexpression of interleukin (IL-6), Il-8, RANTES, and VEGF needs to be further evaluated in light of data showing the involvement of YB-1. The role of growth factors, especially VEGF, with the mTOR pathway through CAF stimulation has yet to be studied in ovarian and cervical cancers. Furthermore, we point towards evidence of the presence of an AKT/mTORC2-mediated process in the hypoxic environment. Especially as YB-1 is implicated to act upon AKT expression, the process and interconnection with mTORC2 must be further investigated. All gynecological cancers have been reported to show an overexpression of HIF in a hypoxic environment, but data suggest that HIF enables specific isoforms of the PKC family to accumulate. As the cascade continues, this leads to an mTORC2-mediated effect currently reported only in cervical cancer [94,95]. Therefore, a further inquiry to be opened by this review is the role played by hypoxia downstream in the mTORC2 cascade. The question arises whether mTORC2 signaling plays a role in all gynecological cancer signaling procedures. Interestingly, research elucidated that the mTOR pathway probably results in alterations due to YB-1 activity and is most likely not impacted by eukaryotic initiation translation factors.

Author Contributions: Conceptualization of the review, M.S., S.B., J.H.; writing of the original draft: M.S., S.B., J.K.; writing—review and editing the manuscript: M.S., J.K., I.T., J.H. All authors have read and agreed to the published version of the manuscript.

References

1. Husseinzadeh, N.; Husseinzadeh, H.D. MTOR inhibitors and their clinical application in cervical, endometrial and ovarian cancers: A critical review. *Gynecol. Oncol.* **2014**, *133*, 375–381. [CrossRef] [PubMed]
2. Dobbin, Z.; Landen, C. The importance of the PI3K/AKT/MTOR pathway in the progression of ovarian cancer. *Int. J. Mol. Sci.* **2013**, *14*, 8213–8227. [CrossRef] [PubMed]
3. Yoshida, Y.; Kurokawa, T.; Horiuchi, Y.; Sawamura, Y.; Shinagawa, A.; Kotsuji, F. Localisation of phosphorylated mTOR expression is critical to tumour progression and outcomes in patients with endometrial cancer. *Eur. J. Cancer* **2010**, *46*, 3445–3452. [CrossRef] [PubMed]
4. Lindquist, J.A.; Mertens, P.R. Cold shock proteins: From cellular mechanisms to pathophysiology and disease. *Cell Commun. Signal.* **2018**, *16*, 1–14. [CrossRef]
5. Nishio, S.; Ushijima, K.; Yamaguchi, T.; Sasajima, Y.; Tsuda, H.; Kasamatsu, T.; Kage, M.; Ono, M.; Kuwano, M.; Kamura, T. Nuclear Y-box-binding protein-1 is a poor prognostic marker and related to epidermal growth factor receptor in uterine cervical cancer. *Gynecol. Oncol.* **2014**, *132*, 703–708. [CrossRef]

6. Hohlfeld, R.; Brandt, S.; Bernhardt, A.; Gorny, X.; Schindele, D.; Jandrig, B.; Schostak, M.; Isermann, B.; Lindquist, J.A.; Mertens, P.R. Crosstalk between Akt signaling and cold shock proteins in mediating invasive cell phenotypes. *Oncotarget* **2018**, *9*, 19039–19049. [CrossRef]

7. Maier, E.; Attenberger, F.; Tiwari, A.; Lettau, K.; Rebholz, S.; Fehrenbacher, B.; Schaller, M.; Gani, C.; Toulany, M. Dual targeting of Y-box binding Protein-1 and Akt inhibits proliferation and enhances the chemosensitivity of colorectal cancer cells. *Cancers* **2019**, *11*, 562. [CrossRef]

8. Darb-Esfahani, S.; Faggad, A.; Noske, A.; Weichert, W.; Buckendahl, A.C.; Müller, B.; Budczies, J.; Röske, A.; Dietel, M.; Denkert, C. Phospho-mTOR and phospho-4EBP1 in endometrial adenocarcinoma: Association with stage and grade in vivo and link with response to rapamycin treatment in vitro. *J. Cancer Res. Clin. Oncol.* **2009**, *135*, 933–941. [CrossRef]

9. Diaz-Padilla, I.; Duran, I.; Clarke, B.A.; Oza, A.M. Biologic rationale and clinical activity of mTOR inhibitors in gynecological cancer. *Cancer Treat. Rev.* **2012**, *38*, 767–775. [CrossRef]

10. Kato, E.; Orisaka, M.; Kurokawa, T.; Chino, Y.; Fujita, Y.; Shinagawa, A.; Yoshida, Y. Relation between outcomes and expression of estrogen receptor-α phosphorylated at Ser167 in endometrioid endometrial cancer. *Cancer Sci.* **2014**, *105*, 1307–1312. [CrossRef]

11. Kassem, L.; Abdel-Rahman, O. Targeting mTOR pathway in gynecological malignancies: Biological rationale and systematic review of published data. *Crit. Rev. Oncol. Hematol.* **2016**, *108*, 1–12. [CrossRef] [PubMed]

12. Silveira, C.G.T.; Krampe, J.; Ruhland, B.; Diedrich, K.; Hornung, D.; Agic, A. Cold-shock domain family member YB-1 expression in endometrium and endometriosis. *Hum. Reprod.* **2012**, *27*, 173–182. [CrossRef] [PubMed]

13. Lu, R.; Yang, Z.; Xu, G.; Yu, S. miR-338 modulates proliferation and autophagy by PI3K/AKT/mTOR signaling pathway in cervical cancer. *Biomed. Pharmacother.* **2018**, *105*, 633–644. [CrossRef] [PubMed]

14. Zhang, X.Y.; Zhang, H.Y.; Zhang, P.N.; Lu, X.; Sun, H. Elevated phosphatidylinositol 3-kinase activation and its clinicopathological significance in cervical cancer. *Eur. J. Obstet. Gynecol. Reprod. Biol.* **2008**, *139*, 237–244. [CrossRef] [PubMed]

15. Ji, J.; Zheng, P.S. Activation of mTOR signaling pathway contributes to survival of cervical cancer cells. *Gynecol. Oncol.* **2010**, *117*, 103–108. [CrossRef]

16. Feng, W.; Duan, X.; Liu, J.; Xiao, J.; Brown, R.E. Morphoproteomic evidence of constitutively activated and overexpressed mTOR pathway in cervical squamous carcinoma and high grade squamous intraepithelial lesions. *Int. J. Clin. Exp. Pathol.* **2009**, *2*, 249–260.

17. De Melo, A.C.; Paulino, E.; Garces, A.H.I. A review of mTOR pathway inhibitors in gynecologic cancer. *Oxid. Med. Cell. Longev.* **2017**, *2017*, 4809751. [CrossRef]

18. Zhang, Y.; Reng, S.R.; Wang, L.; Lu, L.; Zhao, Z.H.; Zhang, Z.K.; Feng, X.D.; Ding, X.D.; Wang, J.; Feng, G.; et al. Overexpression of Y-box binding protein-1 in cervical cancer and its association with the pathological response rate to chemoradiotherapy. *Med. Oncol.* **2012**, *29*, 1992–1997. [CrossRef]

19. Pang, T.; Li, M.; Zhang, Y.; Yong, W.; Kang, H.; Yao, Y.; Hu, X. Y Box-binding protein 1 promotes epithelial-mesenchymal transition, invasion, and metastasis of cervical cancer via enhancing the expressions of snail. *Int. J. Gynecol. Cancer* **2017**, *27*, 1753–1760. [CrossRef]

20. Smolle, E.; Taucher, V.; Pichler, M.; Petru, E.; Lax, S.; Haybaeck, J. Targeting signaling pathways in epithelial ovarian cancer. *Int. J. Mol. Sci.* **2013**, *14*, 9536–9555. [CrossRef]

21. MacKay, H.J.; Eisenhauer, E.A.; Kamel-Reid, S.; Tsao, M.; Clarke, B.; Karakasis, K.; Werner, H.M.J.; Trovik, J.; Akslen, L.A.; Salvesen, H.B.; et al. Molecular determinants of outcome with mammalian target of rapamycin inhibition in endometrial cancer. *Cancer* **2014**, *120*, 603–610. [CrossRef] [PubMed]

22. Rohr, I.; Braicu, E.I.; En-Nia, A.; Heinrich, M.; Richter, R.; Chekerov, R.; Dechend, R.; Heidecke, H.; Dragun, D.; Schäfer, R.; et al. Y-box protein-1/p18 as novel serum marker for ovarian cancer diagnosis: A study by the Tumor Bank Ovarian Cancer (TOC). *Cytokine* **2016**, *85*, 157–164. [CrossRef] [PubMed]

23. Liu, S.; Marneth, A.E.; Alexe, G.; Walker, S.R.; Gandler, H.I.; Ye, D.Q.; Labella, K.; Mathur, R.; Toniolo, P.A.; Tillgren, M.; et al. The kinases IKBKE and TBK1 regulate MYC-dependent survival pathways through YB-1 in AML and are targets for therapy. *Blood Adv.* **2018**, *2*, 3428–3442. [CrossRef] [PubMed]

24. Jin, X.; Jiao, X.; Jiao, J.; Zhang, T.; Cui, B. Increased expression of FHL2 promotes tumorigenesis in cervical cancer and is correlated with poor prognosis. *Gene* **2018**, *669*, 99–106. [CrossRef] [PubMed]

25. Xu, K.; Liu, P.; Wei, W. mTOR signaling in tumorigenesis. *Biochim. Biophys. Acta Rev. Cancer* **2014**, *1846*, 638–654. [CrossRef] [PubMed]

26. Pópulo, H.; Lopes, J.M.; Soares, P. The mTOR signalling pathway in human cancer. *Int. J. Mol. Sci.* **2012**, *13*, 1886–1918. [CrossRef]

27. Montero, J.C.; Chen, X.; Ocaña, A.; Pandiella, A. Predominance of mTORC1 over mTORC2 in the regulation of proliferation of ovarian cancer cells: Therapeutic implications. *Mol. Cancer Ther.* **2012**, *11*, 1342–1352. [CrossRef]

28. Noske, A.; Lindenberg, J.L.; Darb-Esfahani, S.; Weichert, W.; Buckendahl, A.-C.; Röske, A.; Sehouli, J.; Dietel, M.; Denkert, C. Activation of mTOR in a subgroup of ovarian carcinomas: Correlation with p-eIF-4E and prognosis. *Oncol. Rep.* **2008**, *20*, 1409–1417. [CrossRef]

29. Liu, P.; Gan, W.; Inuzuka, H.; Lazorchak, A.S.; Gao, D.; Arojo, O.; Liu, D.; Wan, L.; Zhai, B.; Yu, Y.; et al. Sin1 phosphorylation impairs mTORC2 complex integrity and inhibits downstream Akt signalling to suppress tumorigenesis. *Nat. Cell Biol.* **2013**, *15*, 1340–1350. [CrossRef]

30. Lyabin, D.N.; Ovchinnikov, L.P. Selective regulation of YB-1 mRNA translation by the mTOR signaling pathway is not mediated by 4E-binding protein. *Sci. Rep.* **2016**, *6*, 22502. [CrossRef]

31. Iglesias, D.A.; Zhang, Q.; Celestino, J.; Sun, C.C.; Yates, M.S.; Schmandt, R.E.; Lu, K.H. Lean body weight and metformin are insufficient to prevent endometrial hyperplasia in mice harboring inactivating mutations in PTEN. *Oncology* **2017**, *92*, 109–114. [CrossRef] [PubMed]

32. Sahoo, S.S.; Lombard, J.M.; Ius, Y.; O'Sullivan, R.; Wood, L.G.; Nahar, P.; Jaaback, K.; Tanwar, P.S. Adipose-derived VEGF–mTOR signaling promotes endometrial hyperplasia and cancer: Implications for obese women. *Mol. Cancer Res.* **2018**, *16*, 309–321. [CrossRef] [PubMed]

33. Zhu, Y.; Shen, J.; Gao, L.; Feng, Y. Estrogen promotes fat mass and obesity-associated protein nuclear localization and enhances endometrial cancer cell proliferation via the mTOR signaling pathway. *Oncol. Rep.* **2016**, *35*, 2391–2397. [CrossRef] [PubMed]

34. Han, J.; Zhang, L.; Guo, H.; Wysham, W.Z.; Roque, D.R.; Willson, A.K.; Sheng, X.; Zhou, C.; Bae-Jump, V.L. Glucose promotes cell proliferation, glucose uptake and invasion in endometrial cancer cells via AMPK/mTOR/S6 and MAPK signaling. *Gynecol. Oncol.* **2015**, *138*, 668–675. [CrossRef]

35. Zhang, L.; Wu, J.; Ling, M.T.; Zhao, L.; Zhao, K.N. The role of the PI3K/Akt/mTOR signalling pathway in human cancers induced by infection with human papillomaviruses. *Mol. Cancer.* **2015**, *14*, 1–13. [CrossRef]

36. Narisawa-Saito, M.; Inagawa, Y.; Yoshimatsu, Y.; Haga, K.; Tanaka, K.; Egawa, N.; Ohno, S.I.; Ichikawa, H.; Yugawa, T.; Fujita, M.; et al. A critical role of MYC for transformation of human cells by HPV16 E6E7 and oncogenic HRAS. *Carcinogenesis* **2012**, *33*, 910–917. [CrossRef]

37. Molinolo, A.A.; Marsh, C.; El Dinali, M.; Gangane, N.; Jennison, K.; Hewitt, S.; Patel, V.; Seiwert, T.Y.; Gutkind, J.S. mTOR as a molecular target in HPV-associated oral and cervical squamous carcinomas. *Clin. Cancer Res.* **2012**, *18*, 2558–2568. [CrossRef]

38. Rabachini, T.; Boccardo, E.; Andrade, R.; Perez, K.R.; Nonogaki, S.; Cuccovia, I.M.; Villa, L.L. HPV-16 E7 expression up-regulates phospholipase D activity and promotes rapamycin resistance in a pRB-dependent manner. *BMC Cancer* **2018**, *18*, 3–10. [CrossRef]

39. Ueno, S.; Sudo, T.; Oka, N.; Wakahashi, S.; Yamaguchi, S.; Fujiwara, K.; Mikami, Y.; Nishimura, R. Absence of human papillomavirus infection and activation of pi3k-akt pathway in cervical clear cell carcinoma. *Int. J. Gynecol. Cancer* **2013**, *23*, 1084–1091. [CrossRef]

40. Roche, E.; Lascombe, I.; Bittard, H.; Mougin, C.; Fauconnet, S. The PPARβ agonist L-165041 promotes VEGF mRNA stabilization in HPV18-harboring HeLa cells through a receptor-independent mechanism. *Cell. Signal.* **2014**, *26*, 433–443. [CrossRef]

41. Grassi, M.L.; de Souza Palma, C.; Thomé, C.H.; Lanfredi, G.P.; Poersch, A.; Faça, V.M. Proteomic analysis of ovarian cancer cells during epithelial-mesenchymal transition (EMT) induced by epidermal growth factor (EGF) reveals mechanisms of cell cycle control. *J. Proteom.* **2017**, *151*, 2–11. [CrossRef] [PubMed]

42. Trinh, X.B.; Tjalma, W.A.A.; Vermeulen, P.B.; Van den Eynden, G.; Van der Auwera, I.; Van Laere, S.J.; Helleman, J.; Berns, E.M.J.J.; Dirix, L.Y.; van Dam, P.A. The VEGF pathway and the AKT/mTOR/p70S6K1 signalling pathway in human epithelial ovarian cancer. *Br. J. Cancer* **2009**, *100*, 971–978. [CrossRef] [PubMed]

43. Lau, M.T.; Leung, P.C. The PI3K/Akt/mTOR signaling pathway mediates insulin-like growth factor 1-induced E-cadherin down-regulation and cell proliferation in ovarian cancer cells. *Cancer Lett.* **2012**, *326*, 191–198. [CrossRef] [PubMed]

44. Griner, S.E.; Joshi, J.P.; Nahta, R. Growth differentiation factor 15 stimulates rapamycin-sensitive ovarian

cancer cell growth and invasion. *Biochem. Pharmacol.* **2013**, *85*, 46–58. [CrossRef] [PubMed]

45. Lee, K.B.; Byun, H.J.; Park, S.H.; Park, C.Y.; Lee, S.H.; Rho, S.B. CYR61 controls p53 and NF-κB expression through PI3K/Akt/mTOR pathways in carboplatin-induced ovarian cancer cells. *Cancer Lett.* **2012**, *315*, 86–95. [CrossRef] [PubMed]

46. Chen, B.; Zhang, C.; Dong, P.; Guo, Y.; Mu, N. Molecular regulation of cervical cancer growth and invasion by VEGFa. *Tumor Biol.* **2014**, *35*, 11587–11593. [CrossRef] [PubMed]

47. Kleinschmidt, E.G.; Schlaepfer, D.D. Focal adhesion kinase signaling in unexpected places. *Curr. Opin. Cell Biol.* **2017**, *45*, 24–30. [CrossRef]

48. Aust, S.; Auer, K.; Bachmayr-Heyda, A.; Denkert, C.; Sehouli, J.; Braicu, I.; Mahner, S.; Lambrechts, S.; Vergote, I.; Grimm, C.; et al. Ambivalent role of pFAK-Y397 in serous ovarian cancer-a study of the OVCAD consortium. *Mol. Cancer* **2014**, *13*, 1–11. [CrossRef]

49. Sato, M.; Kawana, K.; Adachi, K.; Fujimoto, A.; Yoshida, M.; Nakamura, H.; Nishida, H.; Inoue, T.; Taguchi, A.; Ogishima, J.; et al. Targeting glutamine metabolism and the focal adhesion kinase additively inhibits the mammalian target of the rapamycin pathway in spheroid cancer stem-like properties of ovarian clear cell carcinoma in Vitro. *Int. J. Oncol.* **2017**, *50*, 1431–1438. [CrossRef]

50. Subramaniam, K.S.; Tham, S.T.; Mohamed, Z.; Woo, Y.L.; Adenan, N.A.M.; Chung, I. Cancer-associated fibroblasts promote proliferation of endometrial cancer cells. *PLoS ONE* **2013**, *8*, 1–16. [CrossRef]

51. Gozgit, J.M.; Squillace, R.M.; Wongchenko, M.J.; Miller, D.; Wardwell, S.; Mohemmad, Q.; Narasimhan, N.I.; Wang, F.; Clackson, T.; Rivera, V.M. Combined targeting of FGFR2 and mTOR by ponatinib and ridaforolimus results in synergistic antitumor activity in FGFR2 mutant endometrial cancer models. *Cancer Chemother Pharmacol.* **2013**, *71*, 1315–1323. [CrossRef] [PubMed]

52. Wei, R.; De Vivo, I.; Huang, S.; Zhu, X.; Risch, H.; Moore, J.H.; Yu, H.; Garmire, L.X. Meta-dimensional data integration identifies critical pathways for susceptibility, tumorigenesis and progression of endometrial cancer. *Oncotarget* **2016**, *7*, 55249. [CrossRef] [PubMed]

53. Painter, J.N.; Kaufmann, S.; O'Mara, T.A.; Hillman, K.M.; Sivakumaran, H.; Darabi, H.; Cheng, T.H.T.; Pearson, J.; Kazakoff, S.; Waddell, N.; et al. A Common Variant at the 14q32 Endometrial Cancer Risk Locus Activates AKT1 through YY1 Binding. *Am. J. Hum. Genet.* **2016**, *98*, 1159–1169. [CrossRef] [PubMed]

54. Chang, Y.S.; Huang, H.s.D.; Yeh, K.T.; Chang, J.G. Genetic alterations in endometrial cancer by targeted next-generation sequencing. *Exp. Mol. Pathol.* **2016**, *100*, 8–12. [CrossRef]

55. Altomare, D.A.; Wang, H.Q.; Skele, K.L.; De Rienzo, A.; Klein-Szanto, A.J.; Godwin, A.K.; Testa, J.R. AKT and mTOR phosphorylation is frequently detected in ovarian cancer and can be targeted to disrupt ovarian tumor cell growth. *Oncogene* **2004**, *23*, 5853–5857. [CrossRef]

56. Wang, Y.; Sheng, Q.; Spillman, M.A.; Behbakht, K.; Gu, H. Gab2 regulates the migratory behaviors and E-cadherin expression via activation of the PI3K pathway in ovarian cancer cells. *Oncogene* **2012**, *31*, 2512–2520. [CrossRef]

57. Duckworth, C.; Zhang, L.; Carroll, S.L.; Ethier, S.P.; Cheung, H.W. Overexpression of GAB2 in ovarian cancer cells promotes tumor growth and angiogenesis by upregulating chemokine expression. *Oncogene* **2016**, *35*, 4036–4047. [CrossRef]

58. Cheng, K.; Hao, M. Mammalian Target of Rapamycin (mTOR) Regulates Transforming Growth Factor-β1 (TGF-β1)-Induced Epithelial-Mesenchymal Transition via Decreased Pyruvate Kinase M2 (PKM2) Expression in Cervical Cancer Cells. *Med. Sci. Monit.* **2017**, *23*, 2017–2028. [CrossRef]

59. Li, Y.; Wu, T.; Wang, Y.; Yang, L.; Hu, C.; Chen, L.; Wu, S. γ-Glutamyl cyclotransferase contributes to tumor progression in high grade serous ovarian cancer by regulating epithelial-mesenchymal transition via activating PI3K/AKT/mTOR pathway. *Gynecol. Oncol.* **2018**, *149*, 163–172. [CrossRef]

60. Zhang, H.Y.; Sun, H. Up-regulation of Foxp3 inhibits cell proliferation, migration and invasion in epithelial ovarian cancer. *Cancer Lett.* **2010**, *287*, 91–97. [CrossRef]

61. Zhang, Y.; Huang, B.; Wang, H.Y.; Chang, A.; Zheng, X.F.S. Emerging role of MicroRNAs in mTOR signaling. *Cell. Mol. Life Sci.* **2017**, *74*, 2613–2625. [CrossRef]

62. Srivastava, S.K.; Ahmad, A.; Zubair, H.; Miree, O.; Singh, S.; Rocconi, R.P.; Scalici, J.; Singh, A.P. MicroRNAs in gynecological cancers: Small molecules with big implications. *Cancer Lett.* **2017**, *407*, 123–138. [CrossRef]

63. Nair, V.B.; Manasa, V.G.; Sinto, M.S.; Jayasree, K.; James Francis, V.; Kannan, S. Differential expression of

MicroRNAs in uterine cervical cancer and its implications in carcinogenesis; an integrative approach. *Int. J. Gynecol. Cancer* **2018**, *28*, 553–562. [CrossRef]

64. Zeng, Y.; Wang, K.X.; Xu, H.; Hong, Y. Integrative miRNA analysis identifies hsa-miR-3154, hsa-miR-7-3, and hsa-miR-600 as potential prognostic biomarker for cervical cancer. *J. Cell. Biochem.* **2018**, *119*, 1558–1566. [CrossRef]

65. Torres, A.; Torres, K.; Pesci, A.; Ceccaroni, M.; Paszkowski, T.; Cassandrini, P.; Zamboni, G.; Maciejewski, R. Deregulation of miR-100, miR-99a and miR-199b in tissues and plasma coexists with increased expression of mTOR kinase in endometrioid endometrial carcinoma. *BMC Cancer* **2012**, *12*, 369. [CrossRef]

66. Zhang, S.; Wang, M.; Li, Q.; Zhu, P. MiR-101 reduces cell proliferation and invasion and enhances apoptosis in endometrial cancer via regulating PI3K/Akt/mTOR. *Cancer Biomark.* **2017**, *21*, 189–196. [CrossRef]

67. Zhuo, Z.; Yu, H. miR-205 inhibits cell growth by targeting AKT-mTOR signaling in progesterone-resistant endometrial cancer Ishikawa cells. *Oncotarget* **2017**, *8*, 28042–28051. [CrossRef]

68. Li, Y.; Zhang, Z.; Zhang, X.; Lin, Y.; Luo, T.; Xiao, Z.; Zhou, Q. A dual PI3K/AKT/mTOR signaling inhibitor miR-99a suppresses endometrial carcinoma. *Am. J. Transl. Res.* **2016**, *8*, 719–731.

69. Wu, D.; Huang, H.-J.; He, C.-N.; Wang, K.-Y. MicroRNA-199a-3p regulates endometrial cancer cell proliferation by targeting mammalian target of rapamycin (mTOR). *Int. J. Gynecol. Cancer* **2013**, *23*, 1191–1197. [CrossRef]

70. Tsuruta, T.; Kozaki, K.I.; Uesugi, A.; Furuta, M.; Hirasawa, A.; Imoto, I.; Susumu, N.; Aoki, D.; Inazawa, J. miR-152 is a tumor suppressor microRNA that is silenced by DNA hypermethylation in endometrial cancer. *Cancer Res.* **2011**, *71*, 6450–6462. [CrossRef]

71. Liu, Z.; Xu, W.; Huang, N.; Yang, B.B.; Cui, K.; Wan, G.; Liao, M.; He, J.; Xu, H.; Lao, Y.; et al. Hypoxia-induced MIR155 is a potent autophagy inducer by targeting multiple players in the MTOR pathway. *Autophagy* **2013**, *10*, 70–79. [CrossRef]

72. Wang, F.; Shan, S.; Huo, Y.; Xie, Z.; Fang, Y.; Qi, Z.; Chen, F.; Li, Y.; Sun, B. MiR-155-5p inhibits PDK1 and promotes autophagy via the mTOR pathway in cervical cancer. *Int. J. Biochem. Cell Biol.* **2018**, *99*, 91–99. [CrossRef]

73. Wang, L.; Chang, L.; Li, Z.; Gao, Q.; Cai, D.; Tian, Y.; Zeng, L.; Li, M. MiR-99a and -99b inhibit cervical cancer cell proliferation and invasion by targeting mTOR signaling pathway. *Med. Oncol.* **2014**, *31*, 934. [CrossRef]

74. Cong, J.; Liu, R.; Wang, X.; Jiang, H.; Zhang, Y. MiR-634 decreases cell proliferation and induces apoptosis by targeting mTOR signaling pathway in cervical cancer cells. *Artif. Cells Nanomed. Biotechnol.* **2016**, *44*, 1694–1701. [CrossRef]

75. Dai, C.; Xie, Y.; Zhuang, X.; Yuan, Z. MiR-206 inhibits epithelial ovarian cancer cells growth and invasion via blocking c-Met/AKT/mTOR signaling pathway. *Biomed. Pharmacother.* **2018**, *104*, 763–770. [CrossRef]

76. Wang, Y.; Zhang, X.; Tang, W.; Lin, Z.; Xu, L.; Dong, R.; Li, Y.; Li, J.; Zhang, Z.; Li, X.; et al. MiR-130a upregulates mTOR pathway by targeting TSC1 and is transactivated by NF-? B in high-grade serous ovarian carcinoma. *Cell Death Differ.* **2017**, *24*, 2089–2100. [CrossRef]

77. Wang, Z.; Ting, Z.; Li, Y.; Chen, G.; Lu, Y.; Hao, X. microRNA-199a is able to reverse cisplatin resistance in human ovarian cancer cells through the inhibition of mammalian target of rapamycin. *Oncol. Lett.* **2013**, *6*, 789–794. [CrossRef]

78. Nagaraja, A.K.; Creighton, C.J.; Yu, Z.; Zhu, H.; Gunaratne, P.H.; Reid, J.G.; Olokpa, E.; Itamochi, H.; Ueno, N.T.; Hawkins, S.M.; et al. A Link between mir-100 and FRAP1/mTOR in Clear Cell Ovarian Cancer. *Mol. Endocrinol.* **2010**, *24*, 447–463. [CrossRef]

79. Wang, J.Y.; Lu, A.Q.; Chen, L.J. LncRNAs in ovarian cancer. *Clin Chim. Acta* **2019**, *490*, 17–27. [CrossRef]

80. Xie, P.; Cao, H.; Li, Y.; Wang, J.; Cui, Z. Knockdown of lncRNA CCAT2 inhibits endometrial cancer cells growth and metastasis via sponging miR-216b. *Cancer Biomark.* **2017**, *21*, 123–133. [CrossRef]

81. Wang, X.; Wang, Z.; Wang, J.; Wang, Y.; Liu, L.; Xu, X. LncRNA MEG3 has anti-activity effects of cervical cancer. *Biomed. Pharmacother.* **2017**, *94*, 636–643. [CrossRef]

82. Xuan, K.; Dan, S.; Wu, D.; Chen, S.; Zhao, Y.; Hong, Z. LncRNA MEG3 inhibit endometrial carcinoma tumorigenesis and progression through PI3K pathway. *Apoptosis* **2017**, *22*, 1543–1552.

83. Xiu, Y.L.; Sun, K.X.; Chen, X.; Chen, S.; Zhao, Y.; Guo, Q.G.; Zong, Z.H. Upregulation of the lncRNA Meg3 induces autophagy to inhibit tumorigenesis and progression of epithelial ovarian carcinoma by regulating activity of ATG3. *Oncotarget* **2017**, *8*, 31714–31725. [CrossRef]

84. Du, Y.; Wang, L.; Chen, S.; Liu, Y.; Zhao, Y. lncRNA DLEU1 contributes to tumorigenesis and development of endometrial carcinoma by targeting mTOR. *Mol. Carcinog.* **2018**, *57*, 1191–1200. [CrossRef]

85. Liu, C.; Tian, X.; Zhang, J.; Jiang, L. Long Non-coding RNA DLEU1 promotes proliferation and invasion by interacting with miR-381 and enhancing HOXA13 expression in cervical cancer. *Front. Genet.* **2018**, *9*, 1–9. [CrossRef]

86. Wang, L.L.; Sun, K.X.; Wu, D.D.; Xiu, Y.L.; Chen, X.; Chen, S.; Zong, Z.H.; Sang, X.B.; Liu, Y.; Zhao, Y. DLEU1 contributes to ovarian carcinoma tumourigenesis and development by interacting with miR-490-3p and altering CDK1 expression. *J. Cell. Mol. Med.* **2017**, *21*, 3055–3065. [CrossRef]

87. Zhang, S.; Leng, T.; Zhang, Q.; Zhao, Q.; Nie, X.; Yang, L. Sanguinarine inhibits epithelial ovarian cancer development via regulating long non-coding RNA CASC2-EIF4A3 axis and/or inhibiting NF-κB signaling or PI3K/AKT/mTOR pathway. *Biomed. Pharmacother.* **2018**, *102*, 302–308. [CrossRef]

88. Gomez-Roman, N.; Sahasrabudhe, N.M.; McGregor, F.; Chalmers, A.J.; Cassidy, J.; Plumb, J. Hypoxia-inducible factor 1 alpha is required for the tumourigenic and aggressive phenotype associated with Rab25 expression in ovarian cancer. *Oncotarget* **2016**, *7*, 22650–22664. [CrossRef]

89. Kim, H.; Woo, D.J.; Kim, S.Y.; Yang, E.G. p21-activated kinase 4 regulates HIF-1α translation in cancer cells. *Biochem. Biophys. Res. Commun.* **2017**, *486*, 270–276. [CrossRef]

90. Ivanova, I.G.; Park, C.V.; Yemm, A.I.; Kenneth, N.S. PERK/eIF2α signaling inhibits HIF-induced gene expression during the unfolded protein response via YB1-dependent regulation of HIF1α translation. *Nucleic Acids Res.* **2018**, *46*, 3878–3890. [CrossRef]

91. Kim, H.; Na, Y.R.; Kim, S.Y.; Yang, E.G. Protein kinase C isoforms differentially regulate hypoxia-inducible factor-1α accumulation in cancer cells. *J. Cell. Biochem.* **2016**, *117*, 647–658. [CrossRef] [PubMed]

92. Sutton, M.N.; Yang, H.; Huang, G.Y.; Fu, C.; Pontikos, M.; Wang, Y.; Mao, W.; Pang, L.; Yang, M.; Liu, J.; et al. RAS-related GTPases DIRAS1 and DIRAS2 induce autophagic cancer cell death and are required for autophagy in murine ovarian cancer cells. *Autophagy* **2018**, *14*, 637–653. [CrossRef] [PubMed]

93. Lu, Z.; Luo, R.Z.; Lu, Y.; Zhang, X.; Yu, Q.; Khare, S.; Kondo, S.; Kondo, Y.; Yu, Y.; Mills, G.B.; et al. The tumor suppressor gene ARHI regulates autophagy and tumour dormancy in human ovarian cancer cells. *Cell Prolif.* **2008**, *118*, 3917–3929.

94. Bossler, F.; Kuhn, B.J.; Günther, T.; Kraemer, S.J.; Khalkar, P.; Adrian, S.; Lohrey, C.; Holzer, A.; Shimobayashi, M.; Dürst, M.; et al. Repression of human papillomavirus oncogene expression under hypoxia is mediated by PI3K/mTORC2/AKT signaling. *MBio* **2019**, *10*, e02323-18. [CrossRef] [PubMed]

95. Bossler, F.; Hoppe-Seyler, K.; Hoppe-Seyler, F. PI3K/AKT/mTOR Signaling Regulates the Virus/Host Cell Crosstalk in HPV-Positive Cervical Cancer Cells. *Int. J. Mol. Sci.* **2019**, *20*, 2188. [CrossRef] [PubMed]

Zoledronic Acid Abrogates Restraint Stress-Induced Macrophage Infiltration, PDGF-AA Expression and Ovarian Cancer Growth

Claudia B. Colon-Echevarria [1], Tatiana Ortiz [1], Lizette Maldonado [1],
Melanie J. Hidalgo-Vargas [1], Jaileene Pérez-Morales [2], Alexandra N. Aquino-Acevedo [1],
Roberto Herrera-Noriega [1], Margarita Bonilla-Claudio [3], Eida M. Castro [4,5] and
Guillermo N. Armaiz-Pena [1,3,6,*]

[1]   Department of Basic Sciences, Pharmacology Division, School of Medicine, Ponce Health Sciences University, Ponce, PR 00716, USA; ccolon13@stu.psm.edu (C.B.C.-E.); tatianaot@gmail.com (T.O.); limaldonado@psm.edu (L.M.); melanie_hidalgo@outlook.com (M.J.H.-V.); aaquino18@stu.psm.edu (A.N.A.-A.); rherrera18@psm.edu (R.H.-N.)

[2]   Department of Cancer Epidemiology, H. Lee Moffitt Cancer Center and Research Institute, Tampa, FL 33612, USA; jaileene.perez-morales@moffitt.org

[3]   Division of Cancer Biology, Ponce Research Institute, Ponce, PR 00716, USA; mbonilla@psm.edu

[4]   Clinical Psychology Program, School of Behavior and Brain Sciences, Ponce Health Sciences University, Ponce, PR 00716, USA; ecastro@psm.edu

[5]   Mental Health Division, Ponce Research Institute, Ponce, PR 00716, USA

[6]   Division of Women's Health, Ponce Research Institute, Ponce, PR 00716, USA

*   Correspondence: garmaiz@psm.edu

Simple Summary: Biobehavioral disorders can negatively impact patients with ovarian cancer. Growing evidence suggests that chronic stress can promote tumor progression, the release of inflammatory mediators, and macrophage infiltration into the tumor. However, the role of stress hormones in regulating cancer cell/macrophage crosstalk remains unclear. This study aimed to assess the role of stress hormone-stimulated macrophages in modulating inflammatory networks and ovarian cancer biology. Our data show that stress hormones induced secretion of inflammatory proteins in ovarian cancer cell/macrophage co-cultures. Furthermore, we show that restraint stress leads to cancer growth, macrophage infiltration, and PDGF-AA protein expression in animal models of ovarian cancer. Conversely, zoledronic acid was able to prevent the effects of restraint stress on ovarian cancer growth. Overall, our data suggest a role for stress hormone-stimulated macrophages in ovarian cancer progression and suggest the involvement of PDGF-AA as a key mediator of this process.

Abstract: Multiple studies suggest that chronic stress accelerates the growth of existing tumors by activating the sympathetic nervous system. Data suggest that sustained adrenergic signaling can induce tumor growth, secretion of pro-inflammatory cytokines, and macrophage infiltration. Our goal was to study the role of adrenergic-stimulated macrophages in ovarian cancer biology. Cytokine arrays were used to assess the effect of adrenergic stimulation in pro-tumoral cytokine networks. An orthotopic model of ovarian cancer was used to assess the in vivo effect of daily restraint stress on tumor growth and adrenergic-induced macrophages. Cytokine analyses showed that adrenergic stimulation modulated pro-inflammatory cytokine secretion in a SKOV3ip1 ovarian cancer cell/U937 macrophage co-culture system. Among these, platelet-derived growth factor AA (PDGF-AA), epithelial cell-derived neutrophil-activating peptide (ENA-78), Angiogenin, vascular endothelial growth factor (VEGF), granulocyte-macrophage colony-stimulating factor (GM-CSF), interleukin-5 (IL-5), Lipocalin-2, macrophage migration inhibitory factor (MIF), and transferrin receptor (TfR) were upregulated. Enriched biological processes included cytokine-mediated signaling pathways and positive regulation of cell proliferation. In addition, daily restraint stress increased ovarian cancer growth, infiltration of CD68+ macrophages, and expression of PDGF-AA in orthotopic models of ovarian cancer (SKOV3ip1 and HeyT30), while zoledronic acid, a macrophage-depleting agent, abrogated this effect. Furthermore, in ovarian cancer patients, high *PDGFA* expression correlated with worse outcomes. Here, it is shown that the adrenergic regulation of macrophages and *PDGFA* might play a role in ovarian cancer progression.

Keywords: ovarian cancer; adrenergic; macrophages; cytokines; inflammation; *PDGFA*

1. Introduction

Ovarian cancer is the fifth leading cause of cancer death among women in the United States. It also has the highest mortality rate of female reproductive cancers [1,2]. Previous studies have shown that altered psychological states, including chronic stress and depression, contribute to tumor growth and cancer progression [3]. Furthermore, ovarian cancer patients are more likely to suffer from anxiety and depression than the general population [4,5]. This is an important issue to address since psychological stressors contribute to poorer survival and higher mortality of cancer patients [6,7]. Biobehavioral factors have been shown to enhance protumoral factors associated with inflammatory processes [8].

Tumor-associated macrophages (TAMs) are among the most abundant infiltrating immune cells and are key components of the tumor microenvironment. Activated TAMs secrete cytokines, chemokines, proteins, and pro-inflammatory mediators capable of recruiting immune cell populations while ultimately promoting tumor growth [9]. Activation of the sympathetic nervous system and increased levels of catecholamines, epinephrine (Epi), and norepinephrine (NE) in the tumor microenvironment also activate pro-tumoral and pro-inflammatory pathways, induce macrophage infiltration, and promote tumor growth [10]. Several studies have shown that β-adrenergic signaling is capable of mediating the effects of chronic stress on ovarian cancer. This includes activation of metastatic cascades, resistance to chemotherapy, and worse patient outcomes [11,12]. In addition, several studies have shown that adrenergic signaling enhances TAM infiltration, recruitment, and leads to worse survival among ovarian cancer patients [9,13]. Although studies have reported that catecholamines induce TAM infiltration into the tumor microenvironment, the role of stress hormones in the regulation of cancer cells/TAM interaction is not entirely clear.

We investigated the role of adrenergic-stimulated macrophages in modulating pro-inflammatory networks and ovarian cancer biology. This study was guided by the hypothesis that adrenergic signaling induces TAMs to upregulate cytokines involved in pro-inflammatory pathways leading to ovarian cancer progression. We report that alterations in pro-inflammatory networks driven by adrenergic-induced macrophages resulted in enhanced infiltration of TAMs and tumor growth. We demonstrated that the effects of restraint stress on ovarian cancer progression are abrogated by zoledronic acid, a clinically available bisphosphonate, that has been shown to target TAMs in multiple tumor models. Furthermore, our data suggest that adrenergic regulation of macrophages and platelet-derived growth factor AA (PDGF-AA) might play a role in ovarian cancer progression.

2. Results

2.1. Adrenergic Stimuli Increase Pro-Inflammatory Cytokine Production

To characterize changes in pro-inflammatory networks induced by adrenergic signaling, we analyzed cytokine/chemokine protein expression in supernatants from an ovarian cancer cell/macrophage (SKOV3ip1/U937) co-culture system exposed to epinephrine (Epi) or norepinephrine (NE) (Figure 1a,b). First, SKOV3ip1 monocultures treated with Epi or NE for 3 h (hrs) showed no significant difference in cytokine expression from their respective untreated controls. However, longer exposure of monocultures to stress hormones demonstrated significant changes in cytokines expression compared to untreated controls. SKOV3ip1 monoculture exposure to Epi and NE for 24 h showed significant upregulation in expression, 63, and 95 cytokines, respectively (Table S1).

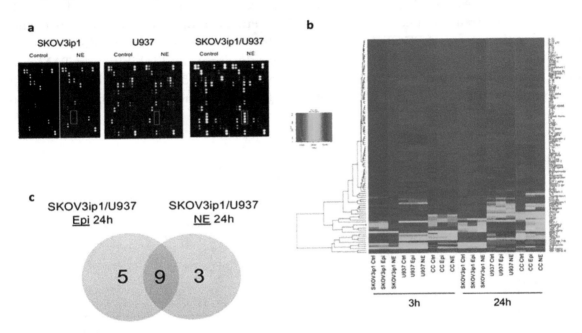

Figure 1. Adrenergic stimuli modulate ovarian cancer cells/macrophage co-cultures cytokine networks. (**a**) Cytokine arrays from SKOV3ip1 and U937 cell lines in monocultures and co-culture conditions 24 h after 10 μM NE exposure. Dots represent cytokines, and red boxes show how changes in cytokine expression are seen in films. Red box demonstrating changes in MIP-1 alpha/beta and MIP-3alpha. (**b**) Heatmap of differentially expressed cytokines between ovarian cancer cells, macrophage monocultures, and co-cultures. The degree of expression is indicated by different colors. Blue, low expression; green, medium expression; red, high expression. Heatmap shows mean raw expression values. (**c**) Venn Diagram of upregulated cytokines shared between epinephrine (Epi)- and norepinephrine (NE)-treated co-culture systems.

To understand the influence of macrophages on cancer cell cytokine crosstalk, we evaluated adrenergic-stimulated co-cultures while adjusting for treated monocultures. Short-term (3 h) exposure of SKOV3ip1/U937 co-cultures to Epi and NE resulted in significant upregulation of 12 and 15 cytokines ($p < 0.05$), compared to SKOV3ip1 monoculture conditions. This early response to stress in both conditions resulted in the expression of known macrophage activity modulators such as MCP1, MCP3, macrophage migration inhibitory factor (MIF), uPAR, and matrix metalloprotein 9 (MMP9). Moreover, we observed a more robust cytokine response in SKOV3ip1/U937 co-cultures 24 h after catecholamine exposure. Compared to stimulated SKOV3ip1 monocultures, Epi-treated co-cultures exhibited 45 upregulated cytokines while NE-treated co-cultures had 20 (Table S2). Many of the upregulated cytokines have been shown to be involved in proangiogenic, metastatic, and angiogenic cascades, for example, Chitinase 3-like 1, vascular endothelial growth factor (VEGF), uPAR, RANTES (CCL5), MIP-3alpha, and CD31.

To further characterize the influence of adrenergic stimuli on macrophage-cancer cell crosstalk, we analyzed adrenergic-stimulated co-cultures compared to untreated co-cultures. Co-cultures treated with Epi or NE for 3 h and 24 h exhibited differential expression of pro-inflammatory cytokines compared to untreated co-cultures (Figure 1b). Specifically, at 3 h, neither Epi or NE-treated co-cultures had significantly upregulated cytokines. More importantly, due to the robustness of the effect observed at 24 h, we decided to focus on this time point. Compared to untreated co-cultures, Epi and NE exposure for 24 h differentially upregulated ($p < 0.05$; fold change > 2) 14 and

12 pro-inflammatory cytokines, respectively (Figure 2a,b). Furthermore, nine of these significantly upregulated cytokines overlapped between Epi- and NE-treated groups: PDGF-AA, epithelial cell-derived neutrophil-activating peptide (ENA-78), Lipocalin-2, Angiogenin, interleukin-5 (IL-5), B-cell activating factor (BAFF), MIF, granulocyte-macrophage colony-stimulating factor (GM-CSF), and TfR (Figure 1c). Among these, PDGF-AA and ENA-78 (CXCL5) were found to be the most upregulated in both treatment conditions (Table S3). Furthermore, in order to confirm the role of macrophages in the release of PDGF-AA following adrenergic stimuli, we used Zoledronic acid (ZA) in vitro. ZA, a clinically available bisphosphonate, has demonstrated inhibition of TAMs in culture conditions and multiple tumor models [14,15]. Treatment with 5 μM of ZA blocked NE-induced PDGF-AA release from both SKOV3 cancer cells and U937 differentiated macrophages (Figure 2c).

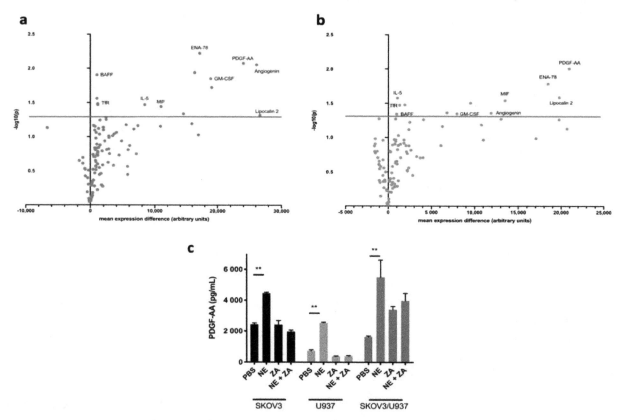

Figure 2. Cytokine profile of adrenergic stimulated ovarian cancer cells/macrophage co-cultures (**a**) Volcano plots showing cytokine changes of SKOV3ip1and U937 co-cultures 24 h after Epi or (**b**) NE treatment. The Y-axis depicts the two-class comparison's statistical significance in –log notation of the t-test's p-value. Thus, the higher the dot, the higher the statistical significance. The X-axis depicts expression compared to monoculture conditions. The farther to the right, the higher the expression. The red line marks the threshold for statistical significance established at $p < 0.05$. Cytokines labeled are shared between Epi and NE groups. (**c**) Zoledronic acid (ZA) prevents NE-induced platelet-derived growth factor AA (PDGF-AA) release in SKOV3 and U937 monocultures and SKOV3/U937 co-cultures. Mean ± SEM. ** $p < 0.01$.

In order to understand the potential role of the different subtypes of macrophages under adrenergic stimuli, we analyzed changes in subsets of cytokine signatures in our U937 monoculture and SKOV3ip1/U937 co-culture systems. Here, we utilized existing data from ovarian carcinoma immune profiling studies [16–18] to determine if there are changes in cytokine signatures suggestive of M1, M2, and TAMs phenotypes (Figure 3a). The results show that NE-treated SKOV3ip1/U937 co-cultures express significantly more factors from a TAMs signature compared to NE-treated U937 macrophages alone. In addition, these robust changes in cytokine expression profiles were not clearly observed in M1 and M2 signatures. (Figure 3b,c).

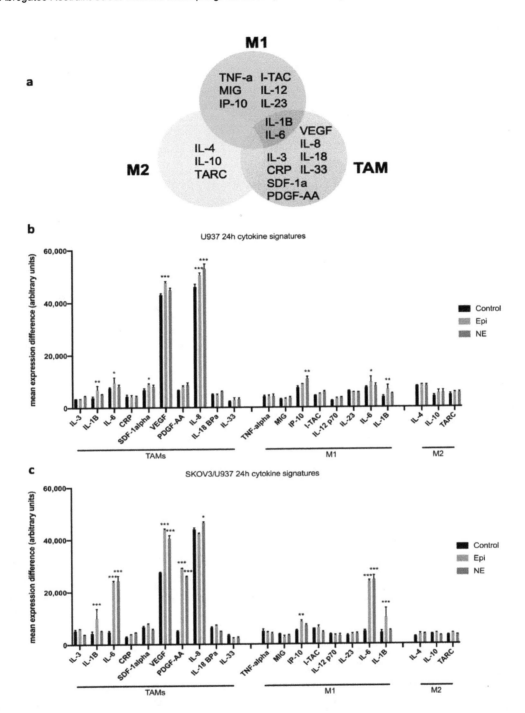

Figure 3. Cytokine signatures associated with Tumor-associated macrophages (TAMs), M1, and M2 phenotypes in U937 monocultures and SKOV3ip1/U937 co-cultures. (**a**) Schematic representation of cytokine signatures categorized by macrophage subsets. (**b**) Cytokine expression signatures in U937 monocultures and (**c**) SKOV3ip1/U937 co-culture conditions after 24-hr exposure to Epi or NE. Mean ± SEM. * $p < 0.05$ ** $p < 0.01$ *** $p < 0.0001$.

2.2. Gene Ontology Biological Process and KEGG Pathway Enrichment Analyses of Differentially Expressed Cytokines

In order to understand the biological processes altered by adrenergic stimuli, we constructed protein-protein interaction (PPI) networks from differentially expressed cytokines identified in adrenergic-induced SKOV3ip1/U937 co-cultures. For this purpose, we used the online STRING database (Search Tool for the Retrieval of Interacting Genes/Proteins; string-db.org/), which provides associations and links between query genes and proteins [19]. The results showed a higher number of interactions among cytokines in the Epi-treated network (node degree: 42, clustering coefficient: 0.786) compared to the NE-treated (node degree: 23, clustering coefficient: 0.576) (Table S4). This difference is also evident as the Epi-treated PPI network demonstrates more interactions than the NE-treated and shared cytokine networks (Figure 4).

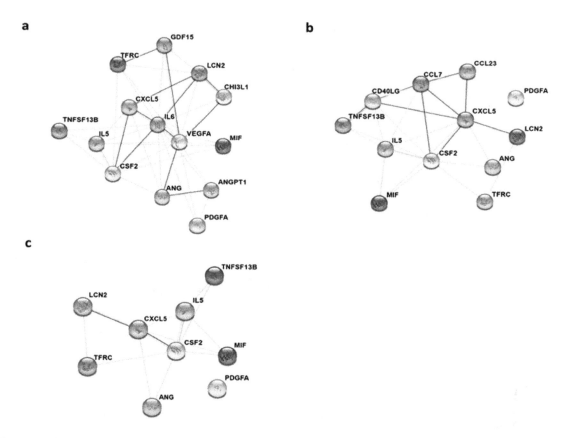

Figure 4. Protein-protein interaction network between differentially expressed cytokines in ovarian cancer–macrophage co-cultures. (**a**) Epi 24 h (**b**) NE 24 h and (**c**) shared cytokines between Epi and NE 24 h treatment. Each node represents a protein, and the edges linking nodes represent known interactions between the two proteins.

For Epi-treated co-cultures, the top five significant gene ontology (GO) biological process enriched were positive regulation of protein phosphorylation (GO:0001934), positive regulation of cell population proliferation (GO:0008284), regulation of signaling receptor activity (GO:00010469), regulation of cell population proliferation (GO:0042127), and positive regulation of response to a stimulus (GO:0048584). NE-treated co-cultures were enriched for regulation of signaling receptor activity (GO:00010469), cytokine-mediated signaling pathway (GO:0019221), cellular response to cytokine stimulus (GO:0071345), positive regulation of cell population proliferation (GO:0008284), and immune response (GO:0006955) (Table S4). Among the three networks, two GO biological processes were shared: positive regulation of cell population proliferation (GO:0008284) and regulation of signaling receptor activity (GO:00010469).

Using the STRING platform, we sought to identify signaling pathways that could be modulated through differentially expressed cytokines in adrenergic stimulated co-cultures. KEGG molecular networks provide molecular interactions representing systemic functions in molecular datasets. KEGG pathway enrichment analyses of shared upregulated cytokines between Epi- and NE-treated co-cultures identified 11 signaling networks (Table S5). These include the IL-17 signaling pathway, the Jak-STAT signaling pathway, TNF signaling pathway, and transcriptional misregulation in cancer.

2.3. Zoledronic Acid Abrogates Restraint Stress-Induced Macrophage Infiltration, PDGF-AA Expression and Tumor Growth in Orthotopic Mouse Models of Ovarian Cancer

Next, we investigated the role of macrophages in the promotion of ovarian cancer tumor growth in response to sustained adrenergic signaling. Due to the known relationship between stress and TAMs in cancer, we sought to determine if inhibition of TAM activity could abrogate the effects of stress on ovarian cancer progression. For this purpose, the effect of zoledronic acid in restraint stress-induced cancer growth was determined in two ovarian cancer orthotopic mouse models. To induce sympathetic nervous system activation, we utilized an established restraint stress animal model capable of inducing the molecular effects of chronic stress [3]. Mice inoculated intraperitoneally with SKOV3ip1 or HeyT30 ovarian cancer cell lines and randomized into four groups: Control, Stress, ZA, and Stress/ZA. Stress groups were subjected to daily restraint stress (2 hrs/day) and administered either D-PBS or ZA (Figure 5a). In the SKOV3ip1 model, restraint stress increased tumor growth by 4.07-fold (mean difference 0.834 g) and nodule counts by 3.54-fold (mean difference 14.14), while ZA significantly abrogated this effect (Figure 5b; $p < 0.001$). In the HeyT30 model, stress significantly increased tumor growth by 2.0-fold (mean difference 1.769 g), and nodule counts by 2.5-fold (mean difference 4.5). Similarly to the SKOV3ip1 model, ZA treatment prevented the effects of stress on tumor growth and nodule development in the HeyT30 model (Figure 5c; $p < 0.05$).

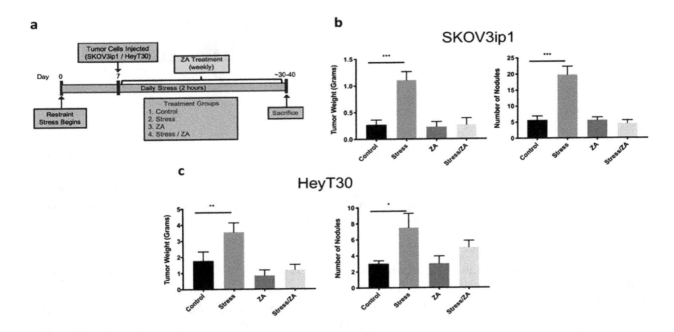

Figure 5. Zoledronic acid (ZA) abrogates restraint stress-induced ovarian cancer tumor growth in an orthotopic Nu/Nu mice model. (**a**) In vivo ovarian cancer orthotopic model timeline (**b**) Tumor weight and tumor nodules in an orthotopic SKOV3ip1 and (**c**) HeyT30 mice model. Stress groups were subjected to daily restraint stress (2 hrs/day), while ZA treatment was administered weekly. Mean ± SEM. * $p < 0.05$ ** $p < 0.01$ *** $p < 0.0001$.

After sacrifice, we proceeded to verify macrophage infiltration in formalin-fixed tumor samples from the restraint stress model through CD68 immunohistochemical staining (Figure 6a; $p < 0.01$). Restraint stress increased CD68+ macrophage infiltration into SKOV3ip1 tumors (21.86 CD68+ cells/high-power field (HPF)), and this effect was abrogated by ZA treatment (4.941 CD68+ cells/HPF). Thus, demonstrating ZA was able to prevent the effects of restraint stress by inhibiting macrophage infiltration.

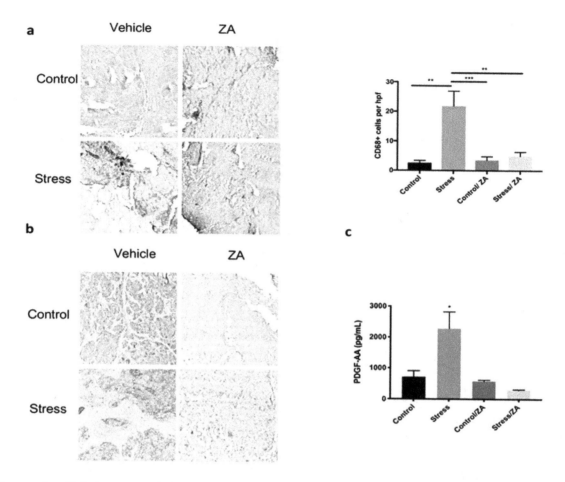

Figure 6. Zoledronic acid (ZA) prevents stress-induced macrophage infiltration and reduces intratumoral PDGF-AA expression in an orthotopic mouse model. Immunohistochemical analysis of SKOV3ip1 tumor samples from mice subjected to restraint stress and ZA showing expression of (**a**) CD68+ and (**b**) PDGF-AA. 20× magnification. (**c**) PDGF-AA protein expression in SKOV3ip1 tumor samples. Mean ± SEM. * $p < 0.05$ ** $p < 0.01$ *** $p < 0.0001$.

Next, we asked if increased adrenergic signaling enhanced PDGF-AA expression in vivo and if ZA was able to block this effect. The results show that restraint stress significantly increased PDGF-AA protein expression in tumors (stress mean 2283 pg/mL ± 1080 SD), while ZA blocked this effect (stress/ZA mean 293.1 pg/mL ± 45.94 SD) (Figure 6b,c; $p < 0.01$). These data confirm our in vitro findings and suggest a role for adrenergic signaling on PDGF-AA expression.

2.4. Elevated Expression of PDGFA Correlates with Poor Outcome in Ovarian Cancer Patients

Next, we sought to understand the prognostic value of the top two significantly upregulated cytokines identified in our in vitro co-culture system, PDGF-AA and ENA-78. The prognostic value of *PDGFA* and *ENA78* mRNA expression in serous ovarian cancer patients was evaluated using the online tool KM plotter, which evaluates the effect of 22,277 genes and their expression [20]. The analysis was restricted to serious histology within the TCGA dataset ($n = 565$). The results showed that high *PDGFA* (Affymetrix ID: 205463_s_at) expression correlated with decreased overall survival (OS) but did not impact progression-free survival (PFS) in ovarian cancer patients (HR 1.54 (95% CI 1.19–1.99); $p < 0.001$ for OS; HR 0.87 (95% CI 0.68–1.11); $p < 0.25$ for PFS). (Figure 7). In contrast, *ENA78* (Affymetrix ID: 215101_s_at) mRNA expression was not associated with prognostic value.

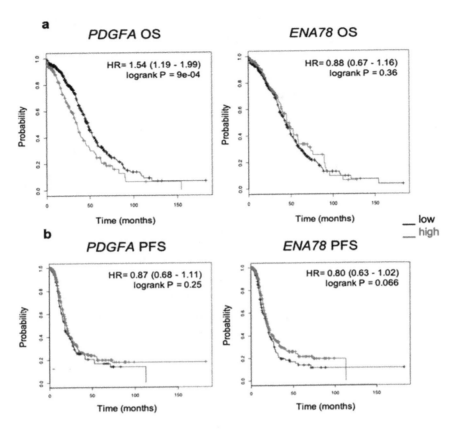

Figure 7. High expression of *PDGFA* correlates with poor outcome in ovarian cancer patients. (**a**) Kaplan–Meier curve of overall survival (OS) ($n = 557$) and (**b**) progression-free survival (PFS) ($n = 522$) in patients with serous epithelial ovarian carcinoma with high or low *PDGFA* and *ENA78* (*CXCL5*) mRNA obtained from KM Plotter using TCGA data. Affymetrix ID: 205463_s_at and 215101_s_at.

3. Discussion

In this study, we investigated the role of adrenergic signaling in the exacerbation of pro-inflammatory networks in ovarian cancer using a combination of molecular and bioinformatic techniques. Using a co-culture system, we were able to dissect the pro-inflammatory signatures exacerbated through macrophage-cancer cell crosstalk in the tumor microenvironment in the context of chronic stress. The results show that exacerbation of pro-inflammatory cytokines by adrenergic stimuli alters the ovarian cancer microenvironment by inducing activation of protumoral pathways. In addition, we show that pharmacological intervention with ZA is able to prevent the effects of stress on cancer progression by targeting TAMs.

Previous work has shown that ovarian cancer cells can recruit macrophages into the tumor through the secretion of MCP1 [13]. However, the role of these TAMs and their tumor-promoting effects on the tumor microenvironment in the context of stress are not well understood. For the last several years, a growing body of literature has studied the role of inflammation in multiple types of cancers [21,22]. In ovarian cancer, chronic inflammation in the tumor microenvironment has been shown to potentiate tumorigenesis, metastasis, and chemoresistance through cytokine networks capable of immune cell recruitment and stimulating the production of growth factors [23]. For example, macrophage production of IL-6 can induce cell proliferation through the STAT3 axis and production of matrix metalloproteins (MMPs) [24,25]. In addition, previous studies have demonstrated that stress promotes the recruitment of TAMs and the production of inflammatory and angiogenic mediators [26,27].

Since cytokine-mediated communication within the tumor microenvironment is mediated by multiple regulatory networks, cellular stimuli, and cytokine production variations, studying the cytokinome patterns provides an informative network of complex interactions [28]. Thus, understanding interactions within the tumor microenvironment and cytokinome crosstalk and functions will provide insight into the progression of inflammation-driven cancers. This work sought to understand if adrenergic-induced cytokines could modulate the tumor microenvironment and lead to ovarian cancer growth. Dissecting the effects of adrenergic signaling on pro-tumoral macrophage function through exacerbation of cytokine networks will provide new opportunities to target the effects of psychological distress on cancer progression. We identified a pro-inflammatory cytokine network composed of PDGF-AA, ENA-78, GM-CSF, MIF, BAFF, Angiogenin, IL-5, Lipocalin 2, and TfR. Most of which have been involved in promoting angiogenesis and metastasis in various cancers [29–32]. This inflammatory exacerbation might promote the perpetuation of inflammation in the tumor microenvironment through stimulation of persistent crosstalk between stroma and tumor cells.

Within the identified pro-inflammatory cytokine network signature, cell proliferation was identified as a possible mechanism for adrenergic-induced regulation, since PDGF-AA was strongly upregulated in both catecholamine treated co-cultures. The platelet-derived growth factor (PDGF) signaling has been identified as a major player in cancer progression as mediators of proliferation, angiogenesis, and metastasis [33,34]. The prognostic value of the PDGF family components has been studied in multiple types of cancers [35,36]. Interestingly Bartoschek et al. detected PDGF-AA and PDGF-BB in the majority of tumor samples evaluated, compared with -CC and -DD. More importantly, high levels of PDGF-AA expression were also correlated with poor survival in cervical squamous cell carcinoma, glioblastoma multiforme, and kidney renal clear cell carcinoma [35]. Recent studies have explored the inflammatory expression signatures in ovarian cancers, in which elevated expression of intratumoral *PDGFA* was found to increase the risk of death and correlate with adverse outcomes [18]. In vitro PDGFRα blockade with IMC-3G3, a specific monoclonal antibody, in combination with docetaxel sensitized HeyA8-MDR ovarian cancer cells and induced apoptosis. This effect was also exhibited in tumor-bearing mice after inhibition of tumor growth [37].

The key observation in our study is that ZA was able to prevent the effects of adrenergic signaling on tumor growth and block the infiltration of macrophages. ZA is a bisphosphonate used clinically as an adjuvant cancer treatment and prevention of bone metastasis due to the ability to inhibit osteoclast function and bone resorption [38]. Due to sharing the same lineage as osteoclasts, macrophages uptake ZA resulting in reducing survival, viability, and differentiation [39]. These results demonstrate an alternative pharmacological approach to prevent the effects of stress on tumor progression that vary from targeting components of the adrenergic pathway. Further research is needed to address whether directly targeting the pro-inflammatory cytokine network, led by PDGF-AA and ENA-78, is an effective way to block the effects of adrenergic signaling in vitro. If proven, this approach could be used as therapies for ovarian cancer patients suffering from chronic stress and biobehavioral disorders.

4. Materials and Methods

4.1. Cell Lines, Treatments, and Co-Culture System

The derivation and source of the established SKOV3, SKOV3ip1, and HeyT30 ovarian cancer cell lines have been reported previously [3,40,41]. SKOV3, SKOV3ip1, HeyT30 ovarian cancer cells, and human U937 monocytic cell line (CRL-1593.2, ATCC, Manassas, VA, USA) were maintained in RPMI 1640 medium, supplemented with 1% antibiotic/antimycotic and 10% fetal bovine serum. All cell lines were grown in 95% O_2 and 5% CO_2 at 37 °C, routinely screened for mycoplasma contamination (30-1012k, ATCC). Cell line authentication was performed using short tandem repeat analysis. All experiments were performed with cultures grown at 70–80% confluence.

Cultures were treated with 10 μM epinephrine or norepinephrine in dH_2O (Sigma-Aldrich, St. Louis, MO, USA) in serum-free media for 3 h and 24 h as necessary. Previous studies have shown 10 μM catecholamine treatment induces oncogenic hallmarks in cancer studies [42,43]. In respective experiments, cultures were pre-treated with 5 µM Zoledronic acid (Sigma-Aldrich, SML0223) diluted in PBS for 48 hrs [15]. Afterward, cultures were treated with 10 µM norepinephrine for 24 h. Control plates were mock-treated with dH_2O and/or PBS for the same amount of time.

In co-culture experiments, indirect co-culture assays were performed where cancer cells and macrophages were separated by a porous membrane, allowing for the exchange of soluble factors, but no direct physical contact was present. For co-cultures, human U937 cells were differentiated into macrophages by 72 h incubation with 200 nM phorbol 12-myristate 13-acetate (PMA), followed by 24 h incubation in RPMI complete medium. During the 72 h incubation with PMA, U937 monocyte to macrophage differentiation was confirmed by visual analysis of macrophage morphology and attachment to culture plates [44]. Ovarian cancer cells were then seeded (1:1 ratio) on 6-well Transwell inserts with 0.4 µm-pore polycarbonate membranes (Corning, #3412, Glendale, AZ, USA). After a 24 h resting period, cultures were treated with hormones as described previously. After respective treatment, co-culture supernatant was stored at −80 °C for cytokine arrays.

4.2. Cytokine Arrays

For cytokine analysis, supernatant from monocultures or co-cultures of ovarian cancer cells/macrophages were used after storage at −80 °C. To measure cytokines, the Proteome Profiler Human XL Cytokine Array kit (ARY022B, R&D Systems, Minneapolis, MN, USA) was used following the manufacturer's instructions. This array is a membrane-based immunoassay that detects changes in 105 human cytokines simultaneously. After chemiluminescent detection, films were quantified using Quick Spots Tool in Western Vision's HLImage++ for Array Analysis Software (Version 22.0, Salt Lake City, UT, USA). The average intensity of negative controls per group was subtracted from each cytokine measure to deduct the background. Cytokine expression was normalized to respective monoculture conditions. Raw cytokine expression data are included in Table S6.

To view relative cytokine expression among all treatment conditions, heatmaps were constructed in RStudio (Version 1.0.153, Boston, MA, USA) with the following R packages: RColorBrewer, d3heatmap, and ggplot2 [45,46]. To identify significant changes in cytokine patterns, cytokine expression analysis and volcano plots were constructed using GraphPad Prism (version 8.1.0, San Diego, CA, USA) and Multiexperiment viewer (MeV) program, version 10.2 (Rockville, MD, USA) [47].

4.3. Protein-Protein Interaction (PPI) Network Construction

The Search Tool for the Retrieval of Interacting Genes/Proteins (STRING; string-db.org/, Zurich, Switzerland) database provides associations and links between query genes and proteins, creating a PPI network. This network and gene enrichment of differentially expressed cytokines identified previously were constructed with the STRING free online platform (version 11.0) [19]. Network properties include edges: number of interactions; nodes: number of proteins in the network; node degree: average number of interactions; clustering coefficient: the tendency of the network to form clusters. The closer the coefficient is to 1, the more likely the network will form clusters; PPI enrichment p-value: statistical significance.

4.4. Animal Experiments

For animal studies, 8 to 12-week-old female athymic nude (Nu/Nu) mice were obtained from Taconic Laboratories. All experiments were approved by the Institutional Animal Care and Use Committee at Ponce Health Sciences University (IACUC Protocol #240). Animals were assigned randomly into each group (4 groups of 10 mice): (1) Control (intraperitoneal vehicle injection/once per week), (2) Stress (restraint stress/intraperitoneal vehicle injection/once per week), (3) ZA (1 mg/kg ZA/once per week) and (4) Stress/ZA (restraint stress/1 mg/kg ZA/once per week).

To induce chronic stress, we used a daily physical-restraint-stress model, as previously described [3]. Mice were subjected daily to 2 hrs of restraint-stress. Access to food and water was restricted to all groups during chronic stress protocol. HeyT30 (2.5×10^5 cells/200 µL HBSS, Thermo, Rockford,

IL, USA) or SKOV3ip1 (1×10^6 cells/200 μL HBSS) tumor cells were injected intraperitoneally into mice in all groups 7 days after chronic stress protocol began. Mice in experimental groups were treated with 1 mg/kg/once per week ZA until sacrifice. Each group had the following tumor incidence: SKOV3ip1; Control ($n = 7$), Stress ($n = 7$), ZA ($n = 8$), and Stress/ZA ($n = 8$). HeyT30; Control ($n = 8$), Stress ($n = 8$), ZA ($n = 6$), and Stress/ZA ($n = 9$). Animals were sacrificed 30–40 days after tumor cell injection, depending on the tumor burden induced by each cell line. Tumor weight, number of nodules, and nodule location were recorded for each animal immediately after sacrifice. Tumor burden was evaluated by inspecting the peritoneal cavity, removing tumor nodules present, and determining combined tumor weight per mouse. Tumor samples were formalin-fixed and mounted in paraffin blocks for immunohistochemistry analysis. Additional tumor samples were flash-frozen in liquid nitrogen and stored at −80 °C until further processing for ELISA.

4.5. Immunohistochemistry

Immunohistochemistry (IHC) was performed on formalin-fixed, paraffin-embedded tumor samples sliced at 4 μm. Samples were stained for CD68 (1:200; MCA1957, BioRad, Hercules, CA, USA), and PDGF-AA (1:250; sc-9974, Santa Cruz Biotechnology, Dallas, TX, USA) following protocol by Pérez-Morales et al., 2018 [48]. Briefly, slides were heated at 65 °C for 30 min and then deparaffinized using graded xylenes. Endogenous peroxidase activity was blocked by incubation in 3% hydrogen peroxide for 15 min. Antigen retrieval was performed using citrate buffer solution for 40 min in a preheated water bath (95–99 °C) and followed by a 30-min cool-down. Protein block solution was added for one hrs at room temperature. Tissues were incubated overnight in the primary antibody at 4–8 °C in a humidity chamber. Protein block, secondary antibody, and 3,3'-Diaminobenzidine (DAB) in the Super Sensitive Link Label IHC kit (LP000-ULE, BioGenex, Fremont, CA, USA) were used for visualization per manufacturer's instructions. Counterstain was performed using hematoxylin for 20 s, followed by washing with running tap water for five minutes. Slides were dried, mounted, and then blindly scored by two independent investigators. CD68 counts were determined by the amount of CD68+ cells per high power field (HPF) using ImageJ software (Bethesda, MD, USA).

4.6. ELISA

Flash-frozen tumor samples were lysed using Bullet Blender Bead Lysis Kit (Next Advance, Pink5E100, Troy, NY, USA). PDGF-AA levels from in vivo tumor lysates were analyzed by ELISA using the Human PDGF-AA ELISA kit (Thermo; EHPDGFA) according to manufacturer's protocol. Samples were assayed in triplicate, and results represent average mean concentration over triplicate experiments.

4.7. Kaplan–Meier Survival Analysis

Kaplan–Meier Plotter Online Tool (KMPlotter; http://kmplot.com, Budapest, Hungary) was used to analyze the relationship between gene expression and ovarian cancer patient clinical outcomes [20]. We investigated overall survival (OS) and progression-free survival (PFS) in patients with high and low expression of *PDGFA* and *ENA78* (*CXCL5*) (Affymetrix IDs: 205463_s_at and 215101_s_at, Thermo). The analysis was restricted to ovarian cancer serous subtype and TCGA database. Hazard ratio (HR) with 95% confidence interval (CI) and log-rank p-value were retrieved from the online analysis. The threshold for significance was established at $p < 0.05$. HR = 1 indicates that there is no difference in survival between the two groups. HR > 1 or < 1 indicates that one of the groups had better survival than the other.

4.8. Statistical Analysis

Statistical analyses were performed using GraphPad Prism (version 8.1.0). Cytokine expression analysis was performed using raw expression values (arbitrary units). The student's t-test with Welch's approximation for unequal variances was performed to identify significant differences in cytokine expression between groups. One-way ANOVA with Dunnett's multiple comparison test was performed to analyze differences in tumor weight and nodules, CD68, and PDGF-AA expression in tumors. Two-way ANOVA with Dunnett's multiple comparison test was performed for PDGF-AA expression in vitro and macrophage signature expression analysis. The log-rank test was obtained from KM Plotter. The statistical significance threshold was established at $p < 0.05$.

5. Conclusions

In conclusion, we demonstrated that adrenergic signaling is able to exacerbate TAM infiltration, and promote a pro-inflammatory tumor microenvironment, while ZA abrogated this effect. These results provide new insights into the pro-inflammatory profile of the tumor microenvironment and the role of adrenergic signaling in ovarian cancer. Further studies are needed to fully understand the signaling cascades activated by the inflammatory cytokines exacerbated by adrenergic signaling and how ZA affects them. In addition, cytokine profiling provides new opportunities to identify potential biomarkers for early detection and understanding of the damaging effects of behavioral stress on tumoral profiles.

Supplementary Materials:
Table S1: Significantly upregulated cytokines in 24 h Epi- or NE-treated SKOV3ip1 monocultures (adjusted for untreated monocultures), Table S2: Significantly upregulated cytokines in 24 h Epi- or NE-treated co-cultures (adjusted for treated monocultures), Table S3: Significantly upregulated cytokines in 24 h Epi- or NE-treated ovarian cancer cell/macrophage co-cultures, Table S4: Top five gene ontology biological processes enriched from differentially regulated cytokines after adrenergic stimuli, Table S5: KEGG pathway analysis of enriched signaling networks from differentially regulated cytokines after adrenergic stimuli, Table S6: Raw cytokine expression data for monoculture and co-cultures.

Author Contributions: Conceptualization, E.M.C. and G.N.A.-P.; data curation, C.B.C.-E. and J.P.-M.; formal analysis, C.B.C.-E. and J.P.-M.; funding acquisition, G.N.A.-P.; investigation, C.B.C.-E., T.O., M.J.H.-V., A.N.A.-A., R.H.-N. and M.B.-C.; methodology, C.B.C.-E., T.O., L.M., M.J.H.-V., A.N.A.-A., R.H.-N. and M.B.-C.; project administration, L.M. and G.N.A.-P.; resources, T.O., L.M.; software, J.P.-M.; supervision, E.M.C. and G.N.A.-P.; validation, T.O.; visualization, C.B.C.-E. and J.P.-M.; writing–original draft, C.B.C.-E. and G.N.A.P.; writing–review & editing, C.B.C.-E. and G.N.A.-P. All authors have read and agreed to the published version of the manuscript.

Acknowledgments: We would like to acknowledge Camille Chardón-Colón and Jennifer Cabán-Rivera for assistance with tumor immunohistochemistry.

Abbreviations

DAB	3,3'-Diaminobenzidine
Epi	epinephrine
NE	norepinephrine
ZA	zoledronic acid
hrs	hours
BAFF	B-cell activating factor
ENA-78	epithelial cell-derived neutrophil-activating peptide
GM-CSF	granulocyte-macrophage colony-stimulating factor
GO	gene ontology
HR	hazard ratio
HPF	high-power field
IL	interleukin
MIF	macrophage migration inhibitory factor
OS	overall survival
PDGF-AA	platelet-derived growth factor AA
PFS	progression-free survival

TAMs	tumor-associated macrophages
TfR	transferrin receptor
VEGF	vascular endothelial growth factor
PPI	protein-protein interaction
KEGG	Kyoto Encyclopedia of Genes and Genomes
TNF	tumor necrosis factor
STRING	Search Tool for the Retrieval of Interacting Genes/Proteins
KM	Kaplan–Meier
MMP	matrix metalloprotein
PMA	phorbol 12-myristate 13-acetate
MeV	Multiexperiment viewer
IHC	immunohistochemistry
CI	confidence interval

References

1. Howlader, N.; Noone, A.; Krapcho, M.; Miller, D.; Bishop, K.; Altekruse, S.; Kosary, C.; Yu, M.; Ruhl, J.; Tatalovich, Z.; et al. *SEER Cancer Statistics Review, 1975–2013*; National Cancer Institute: Bethesda, MD, USA, 2016; p. 19.

2. Tortolero-Luna, G.; Zavala-Zegarra, D.; Pérez-Ríos, N.; Torres-Cintrón, C.; Ortiz-Ortiz, K.; Traverso-Ortiz, M.; Román-Ruiz, Y.; Veguilla-Rosario, I.; Vázquez-Cubano, N.; Merced-Vélez, M.; et al. *Cancer in Puerto Rico, 2006–2010*; Puerto Rico Central Cancer Registry: San Juan, PR, USA, 2013; p. 107.

3. Thaker, P.H.; Han, L.Y.; Kamat, A.A.; Arevalo, J.M.; Takahashi, R.; Lu, C.; Jennings, N.B.; Armaiz-Pena, G.; Bankson, J.A.; Ravoori, M.; et al. Chronic stress promotes tumor growth and angiogenesis in a mouse model of ovarian carcinoma. *Nat. Med.* **2006**, *12*, 939–944. [CrossRef] [PubMed]

4. Bodurka-Bevers, D.; Basen-Engquist, K.; Carmack, C.L.; Fitzgerald, M.A.; Wolf, J.K.; de Moor, C.; Gershenson, D.M. Depression, anxiety, and quality of life in patients with epithelial ovarian cancer. *Gynecol. Oncol.* **2000**, *78*, 302–308. [CrossRef] [PubMed]

5. Watkins, J.L.; Thaker, P.H.; Nick, A.M.; Ramondetta, L.M.; Kumar, S.; Urbauer, D.L.; Matsuo, K.; Squires, K.C.; Coleman, R.L.; Lutgendorf, S.K.; et al. Clinical impact of selective and nonselective beta-blockers on survival in patients with ovarian cancer. *Cancer* **2015**, *121*, 3444–3451. [CrossRef] [PubMed]

6. Chida, Y.; Hamer, M.; Wardle, J.; Steptoe, A. Do stress-related psychosocial factors contribute to cancer incidence and survival? *Nat. Clin. Pract. Oncol.* **2008**, *5*, 466–475. [CrossRef] [PubMed]

7. Hill, E.M. Quality of life and mental health among women with ovarian cancer: Examining the role of emotional and instrumental social support seeking. *Psychol. Health Med.* **2016**, *21*, 551–561. [CrossRef]

8. Lutgendorf, S.K.; Andersen, B.L. Biobehavioral approaches to cancer progression and survival: Mechanisms and interventions. *Am. Psychol.* **2015**, *70*, 186–197. [CrossRef]

9. Qian, B.Z.; Pollard, J.W. Macrophage diversity enhances tumor progression and metastasis. *Cell* **2010**, *141*, 39–51. [CrossRef]

10. Cole, S.W.; Nagaraja, A.S.; Lutgendorf, S.K.; Green, P.A.; Sood, A.K. Sympathetic nervous system regulation of the tumour microenvironment. *Nat. Rev. Cancer* **2015**, *15*, 563–572. [CrossRef]

11. Nagaraja, A.S.; Dorniak, P.L.; Sadaoui, N.C.; Kang, Y.; Lin, T.; Armaiz-Pena, G.; Wu, S.Y.; Rupaimoole, R.; Allen, J.K.; Gharpure, K.M.; et al. Sustained adrenergic signaling leads to increased metastasis in ovarian cancer via increased PGE2 synthesis. *Oncogene* **2016**, *35*, 2390–2397. [CrossRef]

12. Kang, Y.; Nagaraja, A.S.; Armaiz-Pena, G.N.; Dorniak, P.L.; Hu, W.; Rupaimoole, R.; Liu, T.; Gharpure, K.M.; Previs, R.A.; Hansen, J.M.; et al. Adrenergic Stimulation of DUSP1 Impairs Chemotherapy Response in Ovarian Cancer. *Clin. Cancer Res.* **2016**, *22*, 1713–1724. [CrossRef]

13. Armaiz-Pena, G.N.; Gonzalez-Villasana, V.; Nagaraja, A.S.; Rodriguez-Aguayo, C.; Sadaoui, N.C.; Stone, R.L.; Matsuo, K.; Dalton, H.J.; Previs, R.A.; Jennings, N.B.; et al. Adrenergic regulation of monocyte chemotactic protein 1 leads to enhanced macrophage recruitment and ovarian carcinoma growth. *Oncotarget* **2015**, *6*, 4266–4273. [CrossRef]

14. Jia, X.H.; Du, Y.; Mao, D.; Wang, Z.L.; He, Z.Q.; Qiu, J.D.; Ma, X.B.; Shang, W.T.; Ding, D.; Tian, J. Zoledronic acid prevents the tumor-promoting effects of mesenchymal stem cells via MCP-1 dependent recruitment of macrophages. *Oncotarget* **2015**, *6*, 26018–26028. [CrossRef] [PubMed]

15. Gonzalez-Villasana, V.; Rodriguez-Aguayo, C.; Arumugam, T.; Cruz-Monserrate, Z.; Fuentes-Mattei, E.; Deng, D.; Hwang, R.F.; Wang, H.; Ivan, C.; Garza, R.J.; et al. Bisphosphonates inhibit stellate cell activity and enhance antitumor effects of nanoparticle albumin-bound paclitaxel in pancreatic ductal adenocarcinoma. *Mol. Cancer* **2014**, *13*, 2583–2594. [CrossRef] [PubMed]

16. Kulbe, H.; Chakravarty, P.; Leinster, D.A.; Charles, K.A.; Kwong, J.; Thompson, R.G.; Coward, J.I.; Schioppa, T.; Robinson, S.C.; Gallagher, W.M.; et al. A dynamic inflammatory cytokine network in the human ovarian cancer microenvironment. *Cancer Res.* **2012**, *72*, 66–75. [CrossRef] [PubMed]

17. Reinartz, S.; Finkernagel, F.; Adhikary, T.; Rohnalter, V.; Schumann, T.; Schober, Y.; Nockher, W.A.; Nist, A.; Stiewe, T.; Jansen, J.M.; et al. A transcriptome-based global map of signaling pathways in the ovarian cancer microenvironment associated with clinical outcome. *Genome Biol.* **2016**, *17*, 108. [CrossRef]

18. Nakamura, M.; Bax, H.J.; Scotto, D.; Souri, E.A.; Sollie, S.; Harris, R.J.; Hammar, N.; Walldius, G.; Winship, A.; Ghosh, S.; et al. Immune mediator expression signatures are associated with improved outcome in ovarian carcinoma. *Oncoimmunology* **2019**, *8*, e1593811. [CrossRef]

19. Szklarczyk, D.; Gable, A.L.; Lyon, D.; Junge, A.; Wyder, S.; Huerta-Cepas, J.; Simonovic, M.; Doncheva, N.T.; Morris, J.H.; Bork, P.; et al. STRING v11: Protein-protein association networks with increased coverage, supporting functional discovery in genome-wide experimental datasets. *Nucleic Acids Res.* **2019**, *47*, D607–D613. [CrossRef]

20. Gyorffy, B.; Lanczky, A.; Szallasi, Z. Implementing an online tool for genome-wide validation of survival-associated biomarkers in ovarian-cancer using microarray data from 1287 patients. *Endocr. Relat. Cancer* **2012**, *19*, 197–208. [CrossRef]

21. Costantini, S.; Capone, F.; Guerriero, E.; Castello, G. An approach for understanding the inflammation and cancer relationship. *Immunol Lett* **2009**, *126*, 91–92. [CrossRef]

22. Hanahan, D.; Weinberg, R.A. Hallmarks of cancer: The next generation. *Cell* **2011**, *144*, 646–674. [CrossRef]

23. Savant, S.S.; Sriramkumar, S.; O'Hagan, H.M. The Role of Inflammation and Inflammatory Mediators in the Development, Progression, Metastasis, and Chemoresistance of Epithelial Ovarian Cancer. *Cancers* **2018**, *10*, 251. [CrossRef] [PubMed]

24. Takaishi, K.; Komohara, Y.; Tashiro, H.; Ohtake, H.; Nakagawa, T.; Katabuchi, H.; Takeya, M. Involvement of M2-polarized macrophages in the ascites from advanced epithelial ovarian carcinoma in tumor progression via Stat3 activation. *Cancer Sci.* **2010**, *101*, 2128–2136. [CrossRef] [PubMed]

25. Rabinovich, A.; Medina, L.; Piura, B.; Segal, S.; Huleihel, M. Regulation of ovarian carcinoma SKOV-3 cell proliferation and secretion of MMPs by autocrine IL-6. *Anticancer Res.* **2007**, *27*, 267–272. [PubMed]

26. Sloan, E.K.; Priceman, S.J.; Cox, B.F.; Yu, S.; Pimentel, M.A.; Tangkanangnukul, V.; Arevalo, J.M.; Morizono, K.; Karanikolas, B.D.; Wu, L.; et al. The sympathetic nervous system induces a metastatic switch in primary breast cancer. *Cancer Res.* **2010**, *70*, 7042–7052. [CrossRef]

27. Kim, M.H.; Gorouhi, F.; Ramirez, S.; Granick, J.L.; Byrne, B.A.; Soulika, A.M.; Simon, S.I.; Rivkah Isseroff, R. Catecholamine stress alters neutrophil trafficking and impairs wound healing by beta2-adrenergic receptor-mediated upregulation of IL-6. *J. Investig. Dermatol.* **2014**, *134*, 809–817. [CrossRef]

28. Costantini, S.; Sharma, A.; Colonna, G. The Value of the Cytokinome Profile. In *Inflammatory Diseases—A Modern Perspective*; Nagal, A., Ed.; InTech: London, UK, 2011.

29. Shikada, Y.; Yonemitsu, Y.; Koga, T.; Onimaru, M.; Nakano, T.; Okano, S.; Sata, S.; Nakagawa, K.; Yoshino, I.; Maehara, Y.; et al. Platelet-derived growth factor-AA is an essential and autocrine regulator of vascular endothelial growth factor expression in non-small cell lung carcinomas. *Cancer Res.* **2005**, *65*, 7241–7248. [CrossRef]

30. Zaynagetdinov, R.; Sherrill, T.P.; Gleaves, L.A.; McLoed, A.G.; Saxon, J.A.; Habermann, A.C.; Connelly, L.; Dulek, D.; Peebles, R.S., Jr.; Fingleton, B.; et al. Interleukin-5 facilitates lung metastasis by modulating the immune microenvironment. *Cancer Res.* **2015**, *75*, 1624–1634. [CrossRef]

31. Yang, J.; McNeish, B.; Butterfield, C.; Moses, M.A. Lipocalin 2 is a novel regulator of angiogenesis in human breast cancer. *FASEB J.* **2013**, *27*, 45–50. [CrossRef]

32. Simpson, K.D.; Templeton, D.J.; Cross, J.V. Macrophage migration inhibitory factor promotes tumor growth and metastasis by inducing myeloid-derived suppressor cells in the tumor microenvironment. *J. Immunol.* **2012**, *189*, 5533–5540. [CrossRef]

33. Jansson, S.; Aaltonen, K.; Bendahl, P.O.; Falck, A.K.; Karlsson, M.; Pietras, K.; Ryden, L. The PDGF pathway in breast cancer is linked to tumour aggressiveness, triple-negative subtype and early recurrence. *Breast Cancer Res. Treat.* **2018**, *169*, 231–241. [CrossRef]

34. Yang, Y.; Andersson, P.; Hosaka, K.; Zhang, Y.; Cao, R.; Iwamoto, H.; Yang, X.; Nakamura, M.; Wang, J.; Zhuang, R.; et al. The PDGF-BB-SOX7 axis-modulated IL-33 in pericytes and stromal cells promotes metastasis through tumour-associated macrophages. *Nat. Commun.* **2016**, *7*, 11385. [CrossRef] [PubMed]

35. Bartoschek, M.; Pietras, K. PDGF family function and prognostic value in tumor biology. *Biochem. Biophys. Res. Commun.* **2018**, *503*, 984–990. [CrossRef] [PubMed]

36. Carvalho, I.; Milanezi, F.; Martins, A.; Reis, R.M.; Schmitt, F. Overexpression of platelet-derived growth factor receptor alpha in breast cancer is associated with tumour progression. *Breast Cancer Res.* **2005**, *7*, R788–R795. [CrossRef] [PubMed]

37. Matsuo, K.; Nishimura, M.; Komurov, K.; Shahzad, M.M.; Ali-Fehmi, R.; Roh, J.W.; Lu, C.; Cody, D.D.; Ram, P.T.; Loizos, N.; et al. Platelet-derived growth factor receptor alpha (PDGFRalpha) targeting and relevant biomarkers in ovarian carcinoma. *Gynecol. Oncol.* **2014**, *132*, 166–175. [CrossRef]

38. Coleman, R.E.; Collinson, M.; Gregory, W.; Marshall, H.; Bell, R.; Dodwell, D.; Keane, M.; Gil, M.; Barrett-Lee, P.; Ritchie, D.; et al. Benefits and risks of adjuvant treatment with zoledronic acid in stage II/III breast cancer. 10 years follow-up of the AZURE randomized clinical trial (BIG 01/04). *J. Bone Oncol.* **2018**, *13*, 123–135. [CrossRef]

39. Patntirapong, S.; Poolgesorn, M. Alteration of macrophage viability, differentiation, and function by bisphosphonates. *Oral Dis.* **2018**, *24*, 1294–1302. [CrossRef]

40. Huang, G.S.; Brouwer-Visser, J.; Ramirez, M.J.; Kim, C.H.; Hebert, T.M.; Lin, J.; Arias-Pulido, H.; Qualls, C.R.; Prossnitz, E.R.; Goldberg, G.L.; et al. Insulin-like growth factor 2 expression modulates Taxol resistance and is a candidate biomarker for reduced disease-free survival in ovarian cancer. *Clin. Cancer Res.* **2010**, *16*, 2999–3010. [CrossRef]

41. Shaw, T.J.; Senterman, M.K.; Dawson, K.; Crane, C.A.; Vanderhyden, B.C. Characterization of intraperitoneal, orthotopic, and metastatic xenograft models of human ovarian cancer. *Mol. Ther.* **2004**, *10*, 1032–1042. [CrossRef]

42. Barbieri, A.; Bimonte, S.; Palma, G.; Luciano, A.; Rea, D.; Giudice, A.; Scognamiglio, G.; La Mantia, E.; Franco, R.; Perdona, S.; et al. The stress hormone norepinephrine increases migration of prostate cancer cells in vitro and in vivo. *Int. J. Oncol.* **2015**, *47*, 527–534. [CrossRef]

43. Lamboy-Caraballo, R.; Ortiz-Sanchez, C.; Acevedo-Santiago, A.; Matta, J.; NA Monteiro, A.; Armaiz-Pena, G.N. Norepinephrine-Induced DNA Damage in Ovarian Cancer Cells. *Int. J. Mol. Sci.* **2020**, *21*, 2250. [CrossRef]

44. Sintiprungrat, K.; Singhto, N.; Sinchaikul, S.; Chen, S.T.; Thongboonkerd, V. Alterations in cellular proteome and secretome upon differentiation from monocyte to macrophage by treatment with phorbol myristate acetate: Insights into biological processes. *J. Proteom.* **2010**, *73*, 602–618. [CrossRef] [PubMed]

45. Warnes, G.R.; Bolker, B.; Bonebakker, L.; Gentleman, R.; Huber, W.; Liaw, A.; Lumley, T.; Maechler, M.; Magnusson, A.; Moeller, S.; et al. Various R Programming Tools for Plotting Data; Version 3.0.4, CRAN Repository. 2020. Available online: https://cran.r-project.org/web/packages/gplots/index.html (accessed on 9 September 2020).

46. Wickham, H. *ggplot2: Elegant Graphics for Data Analysis*; Springer: New York, NY, USA, 2016.

47. Saeed, A.I.; Sharov, V.; White, J.; Li, J.; Liang, W.; Bhagabati, N.; Braisted, J.; Klapa, M.; Currier, T.; Thiagarajan, M.; et al. TM4: A free, open-source system for microarray data management and analysis. *Biotechniques* **2003**, *34*, 374–378. [CrossRef] [PubMed]

48. Pérez-Morales, J.; Mejías-Morales, D.; Rivera-Rivera, S.; González-Flores, J.; González-Loperena, M.; Cordero-Báez, F.Y.; Pedreira-García, W.M.; Chardón-Colón, C.; Cabán-Rivera, J.; Cress, W.D.; et al. Hyper-phosphorylation of Rb S249 together with CDK5R2/p39 overexpression are associated with impaired cell adhesion and epithelial-to-mesenchymal transition: Implications as a potential lung cancer grading and staging biomarker. *PLoS ONE* **2018**, *13*, e0207483. [CrossRef] [PubMed]

The Tumor Microenvironment of Epithelial Ovarian Cancer and its Influence on Response to Immunotherapy

Galaxia M. Rodriguez [1,2], Kristianne J. C. Galpin [1,2], Curtis W. McCloskey [1,2] and Barbara C. Vanderhyden [1,2,*]

1   Cancer Therapeutics Program, Ottawa Hospital Research Institute, 501 Smyth Road, Ottawa, ON K1H 8L6, Canada; garodriguez@toh.ca (G.M.R.); kgalpin@ohri.ca (K.J.C.G.); cmccloskey@ohri.ca (C.W.M.)
2   Department of Cellular and Molecular Medicine, University of Ottawa, 451 Smyth Road, Ottawa, ON K1H 8M5, Canada
*   Correspondence: bvanderhyden@ohri.ca

Abstract: Immunotherapy as a treatment for cancer is a growing field of endeavor but reports of success have been limited for epithelial ovarian cancer. Overcoming the challenges to developing more effective therapeutic approaches lies in a better understanding of the factors in cancer cells and the surrounding tumor microenvironment that limit response to immunotherapies. This article provides an overview of some ovarian cancer cell features such as tumor-associated antigens, ovarian cancer-derived exosomes, tumor mutational burden and overexpression of immunoinhibitory molecules. Moreover, we describe relevant cell types found in epithelial ovarian tumors including immune cells (T and B lymphocytes, Tregs, NK cells, TAMs, MDSCs) and other components found in the tumor microenvironment including fibroblasts and the adipocytes in the omentum. We focus on how those components may influence responses to standard treatments or immunotherapies.

Keywords: epithelial ovarian cancer; tumor microenvironment; tumor infiltrating lymphocytes; tumor-associated antigens; ascites; immunosuppression; prognostic factors; cancer-associated fibroblasts; exosomes; adipocytes

1. Introduction

An increasing body of evidence strongly suggests that the immune system is able to identify, control and eliminate nascent neoplastic cells in a process known as cancer immunosurveillance [1]. Epithelial ovarian cancers (EOCs) are "immunogenic tumors" that produce spontaneous antitumor immune responses detectable in peripheral blood, tumors and ascites of patients [2–4]. The resulting presence of tumor infiltrating lymphocytes (TILs) is associated with improved survival in EOC [5]. Unfortunately, there are a number of factors in the tumor microenvironment (TME) that can impair the presence or activity of TILs, thereby facilitating cancer progression.

Various immunotherapeutic strategies are attempting to address the challenges posed by the highly immunosuppressive EOC TME. Immunotherapies encompass many modalities, including immune checkpoint blockade, antibody-based therapies, cancer vaccines, cytokines, adoptive cell transfer, and chimeric antigen receptor-modified T cells [6]. However, emerging cancer immunotherapies (blocking antibodies for checkpoint inhibitors) have shown low rates of responses in

EOC (reviewed in [2]). Improving this response rate is a major goal, which can only be achieved with a better understanding of the elements in the TME that contribute to treatment failure. Immune cells are the main players in the development of antitumor immunity or tumor progression, but there are also other components in the TME that should be taken into consideration when designing new therapeutic strategies. Those components include EOC-derived exosomes, cancer-associated fibroblasts (CAFs) and adipocytes residing in the omentum.

In this review we will describe those elements of the TME, how they influence the burden of the tumor, the responses to therapies, and their relevance in designing cancer immunotherapies for EOC.

2. Cancer Cells and Tumor Antigens

The success of cancer immunotherapy hinges on the ability to generate cancer-specific antitumor T-cell responses, to both recognize tumor-associated antigens (TAAs) and kill tumor cells, and to generate memory responses. TAAs can be classified into different categories: tissue differentiation, cancer testes antigens (CTAs), neoantigens derived from mutations, overexpressed cellular, splice variant, glycolipid, and viral antigens [7,8].

Ideal TAAs for immunotherapy targets are immunogenic and are expressed or overexpressed in tumor tissue, with restricted expression in associated normal tissues, in a significant percentage of patients [9].

Positive responses to immunotherapies such as immune checkpoint inhibitors [blocking programmed cell death protein 1 (PD-1), programmed death-ligand 1 (PD-L1) and cytotoxic T-lymphocyte-associated antigen 4 (CTLA-4)], have been associated with high mutation/neoantigen burden [10,11]. The initial clinical studies of small numbers of EOC patients treated with immune checkpoint inhibitors have resulted in clinical benefits in less than 20% of patients (Table 1). Unfortunately, little is known about the TME at the start of treatment in most studies, making it impossible to discern the factors that may have blocked any response.

The failure to respond could be related to the neoantigen burden in EOC, which may be insufficient to generate a significant antitumoral response [12,13]. There are currently intense research efforts to understand other TAAs (Table 2) recognized by TILs to design informed immunotherapy targets (Table 3).

Table 1. Human studies using immune checkpoint inhibitors in epithelial ovarian cancers (EOC) (completed or partially completed studies).

Target	Agent	EOC Characteristic	Antitumoral Responses	Immune Related Parameters	Clinical Study
PD-1	Nivolumab (Opdivo, BMS-936558, MDX1106) i.v. infusion every 2 weeks (1 or 3 mg/kg)	Advanced or relapsed platinum-resistant ovarian cancer	A quick antitumor response observed by baseline computed tomographic image, decreased CA-125 blood levels. Overall response: 15%, 2§ pts had a durable CR, disease control rate in all 20 pts was 45%. Median PFS 3.5 months.	Expression of PD-L1 in ovarian cancer tissues was not significantly correlated with objective response but 16/20 patients having a high expression of PDL1 on tumors did not respond to treatment (vs. 2/4 responders in the PD-L1-low expression group).	Phase II UMIN000005714 [14]
	Pembrolizumab (Keytruda, MK-3475) i.v. infusion every 2 weeks (10 mg/kg) for up to 2 years	PD-L1+ advanced ovarian cancer	1 * pt CR, 2 pts PR; 6 pts stable disease. Duration of response ≥24 weeks. Overall response was 11.5%. 6/26 (23.1%) had evidence of tumor reduction; 3 had a tumor reduction of at least 30%.	N/A	Phase Ib trial NCT02054806 Active, not recruiting [15]
PD-L1	Avelumab (Bavencio, MSB0010718C) every 2 weeks (10 mg/kg)	Recurrent or refractory ovarian cancer	4/23 (17.4%) pts achieved an unconfirmed best overall response of PR, 11 pts (47.8%) had stable disease, and 2 pts had >30% tumor shrinkage after progression was reported. Median PFS was 11.9 weeks and the PFS rate at 24 weeks was 33.3%.	Exposure to Avelumab significantly increased the ratio of sCD27/sCD40L #. Some antitumor activity of this antibody may be due to ADCC [16].	Phase Ib study NCT01772004 Active, not recruiting [17]
	BMS-936559 (MDX-1105) i.v. infusion every 2 weeks (10 mg/kg) in 6-week cycles	Advanced ovarian cancer	1 of 17 pts (6%) had a PR, and 3 (18%) had stable disease lasting at least 24 weeks.	N/A	Multicenter phase 1 trial NCT00729664 completed [18]
	Ipilimumab i.v. infusions (10 mg/kg) once every 3 weeks for 4 doses (Induction Phase). Once every 12 weeks (Maintenance Phase), until disease progression or unacceptable toxicity occurs	Recurrent platinum-sensitive ovarian cancer	N/A	N/A	Phase II study (NCT01611558) Active, not recruiting
CTLA-4	Ipilumumab Periodic infusions (3 mg/kg) after vaccination with irradiated, autologous tumor cells engineered to secrete GM-CSF (GVAX)	Stage IV ovarian carcinoma	1/9 pts had reduction in circulating CA-125 levels, regression of metastasis, increased humoral reactions to NY-ESO-1. 3 pts achieved stable disease of >6, 4, and 2 months' duration, as measured by CA-125 levels and radiographic criteria.	The extent of therapy-induced tumor necrosis was linearly related to the natural logarithm of the ratio of intratumoral CD8+ effector T cells to FoxP3+ Tregs in post-treatment biopsies.	[19,20]

§ The tumor was histologically identified as clear cell carcinoma in one of the two patients who experienced a CR. * 1 Patient with CR had a PD-L1 gene rearrangement leading to gain of function of the PD-L1 gene secondary to gene amplification, high PD-L1 expression was observed in cancer epithelial cells, as well as high T lymphocyte infiltration (CD4, CD8), some B cells (CD20) and macrophages (CD68) [21]. # sCD27 is a marker of T-cell activation [22], sCD40L is a measure of immune suppression [23]. Complete response (CR), partial response (PR), patients (pts), progression-free survival (PFS), intravenous (i.v.), antibody-dependent cell-mediated cytotoxicity (ADCC), not available (N/A), Granulocyte-macrophage colony-stimulating factor (GM-CSF), forkhead box P3 (FoxP3), regulatory T cells (Tregs).

Table 2. Type and prevalence of tumor-associated antigens (TAAs) in EOC.

TAA Category	TAA	Prevalence (% Patients)	FIGO Stage	References
CTA	OY-TES-1	69% (All subtypes)	I-IV	[24]
	SCP-1	15% (All subtypes)	I-IV	[25]
	SPAG9 [1]	88% (HGSC)	I-IV	[26]
	AKAP4 [2]	93% (Serous)	I-IV	[27]
	NY-ESO-1	43% (All Subtypes)	I-IV	[28]
	MAGE-A [3]	~7–55% (All subtypes)	I-IV	[29–31]
Oncogene	p53	Mutation (95% HGSC)/Amplification (35% HGSC)	I-IV	[32,33]
	Her2neu [4]	35–45% (All subtypes)	I-IV	[34–37]
	WT1 [5]	71.4% (LGSC)	III/IV	[38,39]
	Mesothelin	~55% (HGSC)	I-IV	[40,41]
	MUC16 [6] (CA-125)	82% (HGSC) 80% (All subtypes)		[42]
Neoantigen	Patient/tumor site specific	Greater number in HR deficient [7] tumors	I-IV	[12,43]

[1] SPAG9: Sperm-associated antigen 9. [2] AKAP4: A-kinase anchoring protein 4. [3] MAGE-A: Melanoma antigen. [4] Her2-neu: human epidermal growth factor receptor 2-neu. [5] WT1: Wilms' tumor 1. [6] MUC16: Mucin-16. [7] BRCA1/BRCA2, Fanconi anemia genes (PALB2, FANCA, FANCI, FANCL, and FANCC), restriction site associated DNA genes (RAD50, RAD51, RAD51C, and RAD54L), DNA damage response genes (ATM, ATR, CHEK1, and CHEK2). High-grade serous ovarian cancer (HGSC), low-grade serous ovarian cancer (LGSC).

Table 3. TAA targeted immunotherapies in EOC.

TAA Category	TAA	Immunotherapy	References
CTA	NY-ESO-1	Recombinant protein vaccine (Epitope ESO$_{157-170}$) + Incomplete Freund's Adjuvant	[44]
		Overlapping long peptides + Montanide/Poly-ICLC adjuvants	[45]
		NY-ESO-1b + Montanide	[46]
		Recombinant vaccinia prime-NY-ESO-1 (rV-NY-ESO-1) + recombinant fowlpox boost-NY-ESO-1 (rF-NY-ESO-1)	[47]
		NY-ESO-1-specific engineered T Cells	(NCT03159585, NCT03017131, NCT02457650)
		NYESO-1(C259) transduced autologous T cells	(NCT01567891)
	MAGE-A	Autologous genetically modified MAGE-A4^{c1032} T cells	(NCT03132922)
Oncogene	p53	Modified vaccinia Ankara vaccine vs. wild-type human p53 (p53MVA) + gemcitabine	[48]
		Synthetic long peptide (SLP) vaccine	[49]
	Her2neu	Her2-neu peptide vaccine	(NCT00194714)
		Exvivo Her2-neu specific T-cell expansion	(NCT00228358)
	WT1	Autologous WT1 T Cells + Cyclophosphamide + Fludarabine	(NCT00562640)
		WT1 peptide vaccine + Montanide + GM-CSF + Nivolumab (PD-1)	(NCT02737787)
		WT1 mRNA-loaded DCs[2]	[50]
		WT1 peptide vaccine + Montanide	[51]
	Mesothelin	Anti-Mesothelin CAR-T[1] cells	[41]/(NCT02580747)
	MUC16 (CA-125)	Antibody therapy (Oregovomab, ACA125/Abagovomab)	[52–55]
		CAR-T Therapy + IL-12	[56,57] (NCT02498912)
Neoantigen	Patient/tumor site specific	Autologous DCs pulsed with oxidized autologous whole-tumor cell lysate + bevacizumab + cyclophosphamide	[58]
		Autologous neoantigen engineered T-Cells	(NCT03412877)

[1] Chimeric antigen receptor T cell (CAR-T). [2] Dendritic cells (DCs).

2.1. Neoantigens

Ovarian cancer has been shown to harbor an intermediate neoantigen load by whole exome sequencing/next generation sequencing [12,59]. Whole exome sequencing of tumor cells from ascites samples of three high-grade serous ovarian cancer (HGSC) patients revealed a tumor mutation burden (TMB) of approximately 20–40 mutations across all patients, however only 1/79 mutations (1.3%) were recognized by autologous tumor-associated T cells [60]. Comprehensive genomic profiling of ovarian cancer revealed low overall TMB among subtypes: HGSC (3.6), low-grade serous (LGSOC) (2.7), endometrioid (2.7), mucinous (2.7), and clear cell (2.7). Only a small percentage of patients had a significant TMB (20 or more mutations per Mb), meaning only a small percentage of patients would be predicted to show favorable response to immune therapy [12]. Consequently, in clinical trials of checkpoint inhibitors in EOC, CTLA-4 inhibitors (Ipilimumab), PD1 inhibitors (Nivolumab and Pembrolizumab), and PD-L1 inhibitors (MS-936559 and Avelumab) had response rates of 5–20% [14,20,61] (Table 1). A notable exception is the highly aggressive small cell carcinoma of the ovary, hypercalcemic type which, despite being a monogenic cancer, has responsiveness to anti-PD1 immunotherapy [62].

Neoantigen depletion [63], intratumoral heterogeneity, and clonal evolution of primary tumors and metastases may influence immunosurveillance and response to immunotherapy [64,65]. Epithelial T-cell rich tumors show the lowest amount of clonal diversity, neoantigen diversity and greatest loss of human leukocyte antigen (HLA) expression, which suggests immunoediting in the TME. T-cell poor tumors or "cold tumors" have a higher predicted and more diverse neoantigen load (unedited) [63].

2.2. Cancer Testes Antigens

CTAs are encoded by ~140 genes that are normally only expressed in germ cells (testes, placenta, fetal ovary) and not normal somatic adult cells, but often highly expressed in tumors. This along with their immunogenicity makes them significant targets for cancer immunotherapy [9,66,67]. Vaccination with recombinant MAGE-A3 antigen has been used in Phase I/II clinical trials for melanoma [68] and non-small-cell lung cancer (NSCLC) [69] with a good safety profile and observed humoral response, but only slight effects on survival.

Several CTAs have been described in EOC (Table 2) and have been proposed as immunotherapy targets (Table 3) based on their tissue specificity and high expression in a significant number of EOCs of all subtypes. NY-ESO-1 ($ESO_{157-165}$) specific CD8+ T cells were found in TILs of 71% of (10/14) vaccination naïve seropositive patients, and ex vivo proliferation of NY-ESO-1 specific peripheral blood lymphocytes in 65% of patients suggested that an adaptive immune response against this CTA can be achieved [70,71]. Clinical trials have subsequently tested the feasibility of generating NY-ESO-1 specific immune responses (Table 3). These approaches have generated humoral and CD4+ and CD8+ antigen specific T-cell responses, and in some cases, long lasting/complete responses [44–47]. NY-ESO-1 was not expressed in some recurrent tumors, raising the possibility of immune escape [44]. Furthermore, NY-ESO-1 reactive CD8+ T cells often express higher levels of inhibitory molecules lymphocyte-activation gene 3 (LAG3), PD-1 and CTLA-4, suggesting immunosuppression as a reason for lack of complete response during clinical trials [71].

Many characteristics of CTA epitopes and all TAAs such as (i) immunogenicity; (ii) restriction to HLA-I or -II; (iii) natural processing; (iv) expression; and (v) role in tumor progression remain to be elucidated and require validation in larger sample sizes. While the expression of CTAs does not often correlate with improved survival, their tissue specificity makes CTAs attractive targets for immunotherapies (Table 3) such as peptide vaccines [44,70], antigen-loaded dendritic cell (DC) vaccines [72], or oncolytic viral platforms, and for combined interventions with immune checkpoint inhibitors [73] or chemotherapy [74], in order to overcome tumor escape mechanisms.

2.3. Other TAAs

Genetic and epigenetic aberrations in cancer cells, resulting from mutations, amplifications or deletions in genes, provide both therapeutic targets and potential TAAs for immunotherapy design (Table 2). However, the greatest hurdles still remain in designing immunotherapeutic targets for a disease in which such aberrations, with the exception of p53 mutation (95% of HGSC [33,75]), are relatively uncommon (<20% frequency in HGSC cases) and lack antigen specificity to the tumor. Immunogenic oncogenes p53, Her2-neu and WT1 are broadly overexpressed in EOC, particularly HGSC, and targeted immunotherapies have been explored in clinical trials (Table 3). Other common but infrequent amplifications, mutations or deletions occur in *CCNE1, NF1, PTEN, KRAS, RB, CDK2NA, PIK3CA* and *AKT1/2* and provide potential therapeutic targets for EOC immunotherapy [33]. The DCs, T-cells, and peptide-based vaccine strategies against proteins described above have largely demonstrated immunological responses including CD4+ and CD8+ T-cell responses in preliminary clinical trials following vaccination, but often in the absence of clinical responses. This is perhaps due to widespread immunosuppression in the TME preventing T-cell activation and proliferation, as well as tumor heterogeneity and immunogenicity that impede proper TAA presentation to the immune cells.

The EOC immunopeptidome was profiled by isolating HLA molecules primarily from HGSC tumors and which were analyzed by mass spectrometry [57]. The analysis identified relevant proteins including CRABP1/2, FOLR1, and KLK10 presented on major histocompatibility complex (MHC) I molecules, and mesothelin, PTPRS and UBB presented on MHC-II molecules [57]. The most abundantly detected protein presented on MHC-I molecules was MUC16 (CA-125), with 113 different peptides expressed in approximately 80% of patients. MUC16-derived peptides were highly immunogenic (85% T-cell responses in vitro), and consequently it was proposed as the top candidate for targeted immunotherapy moving forward [57]. Although CA-125 is immunogenic, the large number of trials with a monoclonal antibody targeting CA-125 (Table 3) have been mostly unsuccessful as a monotherapy [76]. This failure could be explained by the weak magnitude of the immune response generated, the loss of expression or down-regulation of CA-125 on EOC cells to avoid immune recognition, or the overgrowth of CA-125(-) EOC cells as a consequence of cancer immunoediting process.

A single TAA is generally only expressed in a subset of patients, making the design of a universal immunotherapy challenging. The main barrier of targeting a single TAA is cancer immunoediting, which enables the enrichment of neoplastic cells in tumors that do not express the targeted TAA over time. Chimeric antigen receptor T (CAR-T) cells provides the option of combining multiple antigen specificities, and delivering direct cytokine stimulation (GM-CSF, IL-12) to the TME, irrespective of the MHC status of the patient [8].

2.4. Tumor Immunogenicity and Other Immunoinhibitory Molecules

Loss of immunogenicity is an immune hallmark of cancer that is exploited by tumors to evade immune recognition. This can be triggered by down-regulation or loss of expression of MHC-I and -II, and the antigen processing and presentation machinery (APM) [77–80]. Expression of MHC-I genes is altered by 60–90%, depending on the cancer type. These impairments reduce the antigens presented on the cell surface leading to decreased or lack of recognition and elimination by cytotoxic T lymphocytes.

The mechanisms that are related to immune cell infiltration in EOC are dependent on MHC-I and -II status [3,81]. The presence of neoantigen-reactive T cells in patients with EOC can improve survival [82]. However, as mentioned before, since ovarian tumors possess intermediate/low mutation burdens, the incidence of naturally processed and presented neoantigens generating a significant antitumoral response is very low [13]. The expression of APM components and the presence of intratumoral T-cell infiltrates were significantly associated with improved survival [81]. Han. et al. demonstrated that the majority of ovarian carcinomas analyzed had either heterogeneous or positive expression of peptide transporter 1 (TAP1), TAP2, HLA class I heavy chain, and beta-2 microglobulin [81]. Concurrent expression of HLA-DR and CA-125 on cancer cells correlated with higher frequency of CD8+ TILs and increased survival [83]. Similarly, tumor cell expression of HLA-DMB was associated with increased numbers of CD8+ TILs and both were associated with improved survival in advanced-stage serous EOC [84]. The regulation of APM components and MHC molecules in human cancers is a significant area of research but is beyond the scope of this review (reviewed in [85,86]).

The mutational profile of EOC can also predict immunogenicity. Tumors with deficient homologous recombination (HR) machinery occur with a frequency of up to 50% [33]. These include mutations in *BRCA1/BRCA2* (20% frequency) or non-BRCA HR deficiencies (Fanconi anemia genes, restriction site associated DNA genes, and DNA damage response genes) [33]. HR deficient tumors have higher predicted neoantigen load, and infiltrating and peritumoral lymphocytes in these tumors have increased PD-1/PD-L1 expression [43], which may enhance susceptibility to immune checkpoint therapy. *BRCA1/2* mutated HGSC tumors have more CD3+ and CD8+ TILs compared to HR-proficient tumors, a signature associated with higher overall survival [43,87]. p53 mutations are also associated with higher levels of TILs [87,88]. Non-HR deficient tumors therefore have poorer overall survival [43] and may be less immunogenic, making them more difficult to target with immunotherapies. Alternative strategies and TAAs to target this group of EOC tumors need further investigation.

The expression of immunoinhibitory molecules on cancer cells, including PD-L1 and Indoleamine 2,3-dioxygenase (IDO) are associated with patient prognosis. Higher expression of PD-L1 on tumor cells correlates with poorer prognosis, suggesting that the PD-1/PD-L pathway can be a good target for restoring antitumor immunity in EOC [89,90], although others have suggested that high PD-1/PD-L1 expression in primary tumors may be associated with a favorable progression-free survival [91,92]. Increased infiltration of CD8+ T cells is associated with high PD-L1 expression likely as a result of an adaptive response where infiltrating CD8+ T cells secrete interferon gamma (IFNγ) that subsequently induces PD-L1 expression on cancer cells. This in turn inhibits T-cell activation and proliferation, preventing successful targeting and clearance of the tumor. Immune checkpoint inhibitors (anti-PD-L1 and PD-1) have been FDA approved for melanoma and NSCLC, but only a small percentage (10–33%) of ovarian cancers express PD-L1 [61,92,93], thus only a small percentage of patients may respond to anti-PD-L1 immunotherapy (Table 1). The enzyme IDO is often overexpressed by cancer cells, but is also produced by DCs and macrophages [94,95] in the TME. IDO catabolizes tryptophan, which leads to cell cycle arrest or apoptosis in NK and CD4 T cells [96], and skewed differentiation of regulatory T cells (Tregs) induced by plasmacytoid DCs, leading to immunosuppression in the TME [97]. Positive staining for IDO, observed in 24–57% of patient samples, is associated with poor prognosis of HGSC, decreased CD8+ TILs, as well as resistance to chemotherapy [98,99]. Targeting IDO with inhibitors may improve outcome [100,101].

3. Immune Cells

Most solid tumors are infiltrated by myeloid- and lymphoid lineage-derived immune cells that are differentially distributed within the TME with a crucial role in the establishment of antitumoral responses or tumor progression [1]. Growing tumor cells release "danger signals" that enable the recruitment of immune cells into the tumor niche. TILs such as CD4+ and CD8+ T cells, B lymphocytes, Natural Killer (NK)-T cells, as well as innate immune cells such as NK cells, macrophages and DCs, are then recruited in order to eliminate nascent neoplastic cells, acting as an extrinsic tumor suppression mechanism [102]. However, immunosurveillance promotes the selection of poorly immunogenic cancer cells through cancer immunoediting where neoplastic cells that resist the elimination phase can persist in equilibrium with effector CD4+ and CD8+ T cells under a pro-inflammatory milieu. Over time, cancer cells with the most immunoevasive characteristics are selected, enabling them to eventually escape immune attack [102]. Finally, immunoedited tumors become clinically apparent with variants that trigger the establishment of an immunosuppressive TME containing immunosuppressive immune cells such as myeloid-derived suppressor cells (MDSCs), Tregs, and others [2,103].

3.1. Immune Modulators and Adaptive Immune Cells in the Ovarian Cancer TME

3.1.1. TILs

TILs can localize into the tumor islet (intraepithelial) and in the peritumoral space (stromal) [2]. Several studies have shown a positive correlation between the presence of intraepithelial TILs and tumor regression in many solid cancers [4,5,104–107]. T cells can be found in primary tumor tissue and omental metastases [4,104,105,107–111] and their presence has been correlated with positive prognosis. Dadmarz et al. demonstrated that TILs isolated from EOC patients (primary tumor, metastases or ascites) were tumor-specific and could recognize autologous TAAs. Antitumoral responses were mainly characterized by the secretion of tumor necrosis factor-alpha (TNFα) and granulocyte macrophage-colony stimulating factor (GM-CSF) when stimulated with autologous tumor [112]. Later, Zhang and colleagues showed that intraepithelial CD3+ TILs can be found in >50% of advanced-stage EOC with their presence correlating with a five-year overall survival rate of 38% in contrast to 4.5% in patients whose tumors contained no T cells [5]. Even after debulking and platinum-based chemotherapy, the presence of intraepithelial CD3+ TILs increased the five-year overall survival rate (>70%) in comparison to patients whose tumors contained no T cells in islets (11%) [5]. T cell-rich tumors correlated with delayed recurrence or death and were associated with increased expression of Interleukin-2 (IL-2), IFNγ and lymphocyte-attracting chemokines within the tumor such as CXCL9 [113], CCL21, and CCL22 [5]. Conversely, tumors with no T cells in islets were associated with an increased level of vascular endothelial growth factor (VEGF), an angiogenic regulatory factor in the TME associated with early recurrence and short survival [5]. A more recent study showed that intratumoral accumulation of CXCR3 ligands such as CXCL9 and CXCL10, predicts survival in advanced HGSC [113] (Figure 1). This study also identified the cyclooxygenase (**COX**) metabolite Prostaglandin E2 as a negative regulator of chemokine secretion that contributes to tumor progression by impeding TILs recruitment in ovarian cancer [113]. Further investigation showed that expression of both COX-1 and COX-2 were negatively correlated with intraepithelial CD8+ TILs as well as with EOC patient survival [114].

While some studies have reported that the presence of both intraepithelial CD3+ and CD8+ T-cells correlates with improved disease-specific survival for EOC patients [81,87] others have shown that this beneficial characteristic is attributed to intraepithelial CD8+ TILs [4,104,105,107–110,115]. No association was found for CD3+ TILs or other subtypes of intraepithelial or stromal TILs in EOC overall patient survival. Interestingly, the subgroups displaying high versus low intraepithelial CD8+/CD4+ TIL ratios had favorable survival prognosis (median = 58 versus 23 months) [106]. This was due to the unfavorable effect of CD4+ CD25+ forkhead box P3+ (FOXP3) Tregs [88,104,106] that will be discussed later.

In 2012, a meta-analysis of ten studies with 1815 ovarian cancer patients confirmed the prognostic value of intraepithelial CD8+ TILs in EOC specimens regardless of the tumor grade, stage, or histologic subtype studied [111]. Their presence suggests that spontaneously activated antitumoral responses are present in the tumor niche to control tumor outgrowth [111] as observed by the presence of tumor-reactive antibodies and T cells found in the peripheral blood of advanced stage EOC patients [116–118], and oligoclonal tumor-reactive T cells isolated from blood, ascites or tumors [88,119–123]. Conversely, the lack of intraepithelial TILs is significantly associated with poor survival among EOC patients [111]. Thus, immunotherapies aiming to increase the effector functions of pre-existing antitumoral CD8+ TILs and triggering effector T cell-trafficking to the TME are the holy grail of cancer immunotherapy.

CD4+ T cells as well as CD8+ T cells can specifically recognize TAAs from malignant cells. CD4+ T helper (Th) cells provide cytokine support for CD8+ T-cell proliferation and expansion to eliminate cancer cells and trigger antitumoral responses. In an analysis of ovarian tumors, Tsiatas et al. found that a high percentage of CD4+ CD25hi cells and activated CD4+ T cells were significantly associated with improved median overall survival [124]. Two other studies also showed a positive correlation of the high frequency of CD4+ TILs and EOC patient survival [110,125]. Nesbeth et al., using an animal model for EOC, found that tumor-primed CD4+ T cells produce high levels of CCL5 that enables the recruitment and activation of DCs to the TME. Mature DCs were then able to prime tumor-specific CD8+ T cells and confer long-term protection [126]. Hence, immunotherapies stimulating both effector CD4+ and CD8+ T cells could confer synergistic antitumoral responses.

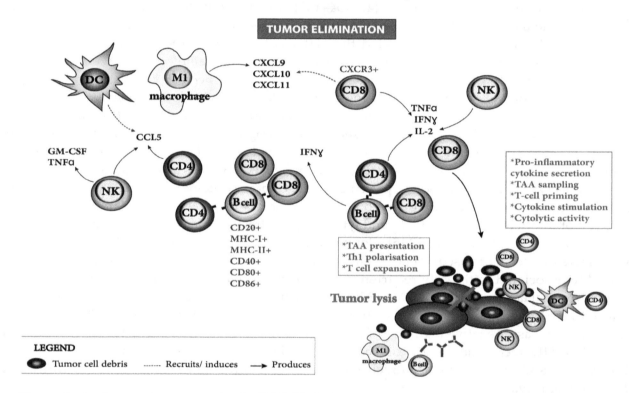

Figure 1. Antitumoral responses in the EOC TME. Immunogenic cell death induces the release of DAMPs mediating the recruitment of innate cells and APCs. Lympho-attracting chemokines produced by APCs such as macrophages enable the recruitment of CD8+ T cells to the tumor niche. DCs are also attracted by the production of CCL5 derived from NK cells and CD4+ T cells. The pro-inflammatory milieu enables TAA sampling and presentation by APCs to T cells to induce their activation and expansion. Pro-inflammatory cytokines released by activated effector T cells, M1 macrophages and DCs allow the amplification of the antitumoral response, enabling the cytolytic death of EOC targeted by CD8+ TILs and NK cells. B cells also participate in antitumor immunity by presenting TAAs to CD8+ T cells, by facilitating Th1 polarization, T-cell expansion and by producing tumor specific antibodies. Danger-associated molecular patterns (DAMPs), Antigen presenting cells (APCs), tumor-associated antigens (TAAs), dendritic cells (DCs), natural killer cells (NKs), CD4+ T helper cell (Th1).

3.1.2. Regulatory T lymphocytes

Tregs negatively regulate antitumoral responses in both a direct and indirect manner, highlighting that Tregs are a fundamental means of tumor immune evasion [127,128]. In healthy tissues, Tregs mediate tolerance by suppressing autoreactive T cells to protect and prevent excessive tissue destruction. Since most TAAs are composed by self-peptides, Tregs are often found in tumors to dampen antitumoral responses. Tregs accumulate and are more frequently present in tumors, with a shift in the median ratio of Tregs to TILs from 3–8% in healthy tissue to 18–25% in all analyzed cancers, including EOC [129]. Curiel et al. analyzed 104 EOC specimens and found that CD4+ CD25+ FOXP3+ Tregs specifically suppress antitumoral T cells in vivo, contributing to tumor growth. In addition, their presence correlates with poor patient outcome [130]. CD4+ Tregs preferentially migrated to tumor and ascites and were rarely found in draining lymph nodes at later cancer stages [131]. Immunotherapies impeding Treg trafficking could release the TME immunosuppression and promote the development of antitumoral responses.

FOXP3+ Tregs express minimal levels of effector cytokines and granzyme B, but are able to induce inhibitory activities through IL-10 and transforming growth factor beta (TGF-β) production [132] and cell–cell interactions [127] (Figure 2). Barnett et al. showed that EOC tumors highly infiltrated by Tregs were associated with poor survival, advanced stage and suboptimal debulking [109]. Investigation of the influence of cytoreduction on the immune system of primary and recurrent EOC found that the ratio of CD4/CD8 is increased in primary but not in recurrent tumors [133]. Primary cytoreduction increased circulating effector CD4+ and CD8+ T cells, but circulating CD4+ Tregs were decreased as well as IL-10 serum levels, but not TGFβ and IL-6 [133]. CD4+ Tregs were also decreased after chemical debulking in patients treated with neoadjuvant chemotherapy. The reduction of the systemic and TME immunosuppression triggered by surgical debulking resulted in an increased capacity of CD8+ T cells to respond to the recall antigens, but not in patients who were previously subjected to chemotherapy or affected by recurrent EOC [133].

Fialová and colleagues studied the dynamics of the tumor-infiltrating immune cells during different stages of EOC [134]. Early stage disease displayed a strong Th17 immune response while stage II patients had responses characterized by the recruitment of Th1 cells. Disseminated disease (stages III and IV) were characterized by high amounts of Tregs, tumor-associated macrophages (TAMs), DCs, and high levels of CCL22, which is secreted by tumor cells, TAMs and DCs to enable further recruitment of Tregs and immunosuppression [134]. Other studies have shown the importance of the TME in facilitating the establishment of tolerance and recruitment of Tregs to sustain tumor growth. Using EOC cell lines in vitro, Facciabene et al. found that tumor hypoxia induces the expression of chemokine ligands such as CCL28, enabling the recruitment of Tregs and triggering angiogenesis [135]. CCL28 overexpression was associated with a poor outcome in patients with EOC [135]. Similarly, CCL22 production by TAMs enabled the recruitment of Tregs [130,134] that induced B7-H4 on antigen-presenting cells including macrophages [136]. CXCR3+ Tregs, able to control type-I T-cell responses, are highly enriched in EOC and represent the majority of Tregs [137]. These Tregs were able to suppress T-cell proliferation and IFNγ secretion [137].

An interesting study analyzed 22 EOC ascites specimens and found significantly elevated levels of IL-6, IL-8, IL-10, IL-15, IP-10, MCP-1, MIP-1β and VEGF and significantly reduced levels of IL-2, IL-5, IL-7, IL-17, PDGF-BB, and CCL5 compared to plasma. Moreover, T cells derived from EOC-associated ascites displayed poor responsiveness when expanded in vitro [138]. The authors claimed that this non-responsiveness could be explained by a high CD4/CD8 ratio that may indicate the presence of Tregs, reduced IL-2 and elevated IL-6 and IL-10 levels triggering a Th2 inhibitory immune response [138]. This high CD4/CD8 ratio was also associated with poor outcome [109,115,136,139], consistent with other studies [124,140,141]. In contrast, a positive correlation between Tregs and patient prognosis has been reported [140]. High tumor grade correlated with higher frequencies of CD3+, CD68+ CD163+ TAMs, and CD25+ FOXP3+ Treg cells, but Treg frequencies were significant predictors of favorable prognosis in patients with familial ovarian cancer (11/73 patients with BRCA mutation) [140]. The presence of FOXP3+ TILs may be linked to positive prognostic factors in optimally debulked HGSC patients [141]. Nevertheless, this disease-specific survival was positively associated along with other TIL markers such as CD8, CD3, TIA-1, CD20 (a B cell surface marker), MHC class I and class II [141].

CD8+ Tregs are also found in EOC [142,143]. They regulate the immunosuppressive TME by limiting immunosurveillance mechanisms and contributing to cancer progression [144]. Recently, Zhang and colleagues showed that CD8+ Tregs are found in the stroma and intraepithelial areas of EOC tumors [143]. CD8+ Tregs are characterized by the expression of FOXP3, CTLA-4, and CD25, but decreased expression of CD28 [143]. CD8+ Tregs were able to convert effector CD8+ T cells into suppressor cells [143]. CD8+ Tregs exert their suppressive function through the secretion of TGF-β1 [142].

Overall, Tregs are considered a critical barrier against antitumoral responses along with tolerance-inducing plasmacytoid DCs, B7-H4+ TAMs, MDSCs, IL-10, TGFβ, and VEGF. All these processes act in concert as a tumor evasion mechanism resulting in tumor progression [145]. Barriers to antitumoral responses are summarized in Figure 2.

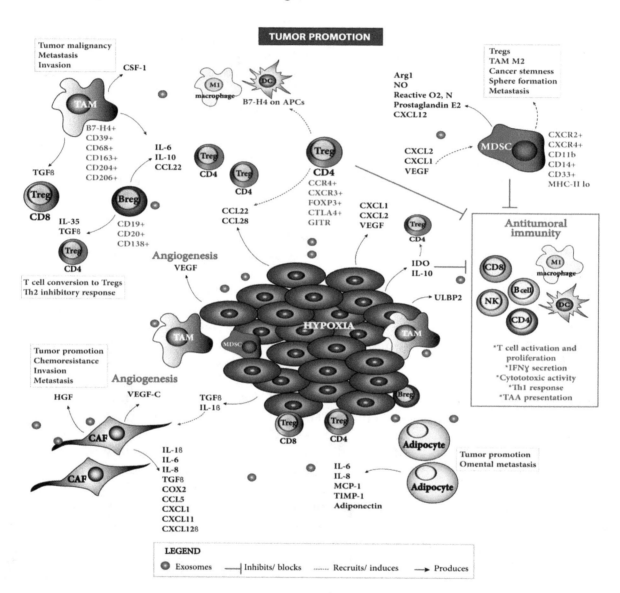

Figure 2. Tumor promoting network in the EOC TME. Outgrowth of EOC provokes hypoxia that induces the expression of chemokines to recruit MDSCs, Tregs, and TAMs. Tregs induce B7-H4 expression on APCs, subsequently blocking cytokine secretion, cytolytic activity, T-cell proliferation and promoting an immunosuppressive TME. EOC cells and MDSCs produce IDO that catabolizes tryptophan, rendering T cells anergic and dysfunctional. MDSCs and TAMs contribute to tumor growth, malignancy, metastasis and stemness. Several tumor promoting cytokines such as IL-6, IL-10 and TGFβ are prominent in the TME. VEGF released by EOC cells and CAFs stimulates angiogenic factors in the TME. CAFs also secrete many factors that mediate tumor cell migration, proliferation, invasion and chemoresistance, and contribute to the immunosuppressive TME. Adipocytes produce FA and cytokines that fuel tumor growth and omental metastasis. Myeloid-derived suppressor cells (MDSCs), tumor-associated macrophages (TAMs), regulatory T cells (Tregs), cancer-associated fibroblasts (CAFs), fatty acids (FA).

3.1.3. B Lymphocytes

B lymphocytes have been reported to have pivotal roles in cancer immunity [146]. Stromal or intraepithelial B lymphocytes have been found in EOC [141]; however their function in tumor development is not yet clear. Their presence is proposed to be associated with a good prognosis depending on the tumor stage and the TME where they are found [4,108,141]. The presence of B cells and CD8+ TILs correlates with increased patient survival compared to CD8+ TILs alone [108]. Nielsen et al. analyzed tumor and serum specimens obtained from patients with HGSC and found that the majority of CD20+ TILs were antigen experienced and suggested to accomplish TAA presentation in the TME since they often co-localized with CD8+ TILs and expressed markers such as MHC-I, MHC-II, CD40, CD80, and CD86 [108]. B cells can achieve antitumor immunity by secreting IFNγ, facilitating CD4+ Th cells to polarize to Th1 responses, and promote T-cell expansion by presenting TAAs [146]. Recently, the positive role of B cells among TILs at metastatic sites from patients with HGSC was reported [147]. B cells were often found in the stroma of metastases and were characterized by a strong memory response against TAAs by production of tumor-specific IgGs (Figure 1). Interestingly, these responses were amplified by chemotherapy [147].

Conversely, a new subset of B cells, regulatory B cells (Bregs), has been recently designated as immunosuppressive cells able to secrete anti-inflammatory mediators such as IL-10, IL-35, and TGF-β, triggering T-cell conversion to Tregs [148] (Figure 2). Indeed, a study that analyzed EOC tumor tissue and omental metastases found that high B cell infiltration negatively correlates with patient survival [149]. High CD20 and CD138 expression correlated with high tumor grade [149]. Analysis of omental specimens from patients with HGSC found that overall survival was 160.6 months in patients with low B-cell expression vs. 47.3 months in those with high B-cell expression, associating increased B-cell infiltration with poorer survival [150]. Similarly, the analysis of post-chemotherapy effusions from ovarian carcinomas revealed that a higher percentage of CD19+ cells (B cell marker) and stage IV disease predicted poor survival for patients [151].

Taken together, it is important to consider that several B-cell subsets with different phenotypes and functions exist, and they may have various roles in modifying the ability of tumors to respond to treatment [146]. Thus, a deep characterization of B-cell subpopulations within the TILs, ascites, and peripheral blood at different stages is crucial in order to provide a better understanding of the capability, importance and therapeutic potential of these cells in EOC.

3.1.4. NK-T Lymphocytes

NK-T cells possess dual-functional capability: as T-cell subsets with a T-cell receptor (TCR)-mediated specific cytotoxicity and as NK cells with acquired killer functions [152,153]. NK-T cells have been found in increased frequencies in EOC tumor ascites compared to blood, but they were decreased at higher tumor grade and in cases of platinum resistance [154]. Moreover, the presence of NK-T cells was inversely correlated with VEGF ascites levels [155]. Since these cells display the most potent cytotoxicity profile, they might be promising agents for adoptive cell immunotherapy [156]. Further studies are needed to better understand the potential antitumoral capacity of these cells and their role in the different EOC TMEs.

3.2. Innate Immune Cells in the Ovarian Cancer TME

3.2.1. NK Cells

Many studies have reported the presence of innate immune cells such as NKs, macrophages and DCs playing important roles in EOC tumorigenesis [103,124,154]. NK cells are crucial effectors in cancer immunosurveillance, recognizing and spontaneously killing virus-infected cells, cancer, and foreign cells hazardous to the host [157]. NK cells mediate antitumoral responses by secreting pro-inflammatory cytokines and chemokines such as IFNγ, TNF, IL-6, GM-CSF and CCL5, which influence antitumor activity and promote innate and adaptive responses in the TME [157–159]

(Figure 1). Tsiatas et al. analyzed 45 fresh specimens from different EOC and found an increased amount of CD56+ NK and NK-T cells along with activated CD4+ and CD8+ CD25+ T cells in serous and endometrioid carcinomas compared with mucinous and clear cell carcinomas [124]. Despite the high concentration of NKs found in ascites compared to peripheral blood, they are functionally impaired [121,160,161]. The influence of infiltrating NK cells on patient outcome is also debated. Analysis of ovarian carcinoma effusions showed that the presence of NK cells at an advanced stage (IV) predicted worse overall survival [151]. However, a positive antitumoral role for NK cells along with effector CD8+ T cells has been reported [162], and NK cell activity of peripheral blood lymphocytes was related to a significant progression-free survival of EOC patients [163]. Importantly, NK cells are activated or not, according to the balance between inhibitory and activating signals through different NK receptors [157]. Like many other cancers, EOC tumors express NK cell receptor ligand ULBP2, which is an indicator of poor prognosis and could promote T-cell dysfunction in the TME [164] (Figure 2). Since NK cells are important players in antitumoral immunity, more studies aiding to characterize their function, phenotypes, incidence and role in the EOC TME are needed to provide new rational for immunotherapies.

3.2.2. Tumor-Associated Macrophages

Both TAMs and MDSCs constitute up to 20% of the EOC TME and are known to maintain and promote an immunosuppressive TME [103] (Figure 2). TAMs are considered the most abundant infiltrating immune cells in EOC tissue and ascites [165,166]. They possess an immunosuppressive M2 phenotype characterized by the expression of CD163, CD204, CD206, and IL-10 [165], and their presence correlates with tumor progression [140,167]. M2 TAMs secrete colony-stimulating factor 1 (CSF-1) that has been found in high levels in malignant EOC [167], and contributes to tumor growth, invasion, and metastasis. Moreover, EOC cells are able to induce an M2 TAM phenotype [168]. TAMs produce the chemokine CCL22 enabling the trafficking of Tregs to the ovarian tumors [130]. EOC cells as well as TAMs are known to express the coinhibitory molecule B7-H4 [169], a member of the B7 family that has a profound inhibitory effect on the growth, cytokine secretion, and development of T-cell cytotoxicity [169]. B7-H4+ TAMs are able to suppress antitumoral responses in EOC [136]. A study of 103 EOC patients showed that enhanced B7-H4 expression in macrophages correlated with Treg cell numbers in the tumor [136]. Tregs and B7-H4+ TAMs were associated with poor patient outcome. Tregs in the TME can induce B7-H4+ TAMs to produce IL-10 and IL-6 [136], further supporting an immunosuppressive milieu. Higher tumor grade correlated with higher frequencies of CD163+ TAMs [140] and worse progression-free survival [170,171]. Importantly, two studies evaluating M1- (HLA-DR, iNOS) and M2-polarization (CD163, VEGF) markers showed that higher M1/M2 TAMs ratio in tumors was associated with a favorable overall survival [172,173], and high serum levels of CD163 predicts poor EOC patient prognosis [174]. In addition, monocyte-derived macrophages in EOC displayed an altered morphology and defective antitumoral functions including defective antibody-dependent cell-mediated cytotoxicity and phagocytosis [175]. Thus, EOC cells and the TME provoke and maintain a strong immunosuppressive M2 phenotype supportive of tumor progression. Immunotherapeutic approaches aiming to switch TAM phenotypes [176] could help the evolution of antitumoral responses and improve patient outcome.

3.2.3. Myeloid-Derived Suppressor Cells

MDSCs are composed of a heterogeneous population of immature myeloid cells that arise in pathologic conditions such as cancer, inflammation and infection, and possess a potent capacity to dampen T-cell responses [177]. MDSCs are considered key inducers of tumor immune evasion and impaired immunity by upregulating arginase-1, nitric oxide, and reactive oxygen species, and by generating reactive nitrogen species [178] (Figure 2). MDSCs also deplete cysteine, induce Tregs, inhibit T-cell activation and proliferation, attenuate the cytolytic ability of NK cells, and trigger a M2 phenotype [103]. Obermajer et al. showed that the frequencies of CD11b+ CD14+ CD33+ CXCR4+

MDSCs in EOC ascites correlated with CXCL12 and prostaglandin E(2) levels [179]. MDSCs derived from EOC patients also increased gene expression of cancer stem cells, sphere formation and metastasis of EOC [180]. Wu et al. characterized typical monocytic CD14+ HLA-DR$^{-/lo}$ MDSCs in peripheral blood and ascites derived from EOC patients and found that MDSCs are enriched in both compartments [181]. Moreover, the density of MDSCs correlated with poor patient prognosis and elevated levels of IL-6 and IL-10 [181,182]. VEGF expression in EOC induced MDSCs recruitment, inhibiting local immunity [182]. A recent study with mouse EOC cells found that *Snail*, a major transcription factor that induces epithelial-mesenchymal transition (EMT), mediates EOC progression by upregulating CXCR2 ligands, enabling the recruitment of MDSCs [183]. EOC cells also attracts myeloid cells by producing adenosine [184]. Hence, strategies targeting MDSCs could release the brakes against antitumoral responses. Metformin, a drug used to treat type 2 diabetes, may trigger EOC clinical benefit by improving antitumoral T-cell responses that are impeded by MDSCs in the TME, since this drug can block MDSC suppressor functions by decreasing CD39 and CD73 expression [185].

4. Exosomes

Highly proliferating cells such as cancer cells produce large amounts of exosomes which are small (40–100 nm) extracellular vesicles [186]. EOC tumor-derived exosomes carry cell membrane proteins and cargo proteins that could be used for diagnostics (EP-CAM) and immunotherapeutic targeting such as neoantigens and TAAs (Her2-neu, CA-125) [186], proteins (TGF-β1) [187], and miRNAs (miR-21) [188] that are involved in disease progression, metastasis, and chemoresistance [186], as well as immunomodulatory proteins (FAS-L) [189]. Exosomes can be taken up by other cancer cells, CAFs, and immune cells, therefore playing an important role in intercellular communication. Thus far, 2035 exosome cargo molecules have been identified from EOC cells in ExoCarta, a database for exosome cargo [190,191]. Exosomes derived from human patient ascites promotes tumor progression in vivo [189,192], and are proposed to have direct and indirect roles in modulating the immune TME, as exosomes could also be taken up by NKs and B cells [192] (Figure 2). In other disease models, such as melanoma and colorectal cancer, exosomes mediate immunosuppression and immune tolerance by suppressing the activation of T and NK cells, monocytes, modulating T-cell inhibitory molecules expression, and inducing CD8+ T-cell apoptosis [193,194]. FAS-L and TRAIL expression on EOC-derived exosomes inhibit activation of peripheral blood mononuclear cells by DCs through induction of apoptosis [189]. EOC-derived exosomes express ligands (MICA/B and ULBP1-3) for the NK receptor NKG2D, acting as a decoy and interfering with NK-mediated targeting of tumor cells [195]. Greater understanding of the complex network of the intercellular communication between EOC cells, CAFs, and immune cells is needed for the rational design of immunotherapeutic interventions, or leveraged for nanomedicine applications such as TAA loaded-DC-derived exosomes [196] and drug delivery systems [186].

5. Cancer-Associated Fibroblasts

CAFs are activated fibroblasts that express α-smooth muscle actin and fibroblast activation protein. They make up 7–85% [197] of the tumor and are the primary stromal cell type in the TME. Cross-talk between epithelial and stromal compartments creates a positive feedback loop, a supportive hyper-activated storm of cytokines, chemokines, angiogenetic factors, and EMT-promoting factors, to promote tumor progression and chemoresistance (Figure 2). CAFs from ovarian cancer patients secrete high levels of hepatocyte growth factor (HGF) that promotes cancer cell proliferation, chemoresistance, invasion, and migration though constitutive activation of cMet/PI3K/Akt pathways and glucose-regulated protein 78 (GRP78) [198,199]. CAFs produce pro-inflammatory cytokines COX-2 and CXCL1 [200], CCL5 [201], CXCL11 [202], and IL-6 [203], which can promote proliferation and EMT. In addition to their direct actions on cancer cells, CAFs also produce exosomes with high levels of TGF-β1 that subsequently activates normal fibroblasts [187]. Interestingly, Givel et al. identified four CAFs subsets in HGSC, finding an accumulation of one subset, CAF-S1, in the mesenchymal molecular subtype of HGSC. CAF-S1 is associated with an immunosuppressive TME, due to its high levels of expression of CXCL12β, which recruits Tregs to the tumor. The CAF-S1 cells also express CD73, B7-H3 and IL-6, which subsequently promote survival and proliferation of Tregs [204]. Thus, CAFs can make major contributions to the creation of an immunosuppressive TME.

On the other hand, EOC cells can stimulate the activation of CAFs by producing high levels of interleukin-1β (IL-1β) [205] and TGF-β [206], which subsequently induces secretion of IL-8, IL-6, IL-1β, VEGF, and growth regulated oncogene-alpha (GRO-α) by CAFs to promote tumor progression [205]. EOC cells release exosomes not only to activate tumor cells, but also to reprogram normal fibroblasts into CAFs [207]. Furthermore, CAFs act on endothelial cells via the secretion of VEGF-C [208] or by upregulating genes such as lipoma-preferred partner, to promote angiogenesis, which leads to tumor progression and chemoresistance [209]. Cross-talk between CAFs and cancer cells, as well as endothelial cells and immune cells, suggests that targeting signaling mechanisms in this relationship may combat chemoresistance and immune modulation better than singly targeting the epithelial compartment.

6. Adipocytes and the Omentum

The unique TME of the omentum, a large visceral fat pad that covers the bowel and abdomen cavities [210,211], suggests a two-step model of omental metastasis and tumorigenesis where ovarian cancer cells preferentially and rapidly home to "milky spots" [212] in the omentum, prior to spreading throughout non-"milky spot" areas of the omentum and peritoneal cavity [213–217]. "Milky spots" are highly vascularized regions with aggregates of immune cells, capable of innate and adaptive immune functions, and antigen presentation similar to lymph node structures [212]. The involvement of the omentum and adipose tissue suggests the need to develop intraperitoneal immunotherapy similar to the advances seen with intraperitoneal chemotherapy.

Adipocytes in the omentum produce cytokines and chemokines, including highly secreted IL-6, IL-8, MCP-1, tissue inhibitor of metalloproteinases-1 (TIMP-1) and adiponectin, to promote cancer growth and omental metastases. Adipocytes can alter their lipid metabolism via Fatty acid–binding protein 4 (FAB4) to undergo lipolysis providing fatty acids (FA) to cancer cells as a fuel source for rapid tumor growth [216]. Cancer cells themselves can also alter lipid metabolism, often by upregulating FA receptor CD36 [218] and FAB4 in omental metastases at the tumor/adipocyte interface to promote FA and cholesterol uptake from adipocytes [216] to fuel tumor progression.

Many studies have suggested an association between obesity and the incidence of ovarian cancer as well as an association with poor prognosis [219]. Indeed, in a murine model of ovarian cancer, metastasis and tumor growth is supported in obese mice through altered regulation of FA pathway and increased immunosuppression, demonstrated by a decreased ratio of M1/M2 macrophages [220] (Figure 2). Improved understanding of how adipocytes and the omentum support ovarian cancer growth and promote peritoneal metastases will reveal therapeutic targets for both conventional therapy and immunotherapy. It will be important to consider how age and obesity [221–223] may dictate differences in response to immunotherapy and how current models with young, lean mice may fail to accurately model responses to immunotherapy.

7. Conclusions

In summary, in order to develop better immunotherapies for EOC we need to identify and consider all key elements found in the TME of not only primary tumors but also in ascites and metastases with a focus on how these features affect and are affected by different cancer therapies. It is crucial to take into account the quality of the TME (immune-activating vs. immune-suppressing mechanisms), tumor immunogenicity, tumor burden mutations, tumor stage, patient overall condition, and age, as well as treatment effects on the TME (chemotherapy, neoadjuvant chemotherapy, surgery debulking). Each of these factors may influence the outcome of EOC and the responses to cancer immunotherapies. Moreover, to avoid tumor recurrence, EOC characteristics such as TAA presentation, expression of coinhibitory molecules, production of immunosuppressive cytokines and chemokines should all be considered to find therapeutic combinations that could synergize and achieve maximal benefits to eliminate EOC. Other articles in this special issue will address some of these topics, including the exploration of promising immunotherapies for HGSC that are currently under investigation [224].

Author Contributions: All authors contributed to the research, writing, and editing of this review article.

Acknowledgments: The authors are grateful for the donations and support from the local community of ovarian cancer patients, especially the late Margaret Craig, and the Carol Annibale Ovarian Cancer Foundation.

References

1. Vesely, M.D.; Schreiber, R.D. Cancer immunoediting: Antigens, mechanisms, and implications to cancer immunotherapy. *Ann. N. Y. Acad. Sci.* **2013**, *1284*, 1–5. [CrossRef] [PubMed]

2. Santoiemma, P.P.; Powell, D.J. Tumor infiltrating lymphocytes in ovarian cancer. *Cancer Biol. Ther.* **2015**, *16*, 807–820. [CrossRef] [PubMed]

3. Santoiemma, P.P.; Reyes, C.; Wang, L.-P.; McLane, M.W.; Feldman, M.D.; Tanyi, J.L.; Powell, D.J. Systematic evaluation of multiple immune markers reveals prognostic factors in ovarian cancer. *Gynecol. Oncol.* **2016**, *143*, 120–127. [CrossRef] [PubMed]

4. Stumpf, M.; Hasenburg, A.; Riener, M.-O.; Jütting, U.; Wang, C.; Shen, Y.; Orlowska-Volk, M.; Fisch, P.; Wang, Z.; Gitsch, G.; et al. Intraepithelial CD8-positive T lymphocytes predict survival for patients with serous stage III ovarian carcinomas: Relevance of clonal selection of T lymphocytes. *Br. J. Cancer* **2009**, *101*, 1513–1521. [CrossRef] [PubMed]

5. Zhang, L.; Conejo-Garcia, J.R.; Katsaros, D.; Gimotty, P.A.; Massobrio, M.; Regnani, G.; Makrigiannakis, A.; Gray, H.; Schlienger, K.; Liebman, M.N.; et al. Intratumoral T cells, recurrence, and survival in epithelial ovarian cancer. *N. Engl. J. Med.* **2003**, *348*, 203–213. [CrossRef] [PubMed]

6. Coukos, G.; Tanyi, J.; Kandalaft, L.E. Opportunities in immunotherapy of ovarian cancer. *Ann. Oncol. Off. J. Eur. Soc. Med. Oncol.* **2016**, *27* (Suppl. 1), i11–i15. [CrossRef] [PubMed]

7. Odunsi, K. Immunotherapy in ovarian cancer. *Ann. Oncol. Off. J. Eur. Soc. Med. Oncol.* **2017**, *28*, viii1–viii7. [CrossRef] [PubMed]

8. Wang, R.-F.; Wang, H.Y. Immune targets and neoantigens for cancer immunotherapy and precision medicine. *Cell Res.* **2017**, *27*, 11–37. [CrossRef] [PubMed]

9. Ilyas, S.; Yang, J.C. Landscape of Tumor Antigens in T-Cell Immunotherapy. *J. Immunol.* **2015**, *195*, 5117–5122. [CrossRef] [PubMed]

10. Rizvi, N.A.; Hellmann, M.D.; Snyder, A.; Kvistborg, P.; Makarov, V.; Havel, J.J.; Lee, W.; Yuan, J.; Wong, P.; Ho, T.S.; et al. Cancer immunology. Mutational landscape determines sensitivity to PD-1 blockade in non-small cell lung cancer. *Science* **2015**, *348*, 124–128. [CrossRef] [PubMed]

11. Van Allen, E.M.; Miao, D.; Schilling, B.; Shukla, S.A.; Blank, C.; Zimmer, L.; Sucker, A.; Hillen, U.; Foppen, M.H.G.; Goldinger, S.M.; et al. Genomic correlates of response to CTLA-4 blockade in metastatic melanoma. *Science* **2015**, *350*, 207–211. [CrossRef] [PubMed]

12. Chalmers, Z.R.; Connelly, C.F.; Fabrizio, D.; Gay, L.; Ali, S.M.; Ennis, R.; Schrock, A.; Campbell, B.; Shlien, A.; Chmielecki, J.; et al. Analysis of 100,000 human cancer genomes reveals the landscape of tumor mutational burden. *Genome Med.* **2017**, *9*, 34. [CrossRef] [PubMed]

13. Martin, S.D.; Brown, S.D.; Wick, D.A.; Nielsen, J.S.; Kroeger, D.R.; Twumasi-Boateng, K.; Holt, R.A.; Nelson, B.H. Low mutation burden in ovarian cancer may limit the utility of neoantigen-targeted vaccines. *PLoS ONE* **2016**, *11*, e0155189. [CrossRef] [PubMed]

14. Hamanishi, J.; Mandai, M.; Ikeda, T.; Minami, M.; Kawaguchi, A.; Murayama, T.; Kanai, M.; Mori, Y.; Matsumoto, S.; Chikuma, S.; et al. Safety and antitumor activity of anti-PD-1 antibody, Nivolumab, in patients with platinum-resistant Ovarian Cancer. *J. Clin. Oncol. Off. J. Am. Soc. Clin. Oncol.* **2015**, *33*, 4015–4022. [CrossRef] [PubMed]

15. Varga, A.; Piha-Paul, S.A.; Ott, P.A.; Mehnert, J.M.; Berton-Rigaud, D.; Johnson, E.A.; Cheng, J.D.; Yuan, S.; Rubin, E.H.; Matei, D.E. Antitumor activity and safety of pembrolizumab in patients (pts) with PD-L1 positive advanced ovarian cancer: Interim results from a phase Ib study. *J. Clin. Oncol.* **2015**, *33*, 5510. [CrossRef]

16. Donahue, R.N.; Lepone, L.M.; Grenga, I.; Jochems, C.; Fantini, M.; Madan, R.A.; Heery, C.R.; Gulley, J.L.; Schlom, J. Analyses of the peripheral immunome following multiple administrations of avelumab, a human IgG1 anti-PD-L1 monoclonal antibody. *J. Immunother. Cancer* **2017**, *5*, 20. [CrossRef] [PubMed]

17. Disis, M.L.; Patel, M.R.; Pant, S.; Hamilton, E.P.; Lockhart, A.C.; Kelly, K.; Beck, J.T.; Gordon, M.S.; Weiss, G.J.; Taylor, M.H.; et al. Avelumab (MSB0010718C; anti-PD-L1) in patients with recurrent/refractory ovarian cancer from the JAVELIN Solid Tumor phase Ib trial: Safety and clinical activity. *J. Clin. Oncol.* **2016**, *34*, 5533. [CrossRef]

18. Brahmer, J.R.; Tykodi, S.S.; Chow, L.Q.M.; Hwu, W.-J.; Topalian, S.L.; Hwu, P.; Drake, C.G.; Camacho, L.H.; Kauh, J.; Odunsi, K.; et al. Safety and activity of anti–PD-L1 antibody in patients with advanced cancer. *N. Engl. J. Med.* **2012**, *366*, 2455–2465. [CrossRef] [PubMed]

19. Hodi, F.S.; Mihm, M.C.; Soiffer, R.J.; Haluska, F.G.; Butler, M.; Seiden, M.V.; Davis, T.; Henry-Spires, R.; MacRae, S.; Willman, A.; et al. Biologic activity of cytotoxic T lymphocyte-associated antigen 4 antibody blockade in previously vaccinated metastatic melanoma and ovarian carcinoma patients. *Proc. Natl. Acad. Sci. USA* **2003**, *100*, 4712–4717. [CrossRef] [PubMed]

20. Hodi, F.S.; Butler, M.; Oble, D.A.; Seiden, M.V.; Haluska, F.G.; Kruse, A.; MacRae, S.; Nelson, M.; Canning, C.; Lowy, I.; et al. Immunologic and clinical effects of antibody blockade of cytotoxic T lymphocyte-associated antigen 4 in previously vaccinated cancer patients. *Proc. Natl. Acad. Sci. USA* **2008**, *105*, 3005–3010. [CrossRef] [PubMed]

21. Bellone, S.; Buza, N.; Choi, J.; Zammataro, L.; Gay, L.; Elvin, J.; Rimm, D.L.; Liu, Y.; Ratner, E.S.; Schwartz, P.E.; et al. Exceptional response to Pembrolizumab in a metastatic, chemotherapy/radiation-resistant ovarian cancer patient harboring a PD-L1-genetic rearrangement. *Clin. Cancer Res.* **2018**. [CrossRef] [PubMed]

22. Huang, J.; Jochems, C.; Anderson, A.M.; Talaie, T.; Jales, A.; Madan, R.A.; Hodge, J.W.; Tsang, K.Y.; Liewehr, D.J.; Steinberg, S.M.; et al. Soluble CD27-pool in humans may contribute to T cell activation and tumor immunity. *J. Immunol.* **2013**, *190*, 6250–6258. [CrossRef] [PubMed]

23. Huang, J.; Jochems, C.; Talaie, T.; Anderson, A.; Jales, A.; Tsang, K.Y.; Madan, R.A.; Gulley, J.L.; Schlom, J. Elevated serum soluble CD40 ligand in cancer patients may play an immunosuppressive role. *Blood* **2012**, *120*, 3030–3038. [CrossRef] [PubMed]

24. Tammela, J.; Uenaka, A.; Ono, T.; Noguchi, Y.; Jungbluth, A.A.; Mhawech-Fauceglia, P.; Qian, F.; Schneider, S.; Sharma, S.; Driscoll, D.; et al. OY-TES-1 expression and serum immunoreactivity in epithelial ovarian cancer. *Int. J. Oncol.* **2006**, *29*, 903–910. [CrossRef] [PubMed]

25. Tammela, J.; Jungbluth, A.A.; Qian, F.; Santiago, D.; Scanlan, M.J.; Keitz, B.; Driscoll, D.; Rodabaugh, K.; Lele, S.; Old, L.J.; et al. SCP-1 cancer/testis antigen is a prognostic indicator and a candidate target for immunotherapy in epithelial ovarian cancer. *Cancer Immun.* **2004**, *4*, 10. [PubMed]

26. Garg, M.; Chaurasiya, D.; Rana, R.; Jagadish, N.; Kanojia, D.; Dudha, N.; Kamran, N.; Salhan, S.; Bhatnagar, A.; Suri, S.; et al. Sperm-associated antigen 9, a novel cancer testis antigen, is a potential target for immunotherapy in epithelial ovarian cancer. *Clin. Cancer Res.* **2007**, *13*, 1421–1428. [CrossRef] [PubMed]

27. Agarwal, S.; Saini, S.; Parashar, D.; Verma, A.; Sinha, A.; Jagadish, N.; Batra, A.; Suri, S.; Gupta, A.; Ansari, A.S.; et al. The novel cancer-testis antigen A-kinase anchor protein 4 (AKAP4) is a potential target for immunotherapy of ovarian serous carcinoma. *Oncoimmunology* **2013**, *2*. [CrossRef] [PubMed]

28. Odunsi, K.; Jungbluth, A.A.; Stockert, E.; Qian, F.; Gnjatic, S.; Tammela, J.; Intengan, M.; Beck, A.; Keitz, B.; Santiago, D.; et al. NY-ESO-1 and LAGE-1 Cancer-Testis Antigens Are Potential Targets for Immunotherapy in Epithelial Ovarian Cancer. *Cancer Res.* **2003**, *63*, 6076–6083. [PubMed]

29. Daudi, S.; Eng, K.H.; Mhawech-Fauceglia, P.; Morrison, C.; Miliotto, A.; Beck, A.; Matsuzaki, J.; Tsuji, T.; Groman, A.; Gnjatic, S.; et al. Expression and immune responses to MAGE antigens predict survival in epithelial ovarian cancer. *PLoS ONE* **2014**, *9*, e104099. [CrossRef] [PubMed]

30. Gillespie, A.M.; Rodgers, S.; Wilson, A.P.; Tidy, J.; Rees, R.C.; Coleman, R.E.; Murray, A.K. MAGE, BAGE and GAGE: Tumour antigen expression in benign and malignant ovarian tissue. *Br. J. Cancer* **1998**, *78*, 816–821. [CrossRef] [PubMed]

31. Yamada, A.; Kataoka, A.; Shichijo, S.; Kamura, T.; Imai, Y.; Nishida, T.; Itoh, K. Expression of MAGE-1, MAGE-2, MAGE-3/-6 and MAGE-4A/-4B genes in ovarian tumors. *Int. J. Cancer* **1995**, *64*, 388–393. [CrossRef] [PubMed]

32. Hardwick, N.; Chung, V.; Cristea, M.; Ellenhorn, J.D.; Diamond, D.J. Overcoming immunosuppression to enhance a p53MVA vaccine. *Oncoimmunology* **2014**, *3*, e958949. [CrossRef] [PubMed]

33. The Cancer Genome Atlas Research Network. Integrated genomic analyses of ovarian carcinoma. *Nature* **2011**, *474*, 609–615. [CrossRef]

34. Fajac, A.; Benard, J.; Lhomme, C.; Rey, A.; Duvillard, P.; Rochard, F.; Bernaudin, J.F.; Riou, G. c-erbB2 gene amplification and protein expression in ovarian epithelial tumors: Evaluation of their respective prognostic significance by multivariate analysis. *Int. J. Cancer* **1995**, *64*, 146–151. [CrossRef] [PubMed]

35. Ioannides, C.G.; Fisk, B.; Fan, D.; Biddison, W.E.; Wharton, J.T.; O'brian, C.A. Cytotoxic T cells isolated from ovarian malignant ascites recognize a peptide derived from the HER-2/neu proto-oncogene. *Cell. Immunol.* **1993**, *151*, 225–234. [CrossRef] [PubMed]

36. Lanitis, E.; Dangaj, D.; Hagemann, I.S.; Song, D.-G.; Best, A.; Sandaltzopoulos, R.; Coukos, G.; Powell, D.J. Primary human ovarian epithelial cancer cells broadly express HER2 at immunologically-detectable levels. *PLoS ONE* **2012**, *7*, e49829. [CrossRef] [PubMed]

37. Nielsen, J.S.; Jakobsen, E.; HOlund, B.; Bertelsen, K.; Jakobsen, A. Prognostic significance of p53, Her-2, and EGFR overexpression in borderline and epithelial ovarian cancer. *Int. J. Gynecol. Cancer* **2004**, *14*, 1086–1096. [CrossRef] [PubMed]

38. Netinatsunthorn, W.; Hanprasertpong, J.; Dechsukhum, C.; Leetanaporn, R.; Geater, A. WT1 gene expression as a prognostic marker in advanced serous epithelial ovarian carcinoma: An immunohistochemical study. *BMC Cancer* **2006**, *6*, 90. [CrossRef] [PubMed]

39. Sallum, L.F.; Andrade, L.; Ramalho, S.; Ferracini, A.C.; de Andrade Natal, R.; Brito, A.B.C.; Sarian, L.O.; Derchain, S. WT1, p53 and p16 expression in the diagnosis of low- and high-grade serous ovarian carcinomas and their relation to prognosis. *Oncotarget* **2018**, *9*, 15818–15827. [CrossRef] [PubMed]

40. Hassan, R.; Kreitman, R.J.; Pastan, I.; Willingham, M.C. Localization of mesothelin in epithelial ovarian cancer. *Appl. Immunohistochem. Mol. Morphol. AIMM* **2005**, *13*, 243–247. [CrossRef] [PubMed]

41. Tanyi, J.L.; Haas, A.R.; Beatty, G.L.; Stashwick, C.J.; O'Hara, M.H.; Morgan, M.A.; Porter, D.L.; Melenhorst, J.J.; Plesa, G.; Lacey, S.F.; et al. Anti-mesothelin chimeric antigen receptor T cells in patients with epithelial ovarian cancer. *J. Clin. Oncol.* **2016**, *34*, 5511. [CrossRef]

42. Felder, M.; Kapur, A.; Gonzalez-Bosquet, J.; Horibata, S.; Heintz, J.; Albrecht, R.; Fass, L.; Kaur, J.; Hu, K.; Shojaei, H.; et al. MUC16 (CA125): Tumor biomarker to cancer therapy, a work in progress. *Mol. Cancer* **2014**, *13*, 129. [CrossRef] [PubMed]

43. Strickland, K.C.; Howitt, B.E.; Shukla, S.A.; Rodig, S.; Ritterhouse, L.L.; Liu, J.F.; Garber, J.E.; Chowdhury, D.; Wu, C.J.; D'Andrea, A.D.; et al. Association and prognostic significance of BRCA1/2-mutation status with neoantigen load, number of tumor-infiltrating lymphocytes and expression of PD-1/PD-L1 in high grade serous ovarian cancer. *Oncotarget* **2016**, *7*, 13587–13598. [CrossRef] [PubMed]

44. Odunsi, K.; Qian, F.; Matsuzaki, J.; Mhawech-Fauceglia, P.; Andrews, C.; Hoffman, E.W.; Pan, L.; Ritter, G.; Villella, J.; Thomas, B.; et al. Vaccination with an NY-ESO-1 peptide of HLA class I/II specificities induces integrated humoral and T cell responses in ovarian cancer. *Proc. Natl. Acad. Sci. USA* **2007**, *104*, 12837–12842. [CrossRef] [PubMed]

45. Sabbatini, P.; Tsuji, T.; Ferran, L.; Ritter, E.; Sedrak, C.; Tuballes, K.; Jungbluth, A.A.; Ritter, G.; Aghajanian, C.; Bell-McGuinn, K.; et al. Phase I trial of overlapping long peptides from a tumor self-antigen and poly-ICLC shows rapid induction of integrated immune response in ovarian cancer patients. *Clin. Cancer Res.* **2012**, *18*, 6497–6508. [CrossRef] [PubMed]

46. Diefenbach, C.S.M.; Gnjatic, S.; Sabbatini, P.; Aghajanian, C.; Hensley, M.L.; Spriggs, D.R.; Iasonos, A.; Lee, H.; Dupont, B.; Pezzulli, S.; et al. Safety and immunogenicity study of NY-ESO-1b peptide and montanide ISA-51 vaccination of patients with epithelial ovarian cancer in high-risk first remission. *Clin. Cancer Res.* **2008**, *14*, 2740–2748. [CrossRef] [PubMed]

47. Odunsi, K.; Matsuzaki, J.; Karbach, J.; Neumann, A.; Mhawech-Fauceglia, P.; Miller, A.; Beck, A.; Morrison, C.D.; Ritter, G.; Godoy, H.; et al. Efficacy of vaccination with recombinant vaccinia and fowlpox vectors expressing NY-ESO-1 antigen in ovarian cancer and melanoma patients. *Proc. Natl. Acad. Sci. USA* **2012**, *109*, 5797–5802. [CrossRef] [PubMed]

48. Hardwick, N.R.; Frankel, P.; Ruel, C.; Kilpatrick, J.; Tsai, W.; Kos, F.; Kaltcheva, T.; Leong, L.; Morgan, R.; Chung, V.; et al. p53-reactive T cells are associated with clinical benefit in patients with platinum-resistant epithelial ovarian cancer after treatment with a p53 vaccine and Gemcitabine chemotherapy. *Clin. Cancer Res.* **2018**. [CrossRef] [PubMed]

49. Leffers, N.; Vermeij, R.; Hoogeboom, B.-N.; Schulze, U.R.; Wolf, R.; Hamming, I.E.; van der Zee, A.G.;

Melief, K.J.; van der Burg, S.H.; Daemen, T.; et al. Long-term clinical and immunological effects of p53-SLP® vaccine in patients with ovarian cancer. *Int. J. Cancer* **2012**, *130*, 105–112. [CrossRef] [PubMed]

50. Coosemans, A.; Vanderstraeten, A.; Tuyaerts, S.; Verschuere, T.; Moerman, P.; Berneman, Z.; Vergote, I.; Amant, F.; Gool, S.W.V. Immunological response after WT1 mRNA-loaded dendritic cell immunotherapy in ovarian carcinoma and carcinosarcoma. *Anticancer Res.* **2013**, *33*, 3855–3859. [PubMed]

51. Miyatake, T.; Ueda, Y.; Morimoto, A.; Enomoto, T.; Nishida, S.; Shirakata, T.; Oka, Y.; Tsuboi, A.; Oji, Y.; Hosen, N.; et al. WT1 peptide immunotherapy for gynecologic malignancies resistant to conventional therapies: A phase II trial. *J. Cancer Res. Clin. Oncol.* **2013**, *139*, 457–463. [CrossRef] [PubMed]

52. Sabbatini, P.; Harter, P.; Scambia, G.; Sehouli, J.; Meier, W.; Wimberger, P.; Baumann, K.H.; Kurzeder, C.; Schmalfeldt, B.; Cibula, D.; et al. Abagovomab as maintenance therapy in patients with epithelial ovarian cancer: A phase III trial of the AGO OVAR, COGI, GINECO, and GEICO—The MIMOSA study. *J. Clin. Oncol. Off. J. Am. Soc. Clin. Oncol.* **2013**, *31*, 1554–1561. [CrossRef] [PubMed]

53. Braly, P.; Nicodemus, C.F.; Chu, C.; Collins, Y.; Edwards, R.; Gordon, A.; McGuire, W.; Schoonmaker, C.; Whiteside, T.; Smith, L.M.; et al. The immune adjuvant properties of front-line carboplatin-paclitaxel: A randomized phase 2 study of alternative schedules of intravenous oregovomab chemoimmunotherapy in advanced ovarian cancer. *J. Immunother.* **2009**, *32*, 54–65. [CrossRef] [PubMed]

54. Berek, J.; Taylor, P.; McGuire, W.; Smith, L.M.; Schultes, B.; Nicodemus, C.F. Oregovomab maintenance monoimmunotherapy does not improve outcomes in advanced ovarian cancer. *J. Clin. Oncol. Off. J. Am. Soc. Clin. Oncol.* **2009**, *27*, 418–425. [CrossRef] [PubMed]

55. Reinartz, S.; Köhler, S.; Schlebusch, H.; Krista, K.; Giffels, P.; Renke, K.; Huober, J.; Möbus, V.; Kreienberg, R.; DuBois, A.; et al. Vaccination of patients with advanced ovarian carcinoma with the anti-idiotype ACA125: Immunological response and survival (phase Ib/II). *Clin. Cancer Res.* **2004**, *10*, 1580–1587. [CrossRef] [PubMed]

56. Koneru, M.; O'Cearbhaill, R.; Pendharkar, S.; Spriggs, D.R.; Brentjens, R.J. A phase I clinical trial of adoptive T cell therapy using IL-12 secreting MUC-16(ecto) directed chimeric antigen receptors for recurrent ovarian cancer. *J. Transl. Med.* **2015**, *13*, 102. [CrossRef] [PubMed]

57. Schuster, H.; Peper, J.K.; Bösmüller, H.-C.; Röhle, K.; Backert, L.; Bilich, T.; Ney, B.; Löffler, M.W.; Kowalewski, D.J.; Trautwein, N.; et al. The immunopeptidomic landscape of ovarian carcinomas. *Proc. Natl. Acad. Sci. USA* **2017**, *114*, E9942–E9951. [CrossRef] [PubMed]

58. Tanyi, J.L.; Bobisse, S.; Ophir, E.; Tuyaerts, S.; Roberti, A.; Genolet, R.; Baumgartner, P.; Stevenson, B.J.; Iseli, C.; Dangaj, D.; et al. Personalized cancer vaccine effectively mobilizes antitumor T cell immunity in ovarian cancer. *Sci. Transl. Med.* **2018**, *10*, eaao5931. [CrossRef] [PubMed]

59. Alexandrov, L.B.; Nik-Zainal, S.; Wedge, D.C.; Aparicio, S.A.J.R.; Behjati, S.; Biankin, A.V.; Bignell, G.R.; Bolli, N.; Borg, A.; Børresen-Dale, A.-L.; et al. Signatures of mutational processes in human cancer. *Nature* **2013**, *500*, 415–421. [CrossRef] [PubMed]

60. Wick, D.A.; Webb, J.R.; Nielsen, J.S.; Martin, S.D.; Kroeger, D.R.; Milne, K.; Castellarin, M.; Twumasi-Boateng, K.; Watson, P.H.; Holt, R.A.; et al. Surveillance of the tumor mutanome by T cells during progression from primary to recurrent ovarian cancer. *Clin. Cancer Res.* **2014**, *20*, 1125–1134. [CrossRef] [PubMed]

61. Hamanishi, J.; Mandai, M.; Konishi, I. Immune checkpoint inhibition in ovarian cancer. *Int. Immunol.* **2016**, *28*, 339–348. [CrossRef] [PubMed]

62. Jelinic, P.; Ricca, J.; Van Oudenhove, E.; Olvera, N.; Merghoub, T.; Levine, D.A.; Zamarin, D. Immune-active microenvironment in Small Cell Carcinoma of the Ovary, Hypercalcemic Type: Rationale for immune checkpoint blockade. *JNCI J. Natl. Cancer Inst.* **2018**. [CrossRef] [PubMed]

63. Zhang, A.W.; McPherson, A.; Milne, K.; Kroeger, D.R.; Hamilton, P.T.; Miranda, A.; Funnell, T.; Little, N.; de Souza, C.P.E.; Laan, S.; et al. Interfaces of malignant and immunologic clonal dynamics in ovarian cancer. *Cell* **2018**, *173*, 1755–1769. [CrossRef] [PubMed]

64. McGranahan, N.; Swanton, C. Clonal heterogeneity and tumor evolution: Past, present, and the future. *Cell* **2017**, *168*, 613–628. [CrossRef] [PubMed]

65. Bashashati, A.; Ha, G.; Tone, A.; Ding, J.; Prentice, L.M.; Roth, A.; Rosner, J.; Shumansky, K.; Kalloger, S.; Senz, J.; et al. Distinct evolutionary trajectories of primary high-grade serous ovarian cancers revealed through spatial mutational profiling. *J. Pathol.* **2013**, *231*, 21–34. [CrossRef] [PubMed]

66. Caballero, O.L.; Chen, Y.-T. Cancer/testis (CT) antigens: Potential targets for immunotherapy. *Cancer Sci.* **2009**, *100*, 2014–2021. [CrossRef] [PubMed]

67. Want, M.Y.; Lugade, A.A.; Battaglia, S.; Odunsi, K. Nature of tumor rejection antigens in ovarian cancer. *Immunology* **2018**. [CrossRef] [PubMed]

68. Grob, J.-J.; Mortier, L.; D'Hondt, L.; Grange, F.; Baurain, J.F.; Dréno, B.; Lebbe, C.; Robert, C.; Dompmartin, A.; Neyns, B.; et al. Safety and immunogenicity of MAGE-A3 cancer immunotherapeutic with dacarbazine in patients with MAGE-A3-positive metastatic cutaneous melanoma: An open phase I/II study with a first assessment of a predictive gene signature. *ESMO Open* **2017**, *2*, e000203. [CrossRef] [PubMed]

69. Vansteenkiste, J.; Zielinski, M.; Linder, A.; Dahabreh, J.; Gonzalez, E.E.; Malinowski, W.; Lopez-Brea, M.; Vanakesa, T.; Jassem, J.; Kalofonos, H.; et al. Adjuvant MAGE-A3 immunotherapy in resected non-small-cell lung cancer: Phase II randomized study results. *J. Clin. Oncol. Off. J. Am. Soc. Clin. Oncol.* **2013**, *31*, 2396–2403. [CrossRef] [PubMed]

70. Matsuzaki, J.; Qian, F.; Luescher, I.; Lele, S.; Ritter, G.; Shrikant, P.A.; Gnjatic, S.; Old, L.J.; Odunsi, K. Recognition of naturally processed and ovarian cancer reactive CD8+ T cell epitopes within a promiscuous HLA class II T-helper region of NY-ESO-1. *Cancer Immunol. Immunother. CII* **2008**, *57*, 1185–1195. [CrossRef] [PubMed]

71. Matsuzaki, J.; Gnjatic, S.; Mhawech-Fauceglia, P.; Beck, A.; Miller, A.; Tsuji, T.; Eppolito, C.; Qian, F.; Lele, S.; Shrikant, P.; et al. Tumor-infiltrating NY-ESO-1–specific CD8+ T cells are negatively regulated by LAG-3 and PD-1 in human ovarian cancer. *Proc. Natl. Acad. Sci. USA* **2010**, *107*, 7875–7880. [CrossRef] [PubMed]

72. Hanlon, D.J.; Aldo, P.B.; Devine, L.; Alvero, A.B.; Engberg, A.K.; Edelson, R.; Mor, G. Enhanced stimulation of anti-ovarian cancer CD8(+) T cells by dendritic cells loaded with nanoparticle encapsulated tumor antigen. *Am. J. Reprod. Immunol.* **2011**, *65*, 597–609. [CrossRef] [PubMed]

73. Xue, W.; Metheringham, R.L.; Brentville, V.A.; Gunn, B.; Symonds, P.; Yagita, H.; Ramage, J.M.; Durrant, L.G. SCIB2, an antibody DNA vaccine encoding NY-ESO-1 epitopes, induces potent antitumor immunity which is further enhanced by checkpoint blockade. *Oncoimmunology* **2016**, *5*, e1169353. [CrossRef] [PubMed]

74. Odunsi, K.; Matsuzaki, J.; James, S.R.; Mhawech-Fauceglia, P.; Tsuji, T.; Miller, A.; Zhang, W.; Akers, S.N.; Griffiths, E.A.; Miliotto, A.; et al. Epigenetic potentiation of NY-ESO-1 vaccine therapy in human ovarian cancer. *Cancer Immunol. Res.* **2014**, *2*, 37–49. [CrossRef] [PubMed]

75. Reid, B.M.; Permuth, J.B.; Sellers, T.A. Epidemiology of ovarian cancer: A review. *Cancer Biol. Med.* **2017**, *14*, 9–32. [CrossRef] [PubMed]

76. Leffers, N.; Daemen, T.; Helfrich, W.; Boezen, H.M.; Cohlen, B.J.; Melief, C.J.; Nijman, H.W. Antigen-specific active immunotherapy for ovarian cancer. In *The Cochrane Library*; John Wiley & Sons, Ltd.: Hoboken, NJ, USA, 2014.

77. Marincola, F.M.; Jaffee, E.M.; Hicklin, D.J.; Ferrone, S. Escape of human solid tumors from T-cell recognition: Molecular mechanisms and functional significance. *Adv. Immunol.* **2000**, *74*, 181–273. [PubMed]

78. Campoli, M.; Chang, C.-C.; Ferrone, S. HLA class I antigen loss, tumor immune escape and immune selection. *Vaccine* **2002**, *20* (Suppl. 4), 40–45. [CrossRef]

79. Chang, C.-C.; Campoli, M.; Ferrone, S. Classical and nonclassical HLA class I antigen and NK Cell-activating ligand changes in malignant cells: Current challenges and future directions. *Adv. Cancer Res.* **2005**, *93*, 189–234. [CrossRef] [PubMed]

80. Aptsiauri, N.; Cabrera, T.; Mendez, R.; Garcia-Lora, A.; Ruiz-Cabello, F.; Garrido, F. Role of altered expression of HLA class I molecules in cancer progression. *Adv. Exp. Med. Biol.* **2007**, *601*, 123–131. [PubMed]

81. Han, L.Y.; Fletcher, M.S.; Urbauer, D.L.; Mueller, P.; Landen, C.N.; Kamat, A.A.; Lin, Y.G.; Merritt, W.M.; Spannuth, W.A.; Deavers, M.T.; et al. HLA class I antigen processing machinery component expression and intratumoral T-Cell infiltrate as independent prognostic markers in ovarian carcinoma. *Clin. Cancer Res.* **2008**, *14*, 3372–3379. [CrossRef] [PubMed]

82. Brown, S.D.; Warren, R.L.; Gibb, E.A.; Martin, S.D.; Spinelli, J.J.; Nelson, B.H.; Holt, R.A. Neo-antigens predicted by tumor genome meta-analysis correlate with increased patient survival. *Genome Res.* **2014**, *24*, 743–750. [CrossRef] [PubMed]

83. Matsushita, N.; Ghazizadeh, M.; Konishi, H.; Araki, T. Association of ovarian tumor epithelium coexpressing HLA-DR and CA-125 antigens with tumor infiltrating cytotoxic T lymphocytes. *J. Nippon Med. Sch. Nippon Ika Daigaku Zasshi* **2003**, *70*, 40–44. [CrossRef] [PubMed]

84. Callahan, M.J.; Nagymanyoki, Z.; Bonome, T.; Johnson, M.E.; Litkouhi, B.; Sullivan, E.H.; Hirsch, M.S.; Matulonis, U.A.; Liu, J.; Birrer, M.J.; et al. Increased HLA-DMB expression in the tumor epithelium is associated with increased CTL infiltration and improved prognosis in advanced-stage serous ovarian cancer. *Clin. Cancer Res.* **2008**, *14*, 7667–7673. [CrossRef] [PubMed]

85. Garrido, F.; Perea, F.; Bernal, M.; Sánchez-Palencia, A.; Aptsiauri, N.; Ruiz-Cabello, F. The escape of cancer from T cell-mediated immune surveillance: HLA class I loss and tumor tissue architecture. *Vaccines* **2017**, *5*, 7. [CrossRef] [PubMed]

86. Garrido, F.; Ruiz-Cabello, F.; Aptsiauri, N. Rejection versus escape: The tumor MHC dilemma. *Cancer Immunol. Immunother.* **2017**, *66*, 259–271. [CrossRef] [PubMed]

87. Clarke, B.; Tinker, A.V.; Lee, C.-H.; Subramanian, S.; van de Rijn, M.; Turbin, D.; Kalloger, S.; Han, G.; Ceballos, K.; Cadungog, M.G.; et al. Intraepithelial T cells and prognosis in ovarian carcinoma: Novel associations with stage, tumor type, and BRCA1 loss. *Mod. Pathol.* **2009**, *22*, 393–402. [CrossRef] [PubMed]

88. Shah, C.A.; Allison, K.H.; Garcia, R.L.; Gray, H.J.; Goff, B.A.; Swisher, E.M. Intratumoral T cells, tumor-associated macrophages, and regulatory T cells: Association with p53 mutations, circulating tumor DNA and survival in women with ovarian cancer. *Gynecol. Oncol.* **2008**, *109*, 215–219. [CrossRef] [PubMed]

89. Abiko, K.; Matsumura, N.; Hamanishi, J.; Horikawa, N.; Murakami, R.; Yamaguchi, K.; Yoshioka, Y.; Baba, T.; Konishi, I.; Mandai, M. IFN-γ from lymphocytes induces PD-L1 expression and promotes progression of ovarian cancer. *Br. J. Cancer* **2015**, *112*, 1501–1509. [CrossRef] [PubMed]

90. Hamanishi, J.; Mandai, M.; Iwasaki, M.; Okazaki, T.; Tanaka, Y.; Yamaguchi, K.; Higuchi, T.; Yagi, H.; Takakura, K.; Minato, N.; et al. Programmed cell death 1 ligand 1 and tumor-infiltrating CD8+ T lymphocytes are prognostic factors of human ovarian cancer. *Proc. Natl. Acad. Sci. USA* **2007**, *104*, 3360–3365. [CrossRef] [PubMed]

91. Darb-Esfahani, S.; Kunze, C.A.; Kulbe, H.; Sehouli, J.; Wienert, S.; Lindner, J.; Budczies, J.; Bockmayr, M.; Dietel, M.; Denkert, C.; et al. Prognostic impact of programmed cell death-1 (PD-1) and PD-ligand 1 (PD-L1) expression in cancer cells and tumor-infiltrating lymphocytes in ovarian high grade serous carcinoma. *Oncotarget* **2016**, *7*, 1486–1499. [CrossRef] [PubMed]

92. Webb, J.R.; Milne, K.; Kroeger, D.R.; Nelson, B.H. PD-L1 expression is associated with tumor-infiltrating T cells and favorable prognosis in high-grade serous ovarian cancer. *Gynecol. Oncol.* **2016**, *141*, 293–302. [CrossRef] [PubMed]

93. Drakes, M.L.; Mehrotra, S.; Aldulescu, M.; Potkul, R.K.; Liu, Y.; Grisoli, A.; Joyce, C.; O'Brien, T.E.; Stack, M.S.; Stiff, P.J. Stratification of ovarian tumor pathology by expression of programmed cell death-1 (PD-1) and PD-ligand-1 (PD-L1) in ovarian cancer. *J. Ovarian Res.* **2018**, *11*. [CrossRef] [PubMed]

94. Goyne, H.E.; Stone, P.J.B.; Burnett, A.F.; Cannon, M.J. Ovarian tumor ascites CD14+ cells suppress dendritic cell-activated CD4+ T-cell responses through IL-10 secretion and indoleamine 2,3-dioxygenase. *J. Immunother.* **2014**, *37*, 163–169. [CrossRef] [PubMed]

95. Hennequart, M.; Pilotte, L.; Cane, S.; Hoffmann, D.; Stroobant, V.; Plaen, E.D.; Eynde, B.J.V. den Constitutive IDO1 expression in human tumors is driven by Cyclooxygenase-2 and mediates intrinsic immune resistance. *Cancer Immunol. Res.* **2017**. [CrossRef] [PubMed]

96. Tanizaki, Y.; Kobayashi, A.; Toujima, S.; Shiro, M.; Mizoguchi, M.; Mabuchi, Y.; Yagi, S.; Minami, S.; Takikawa, O.; Ino, K. Indoleamine 2,3-dioxygenase promotes peritoneal metastasis of ovarian cancer by inducing an immunosuppressive environment. *Cancer Sci.* **2014**, *105*, 966–973. [CrossRef] [PubMed]

97. Ino, K. Indoleamine 2,3-dioxygenase and immune tolerance in ovarian cancer. *Curr. Opin. Obstet. Gynecol.* **2011**, *23*, 13–18. [CrossRef] [PubMed]

98. Inaba, T.; Ino, K.; Kajiyama, H.; Yamamoto, E.; Shibata, K.; Nawa, A.; Nagasaka, T.; Akimoto, H.; Takikawa, O.; Kikkawa, F. Role of the immunosuppressive enzyme indoleamine 2,3-dioxygenase in the progression of ovarian carcinoma. *Gynecol. Oncol.* **2009**, *115*, 185–192. [CrossRef] [PubMed]

99. Takao, M.; Okamoto, A.; Nikaido, T.; Urashima, M.; Takakura, S.; Saito, M.; Saito, M.; Okamoto, S.; Takikawa, O.; Sasaki, H.; et al. Increased synthesis of indoleamine-2,3-dioxygenase protein is positively associated with impaired survival in patients with serous-type, but not with other types of, ovarian cancer. *Oncol. Rep.* **2007**, *17*, 1333–1339. [CrossRef] [PubMed]

100. Qian, F.; Villella, J.; Wallace, P.K.; Mhawech-Fauceglia, P.; Tario, J.D.; Andrews, C.; Matsuzaki, J.; Valmori, D.; Ayyoub, M.; Frederick, P.J.; et al. Efficacy of levo-1-methyl tryptophan and dextro-1-methyl tryptophan in reversing indoleamine-2,3-dioxygenase-mediated arrest of T-cell proliferation in human epithelial ovarian cancer. *Cancer Res.* **2009**, *69*, 5498–5504. [CrossRef] [PubMed]

101. Sheridan, C. IDO inhibitors move center stage in immuno-oncology. *Nat. Biotechnol.* **2015**, *33*, 321–322. [CrossRef] [PubMed]

102. Schreiber, R.D.; Old, L.J.; Smyth, M.J. Cancer immunoediting: Integrating immunity's roles in cancer suppression and promotion. *Science* **2011**, *331*, 1565–1570. [CrossRef] [PubMed]

103. Okła, K.; Wertel, I.; Polak, G.; Surówka, J.; Wawruszak, A.; Kotarski, J. Tumor-associated macrophages and myeloid-derived suppressor cells as immunosuppressive mechanism in ovarian cancer patients: Progress and challenges. *Int. Rev. Immunol.* **2016**, *35*, 372–385. [CrossRef] [PubMed]

104. Leffers, N.; Gooden, M.J.M.; de Jong, R.A.; Hoogeboom, B.-N.; ten Hoor, K.A.; Hollema, H.; Boezen, H.M.; van der Zee, A.G.J.; Daemen, T.; Nijman, H.W. Prognostic significance of tumor-infiltrating T-lymphocytes in primary and metastatic lesions of advanced stage ovarian cancer. *Cancer Immunol. Immunother. CII* **2009**, *58*, 449–459. [CrossRef] [PubMed]

105. Raspollini, M.R.; Castiglione, F.; Rossi Degl'innocenti, D.; Amunni, G.; Villanucci, A.; Garbini, F.; Baroni, G.; Taddei, G.L. Tumour-infiltrating gamma/delta T-lymphocytes are correlated with a brief disease-free interval in advanced ovarian serous carcinoma. *Ann. Oncol. Off. J. Eur. Soc. Med. Oncol.* **2005**, *16*, 590–596. [CrossRef] [PubMed]

106. Sato, E.; Olson, S.H.; Ahn, J.; Bundy, B.; Nishikawa, H.; Qian, F.; Jungbluth, A.A.; Frosina, D.; Gnjatic, S.; Ambrosone, C.; et al. Intraepithelial CD8+ tumor-infiltrating lymphocytes and a high CD8+/regulatory T cell ratio are associated with favorable prognosis in ovarian cancer. *Proc. Natl. Acad. Sci. USA* **2005**, *102*, 18538–18543. [CrossRef] [PubMed]

107. Tomsová, M.; Melichar, B.; Sedláková, I.; Steiner, I. Prognostic significance of CD3+ tumor-infiltrating lymphocytes in ovarian carcinoma. *Gynecol. Oncol.* **2008**, *108*, 415–420. [CrossRef] [PubMed]

108. Nielsen, J.S.; Sahota, R.A.; Milne, K.; Kost, S.E.; Nesslinger, N.J.; Watson, P.H.; Nelson, B.H. CD20+ tumor-infiltrating lymphocytes have an atypical CD27- memory phenotype and together with CD8+ T cells promote favorable prognosis in ovarian cancer. *Clin. Cancer Res.* **2012**, *18*, 3281–3292. [CrossRef] [PubMed]

109. Barnett, J.C.; Bean, S.M.; Whitaker, R.S.; Kondoh, E.; Baba, T.; Fujii, S.; Marks, J.R.; Dressman, H.K.; Murphy, S.K.; Berchuck, A. Ovarian cancer tumor infiltrating T-regulatory (T(reg)) cells are associated with a metastatic phenotype. *Gynecol. Oncol.* **2010**, *116*, 556–562. [CrossRef] [PubMed]

110. Hamanishi, J.; Mandai, M.; Abiko, K.; Matsumura, N.; Baba, T.; Yoshioka, Y.; Kosaka, K.; Konishi, I. The comprehensive assessment of local immune status of ovarian cancer by the clustering of multiple immune factors. *Clin. Immunol.* **2011**, *141*, 338–347. [CrossRef] [PubMed]

111. Hwang, W.-T.; Adams, S.F.; Tahirovic, E.; Hagemann, I.S.; Coukos, G. Prognostic significance of tumor-infiltrating T cells in ovarian cancer: A meta-analysis. *Gynecol. Oncol.* **2012**, *124*, 192–198. [CrossRef] [PubMed]

112. Dadmarz, R.D.; Ordoubadi, A.; Mixon, A.; Thompson, C.O.; Barracchini, K.C.; Hijazi, Y.M.; Steller, M.A.; Rosenberg, S.A.; Schwartzentruber, D.J. Tumor-infiltrating lymphocytes from human ovarian cancer patients recognize autologous tumor in an MHC class II-restricted fashion. *Cancer J. Sci. Am.* **1996**, *2*, 263–272. [PubMed]

113. Bronger, H.; Singer, J.; Windmüller, C.; Reuning, U.; Zech, D.; Delbridge, C.; Dorn, J.; Kiechle, M.; Schmalfeldt, B.; Schmitt, M.; et al. CXCL9 and CXCL10 predict survival and are regulated by cyclooxygenase inhibition in advanced serous ovarian cancer. *Br. J. Cancer* **2016**, *115*, 553–563. [CrossRef] [PubMed]

114. Liu, M.; Matsumura, N.; Mandai, M.; Li, K.; Yagi, H.; Baba, T.; Suzuki, A.; Hamanishi, J.; Fukuhara, K.; Konishi, I. Classification using hierarchical clustering of tumor-infiltrating immune cells identifies poor prognostic ovarian cancers with high levels of COX expression. *Mod. Pathol.* **2009**, *22*, 373–384. [CrossRef] [PubMed]

115. Hermans, C.; Anz, D.; Engel, J.; Kirchner, T.; Endres, S.; Mayr, D. Analysis of FoxP3+ T-regulatory cells and CD8+ T-cells in ovarian carcinoma: Location and tumor infiltration patterns are key prognostic markers. *PLoS ONE* **2014**, *9*, e111757. [CrossRef] [PubMed]

116. Shi, J.-X.; Qin, J.-J.; Ye, H.; Wang, P.; Wang, K.-J.; Zhang, J.-Y. Tumor associated antigens or anti-TAA autoantibodies as biomarkers in the diagnosis of ovarian cancer: A systematic review with meta-analysis. *Expert Rev. Mol. Diagn.* **2015**, *15*, 829–852. [CrossRef] [PubMed]

117. Taylor, D.D.; Gercel-Taylor, C.; Parker, L.P. Patient-derived tumor-reactive antibodies as diagnostic markers for ovarian cancer. *Gynecol. Oncol.* **2009**, *115*, 112–120. [CrossRef] [PubMed]

118. Taylor, D.D.; Atay, S.; Metzinger, D.S.; Gercel-Taylor, C. Characterization of humoral responses of ovarian cancer patients: Antibody subclasses and antigenic components. *Gynecol. Oncol.* **2010**, *116*, 213–221. [CrossRef] [PubMed]

119. Jang, M.; Yew, P.-Y.; Hasegawa, K.; Ikeda, Y.; Fujiwara, K.; Fleming, G.F.; Nakamura, Y.; Park, J.-H. Characterization of T cell repertoire of blood, tumor, and ascites in ovarian cancer patients using next generation sequencing. *Oncoimmunology* **2015**, *4*, e1030561. [CrossRef] [PubMed]

120. Landskron, J.; Helland, Ø.; Torgersen, K.M.; Aandahl, E.M.; Gjertsen, B.T.; Bjørge, L.; Taskén, K. Activated regulatory and memory T-cells accumulate in malignant ascites from ovarian carcinoma patients. *Cancer Immunol. Immunother.* **2015**, *64*, 337–347. [CrossRef] [PubMed]

121. Lukesova, S.; Vroblova, V.; Tosner, J.; Kopecky, J.; Sedlakova, I.; Čermáková, E.; Vokurkova, D.; Kopecky, O. Comparative study of various subpopulations of cytotoxic cells in blood and ascites from patients with ovarian carcinoma. *Contemp. Oncol. Poznan Pol.* **2015**, *19*, 290–299. [CrossRef] [PubMed]

122. Martin, S.D.; Wick, D.A.; Nielsen, J.S.; Little, N.; Holt, R.A.; Nelson, B.H. A library-based screening method identifies neoantigen-reactive T cells in peripheral blood prior to relapse of ovarian cancer. *Oncoimmunology* **2017**, *7*, e1371895. [CrossRef] [PubMed]

123. Nelson, B.H. The impact of T-cell immunity on ovarian cancer outcomes. *Immunol. Rev.* **2008**, *222*, 101–116. [CrossRef] [PubMed]

124. Tsiatas, M.L.; Gyftaki, R.; Liacos, C.; Politi, E.; Rodolakis, A.; Dimopoulos, M.-A.; Bamias, A. Study of T lymphocytes infiltrating peritoneal metastases in advanced ovarian cancer: Associations with vascular endothelial growth factor levels and prognosis in patients receiving platinum-based chemotherapy. *Int. J. Gynecol. Cancer Off. J. Int. Gynecol. Cancer Soc.* **2009**, *19*, 1329–1334. [CrossRef] [PubMed]

125. Le Page, C.; Marineau, A.; Bonza, P.K.; Rahimi, K.; Cyr, L.; Labouba, I.; Madore, J.; Delvoye, N.; Mes-Masson, A.-M.; Provencher, D.M.; et al. BTN3A2 expression in epithelial ovarian cancer is associated with higher tumor infiltrating T cells and a better prognosis. *PLoS ONE* **2012**, *7*, e38541. [CrossRef] [PubMed]

126. Nesbeth, Y.C.; Martinez, D.G.; Toraya, S.; Scarlett, U.K.; Cubillos-Ruiz, J.R.; Rutkowski, M.R.; Conejo-Garcia, J.R. CD4+ T cells elicit host immune responses to MHC class II-negative ovarian cancer through CCL5 secretion and CD40-mediated licensing of dendritic cells. *J. Immunol.* **2010**, *184*, 5654–5662. [CrossRef] [PubMed]

127. Hanahan, D.; Coussens, L.M. Accessories to the crime: Functions of cells recruited to the tumor microenvironment. *Cancer Cell* **2012**, *21*, 309–322. [CrossRef] [PubMed]

128. Mittal, D.; Gubin, M.M.; Schreiber, R.D.; Smyth, M.J. New insights into cancer immunoediting and its three component phases–elimination, equilibrium and escape. *Curr. Opin. Immunol.* **2014**, *27*, 16–25. [CrossRef] [PubMed]

129. Sehouli, J.; Loddenkemper, C.; Cornu, T.; Schwachula, T.; Hoffmüller, U.; Grützkau, A.; Lohneis, P.; Dickhaus, T.; Gröne, J.; Kruschewski, M.; et al. Epigenetic quantification of tumor-infiltrating T-lymphocytes. *Epigenetics* **2011**, *6*, 236–246. [CrossRef] [PubMed]

130. Curiel, T.J.; Coukos, G.; Zou, L.; Alvarez, X.; Cheng, P.; Mottram, P.; Evdemon-Hogan, M.; Conejo-Garcia, J.R.; Zhang, L.; Burow, M.; et al. Specific recruitment of regulatory T cells in ovarian carcinoma fosters immune privilege and predicts reduced survival. *Nat. Med.* **2004**, *10*, 942–949. [CrossRef] [PubMed]

131. Woo, E.Y.; Chu, C.S.; Goletz, T.J.; Schlienger, K.; Yeh, H.; Coukos, G.; Rubin, S.C.; Kaiser, L.R.; June, C.H. Regulatory CD4(+)CD25(+) T cells in tumors from patients with early-stage non-small cell lung cancer and late-stage ovarian cancer. *Cancer Res.* **2001**, *61*, 4766–4772. [PubMed]

132. Kryczek, I.; Liu, R.; Wang, G.; Wu, K.; Shu, X.; Szeliga, W.; Vatan, L.; Finlayson, E.; Huang, E.; Simeone, D.; et al. FOXP3 defines regulatory T cells in human tumor and autoimmune disease. *Cancer Res.* **2009**, *69*, 3995–4000. [CrossRef] [PubMed]

133. Napoletano, C.; Bellati, F.; Landi, R.; Pauselli, S.; Marchetti, C.; Visconti, V.; Sale, P.; Liberati, M.; Rughetti, A.; Frati, L.; et al. Ovarian cancer cytoreduction induces changes in T cell population subsets reducing immunosuppression. *J. Cell. Mol. Med.* **2010**, *14*, 2748–2759. [CrossRef] [PubMed]

134. Fialová, A.; Partlová, S.; Sojka, L.; Hromádková, H.; Brtnický, T.; Fučíková, J.; Kocián, P.; Rob, L.; Bartůňková, J.; Spíšek, R. Dynamics of T-cell infiltration during the course of ovarian cancer: The gradual shift from a Th17 effector cell response to a predominant infiltration by regulatory T-cells. *Int. J. Cancer* **2013**, *132*, 1070–1079. [CrossRef] [PubMed]

135. Facciabene, A.; Peng, X.; Hagemann, I.S.; Balint, K.; Barchetti, A.; Wang, L.-P.; Gimotty, P.A.; Gilks, C.B.; Lal, P.; Zhang, L.; et al. Tumour hypoxia promotes tolerance and angiogenesis via CCL28 and T(reg) cells. *Nature* **2011**, *475*, 226–230. [CrossRef] [PubMed]

136. Kryczek, I.; Wei, S.; Zhu, G.; Myers, L.; Mottram, P.; Cheng, P.; Chen, L.; Coukos, G.; Zou, W. Relationship between B7-H4, regulatory T cells, and patient outcome in human ovarian carcinoma. *Cancer Res.* **2007**, *67*, 8900–8905. [CrossRef] [PubMed]

137. Redjimi, N.; Raffin, C.; Raimbaud, I.; Pignon, P.; Matsuzaki, J.; Odunsi, K.; Valmori, D.; Ayyoub, M. CXCR3+ T regulatory cells selectively accumulate in human ovarian carcinomas to limit type I immunity. *Cancer Res.* **2012**, *72*, 4351–4360. [CrossRef] [PubMed]

138. Giuntoli, R.L.; Webb, T.J.; Zoso, A.; Rogers, O.; Diaz-Montes, T.P.; Bristow, R.E.; Oelke, M. Ovarian Cancer-associated Ascites Demonstrates Altered Immune Environment: Implications for Antitumor Immunity. *Anticancer Res.* **2009**, *29*, 2875–2884. [PubMed]

139. Wolf, D.; Wolf, A.M.; Rumpold, H.; Fiegl, H.; Zeimet, A.G.; Muller-Holzner, E.; Deibl, M.; Gastl, G.; Gunsilius, E.; Marth, C. The expression of the regulatory T cell-specific forkhead box transcription factor FoxP3 is associated with poor prognosis in ovarian cancer. *Clin. Cancer Res.* **2005**, *11*, 8326–8331. [CrossRef] [PubMed]

140. Mhawech-Fauceglia, P.; Wang, D.; Ali, L.; Lele, S.; Huba, M.A.; Liu, S.; Odunsi, K. Intraepithelial T cells and tumor-associated macrophages in ovarian cancer patients. *Cancer Immun.* **2013**, *13*, 1. [PubMed]

141. Milne, K.; Köbel, M.; Kalloger, S.E.; Barnes, R.O.; Gao, D.; Gilks, C.B.; Watson, P.H.; Nelson, B.H. Systematic analysis of immune infiltrates in high-grade serous ovarian cancer reveals CD20, FoxP3 and TIA-1 as positive prognostic factors. *PLoS ONE* **2009**, *4*, e6412. [CrossRef] [PubMed]

142. Wu, M.; Chen, X.; Lou, J.; Zhang, S.; Zhang, X.; Huang, L.; Sun, R.; Huang, P.; Wang, F.; Pan, S. TGF-β1 contributes to CD8+ Treg induction through p38 MAPK signaling in ovarian cancer microenvironment. *Oncotarget* **2016**, *7*, 44534–44544. [CrossRef] [PubMed]

143. Zhang, S.; Ke, X.; Zeng, S.; Wu, M.; Lou, J.; Wu, L.; Huang, P.; Huang, L.; Wang, F.; Pan, S. Analysis of CD8+ Treg cells in patients with ovarian cancer: A possible mechanism for immune impairment. *Cell. Mol. Immunol.* **2015**, *12*, 580–591. [CrossRef] [PubMed]

144. Wang, R.-F. CD8+ regulatory T cells, their suppressive mechanisms, and regulation in cancer. *Hum. Immunol.* **2008**, *69*, 811–814. [CrossRef] [PubMed]

145. Yigit, R.; Massuger, L.F.A.G.; Figdor, C.G.; Torensma, R. Ovarian cancer creates a suppressive microenvironment to escape immune elimination. *Gynecol. Oncol.* **2010**, *117*, 366–372. [CrossRef] [PubMed]

146. Sarvaria, A.; Madrigal, J.A.; Saudemont, A. B cell regulation in cancer and anti-tumor immunity. *Cell. Mol. Immunol.* **2017**, *14*, 662–674. [CrossRef] [PubMed]

147. Montfort, A.; Pearce, O.; Maniati, E.; Vincent, B.G.; Bixby, L.; Böhm, S.; Dowe, T.; Wilkes, E.H.; Chakravarty, P.; Thompson, R.; et al. A strong B-cell response is part of the immune landscape in human high-grade serous ovarian metastases. *Clin. Cancer Res.* **2017**, *23*, 250–262. [CrossRef] [PubMed]

148. Rosser, E.C.; Mauri, C. Regulatory B cells: Origin, phenotype, and function. *Immunity* **2015**, *42*, 607–612. [CrossRef] [PubMed]

149. Lundgren, S.; Berntsson, J.; Nodin, B.; Micke, P.; Jirström, K. Prognostic impact of tumour-associated B cells and plasma cells in epithelial ovarian cancer. *J. Ovarian Res.* **2016**, *9*, 21. [CrossRef] [PubMed]

150. Yang, C.; Lee, H.; Jove, V.; Deng, J.; Zhang, W.; Liu, X.; Forman, S.; Dellinger, T.H.; Wakabayashi, M.; Yu, H.; et al. Prognostic significance of B-cells and pSTAT3 in patients with ovarian cancer. *PLoS ONE* **2013**, *8*, e54029. [CrossRef] [PubMed]

151. Dong, H.P.; Elstrand, M.B.; Holth, A.; Silins, I.; Berner, A.; Trope, C.G.; Davidson, B.; Risberg, B. NK- and B-cell infiltration correlates with worse outcome in metastatic ovarian carcinoma. *Am. J. Clin. Pathol.* **2006**, *125*, 451–458. [CrossRef] [PubMed]

152. Lu, P.H.; Negrin, R.S. A novel population of expanded human CD3+CD56+ cells derived from T cells with potent in vivo antitumor activity in mice with severe combined immunodeficiency. *J. Immunol.* **1994**, *153*, 1687–1696. [PubMed]

153. Schmidt-Wolf, I.G.; Lefterova, P.; Mehta, B.A.; Fernandez, L.P.; Huhn, D.; Blume, K.G.; Weissman, I.L.; Negrin, R.S. Phenotypic characterization and identification of effector cells involved in tumor cell recognition of cytokine-induced killer cells. *Exp. Hematol.* **1993**, *21*, 1673–1679. [PubMed]

154. Bamias, A.; Tsiatas, M.L.; Kafantari, E.; Liakou, C.; Rodolakis, A.; Voulgaris, Z.; Vlahos, G.; Papageorgiou, T.;

Tsitsilonis, O.; Bamia, C.; et al. Significant differences of lymphocytes isolated from ascites of patients with ovarian cancer compared to blood and tumor lymphocytes. Association of CD3+CD56+ cells with platinum resistance. *Gynecol. Oncol.* **2007**, *106*, 75–81. [CrossRef] [PubMed]

155. Bamias, A.; Koutsoukou, V.; Terpos, E.; Tsiatas, M.L.; Liakos, C.; Tsitsilonis, O.; Rodolakis, A.; Voulgaris, Z.; Vlahos, G.; Papageorgiou, T.; et al. Correlation of NK T-like CD3+CD56+ cells and CD4+CD25+(hi) regulatory T cells with VEGF and TNFalpha in ascites from advanced ovarian cancer: Association with platinum resistance and prognosis in patients receiving first-line, platinum-based chemotherapy. *Gynecol. Oncol.* **2008**, *108*, 421–427. [CrossRef] [PubMed]

156. Wolf, B.J.; Choi, J.E.; Exley, M.A. Novel approaches to exploiting invariant NKT cells in cancer immunotherapy. *Front. Immunol.* **2018**, *9*, 384. [CrossRef] [PubMed]

157. Guillerey, C.; Huntington, N.D.; Smyth, M.J. Targeting natural killer cells in cancer immunotherapy. *Nat. Immunol.* **2016**, *17*, 1025–1036. [CrossRef] [PubMed]

158. Sungur, C.M.; Murphy, W.J. Positive and negative regulation by NK cells in cancer. *Crit. Rev. Oncog.* **2014**, *19*, 57–66. [CrossRef] [PubMed]

159. Voskoboinik, I.; Smyth, M.J.; Trapani, J.A. Perforin-mediated target-cell death and immune homeostasis. *Nat. Rev. Immunol.* **2006**, *6*, 940–952. [CrossRef] [PubMed]

160. Lai, P.; Rabinowich, H.; Crowley-Nowick, P.A.; Bell, M.C.; Mantovani, G.; Whiteside, T.L. Alterations in expression and function of signal-transducing proteins in tumor-associated T and natural killer cells in patients with ovarian carcinoma. *Clin. Cancer Res.* **1996**, *2*, 161–173. [PubMed]

161. Yunusova, N.V.; Stakheyeva, M.N.; Molchanov, S.V.; Afanas'ev, S.G.; Tsydenova, A.A.; Kolomiets, L.A.; Cherdyntseva, N.V. Functional activity of natural killer cells in biological fluids in patients with colorectal and ovarian cancers. *Cent.-Eur. J. Immunol.* **2018**, *43*, 26–32. [CrossRef] [PubMed]

162. Webb, J.R.; Milne, K.; Watson, P.; Deleeuw, R.J.; Nelson, B.H. Tumor-infiltrating lymphocytes expressing the tissue resident memory marker CD103 are associated with increased survival in high-grade serous ovarian cancer. *Clin. Cancer Res.* **2014**, *20*, 434–444. [CrossRef] [PubMed]

163. Garzetti, G.G.; Cignitti, M.; Ciavattini, A.; Fabris, N.; Romanini, C. Natural killer cell activity and progression-free survival in ovarian cancer. *Gynecol. Obstet. Invest.* **1993**, *35*, 118–120. [CrossRef] [PubMed]

164. Li, K.; Mandai, M.; Hamanishi, J.; Matsumura, N.; Suzuki, A.; Yagi, H.; Yamaguchi, K.; Baba, T.; Fujii, S.; Konishi, I. Clinical significance of the NKG2D ligands, MICA/B and ULBP2 in ovarian cancer: High expression of ULBP2 is an indicator of poor prognosis. *Cancer Immunol. Immunother. CII* **2009**, *58*, 641–652. [CrossRef] [PubMed]

165. Colvin, E.K. Tumor-associated macrophages contribute to tumor progression in ovarian cancer. *Front. Oncol.* **2014**, *4*, 137. [CrossRef] [PubMed]

166. Takaishi, K.; Komohara, Y.; Tashiro, H.; Ohtake, H.; Nakagawa, T.; Katabuchi, H.; Takeya, M. Involvement of M2-polarized macrophages in the ascites from advanced epithelial ovarian carcinoma in tumor progression via Stat3 activation. *Cancer Sci.* **2010**, *101*, 2128–2136. [CrossRef] [PubMed]

167. Kawamura, K.; Komohara, Y.; Takaishi, K.; Katabuchi, H.; Takeya, M. Detection of M2 macrophages and colony-stimulating factor 1 expression in serous and mucinous ovarian epithelial tumors. *Pathol. Int.* **2009**, *59*, 300–305. [CrossRef] [PubMed]

168. Hagemann, T.; Wilson, J.; Burke, F.; Kulbe, H.; Li, N.F.; Plüddemann, A.; Charles, K.; Gordon, S.; Balkwill, F.R. Ovarian cancer cells polarize macrophages toward a tumor-associated phenotype. *J. Immunol.* **2006**, *176*, 5023–5032. [CrossRef] [PubMed]

169. Sica, G.L.; Choi, I.H.; Zhu, G.; Tamada, K.; Wang, S.D.; Tamura, H.; Chapoval, A.I.; Flies, D.B.; Bajorath, J.; Chen, L. B7-H4, a molecule of the B7 family, negatively regulates T cell immunity. *Immunity* **2003**, *18*, 849–861. [CrossRef]

170. Yuan, X.; Zhang, J.; Li, D.; Mao, Y.; Mo, F.; Du, W.; Ma, X. Prognostic significance of tumor-associated macrophages in ovarian cancer: A meta-analysis. *Gynecol. Oncol.* **2017**, *147*, 181–187. [CrossRef] [PubMed]

171. Lan, C.; Huang, X.; Lin, S.; Huang, H.; Cai, Q.; Wan, T.; Lu, J.; Liu, J. Expression of M2-polarized macrophages is associated with poor prognosis for advanced epithelial ovarian cancer. *Technol. Cancer Res. Treat.* **2013**, *12*, 259–267. [CrossRef] [PubMed]

172. He, Y.; Zhang, M.; Wu, X.; Sun, X.; Xu, T.; He, Q.; Di, W. High MUC2 expression in ovarian cancer is inversely associated with the M1/M2 ratio of tumor-associated macrophages and patient survival time. *PLoS ONE* **2013** *8*, e79769. [CrossRef] [PubMed]

173. Zhang, M.; He, Y.; Sun, X.; Li, Q.; Wang, W.; Zhao, A.; Di, W. A high M1/M2 ratio of tumor-associated macrophages is associated with extended survival in ovarian cancer patients. *J. Ovarian Res.* **2014**, *7*, 19. [CrossRef] [PubMed]

174. No, J.H.; Moon, J.M.; Kim, K.; Kim, Y.-B. Prognostic significance of serum soluble CD163 level in patients with epithelial ovarian cancer. *Gynecol. Obstet. Investig.* **2013**, *75*, 263–267. [CrossRef] [PubMed]

175. Gordon, I.O.; Freedman, R.S. Defective antitumor function of monocyte-derived macrophages from epithelial ovarian cancer patients. *Clin. Cancer Res.* **2006**, *12*, 1515–1524. [CrossRef] [PubMed]

176. Genard, G.; Lucas, S.; Michiels, C. Reprogramming of tumor-associated macrophages with anticancer therapies: Radiotherapy versus chemo- and immunotherapies. *Front. Immunol.* **2017**, *8*, 828. [CrossRef] [PubMed]

177. Youn, J.-I.; Gabrilovich, D.I. The biology of myeloid-derived suppressor cells: The blessing and the curse of morphological and functional heterogeneity. *Eur. J. Immunol.* **2010**, *40*, 2969–2975. [CrossRef] [PubMed]

178. Gabrilovich, D.I.; Nagaraj, S. Myeloid-derived suppressor cells as regulators of the immune system. *Nat. Rev. Immunol.* **2009**, *9*, 162–174. [CrossRef] [PubMed]

179. Obermajer, N.; Muthuswamy, R.; Odunsi, K.; Edwards, R.P.; Kalinski, P. PGE(2)-induced CXCL12 production and CXCR4 expression controls the accumulation of human MDSCs in ovarian cancer environment. *Cancer Res.* **2011**, *71*, 7463–7470. [CrossRef] [PubMed]

180. Cui, T.X.; Kryczek, I.; Zhao, L.; Zhao, E.; Kuick, R.; Roh, M.H.; Vatan, L.; Szeliga, W.; Mao, Y.; Thomas, D.G.; et al. Myeloid-derived suppressor cells enhance stemness of cancer cells by inducing microRNA101 and suppressing the corepressor CtBP2. *Immunity* **2013**, *39*, 611–621. [CrossRef] [PubMed]

181. Wu, L.; Deng, Z.; Peng, Y.; Han, L.; Liu, J.; Wang, L.; Li, B.; Zhao, J.; Jiao, S.; Wei, H. Ascites-derived IL-6 and IL-10 synergistically expand CD14+HLA-DR-/low myeloid-derived suppressor cells in ovarian cancer patients. *Oncotarget* **2017**, *8*, 76843–76856. [CrossRef] [PubMed]

182. Horikawa, N.; Abiko, K.; Matsumura, N.; Hamanishi, J.; Baba, T.; Yamaguchi, K.; Yoshioka, Y.; Koshiyama, M.; Konishi, I. Expression of Vascular Endothelial Growth Factor in Ovarian Cancer Inhibits Tumor Immunity through the Accumulation of Myeloid-Derived Suppressor Cells. *Clin. Cancer Res.* **2017**, *23*, 587–599. [CrossRef] [PubMed]

183. Taki, M.; Abiko, K.; Baba, T.; Hamanishi, J.; Yamaguchi, K.; Murakami, R.; Yamanoi, K.; Horikawa, N.; Hosoe, Y.; Nakamura, E.; et al. Snail promotes ovarian cancer progression by recruiting myeloid-derived suppressor cells via CXCR2 ligand upregulation. *Nat. Commun.* **2018**, *9*, 1685. [CrossRef] [PubMed]

184. Montalbán Del Barrio, I.; Penski, C.; Schlahsa, L.; Stein, R.G.; Diessner, J.; Wöckel, A.; Dietl, J.; Lutz, M.B.; Mittelbronn, M.; Wischhusen, J.; et al. Adenosine-generating ovarian cancer cells attract myeloid cells which differentiate into adenosine-generating tumor associated macrophages—A self-amplifying, CD39- and CD73-dependent mechanism for tumor immune escape. *J. Immunother. Cancer* **2016**, *4*, 49. [CrossRef] [PubMed]

185. Li, L.; Wang, L.; Li, J.; Fan, Z.; Yang, L.; Zhang, Z.; Zhang, C.; Yue, D.; Qin, G.; Zhang, T.; et al. Metformin-induced reduction of CD39 and CD73 blocks myeloid-derived suppressor cell activity in patients with ovarian cancer. *Cancer Res.* **2018**, *78*, 1779–1791. [CrossRef] [PubMed]

186. Cheng, L.; Wu, S.; Zhang, K.; Qing, Y.; Xu, T. A comprehensive overview of exosomes in ovarian cancer: Emerging biomarkers and therapeutic strategies. *J. Ovarian Res.* **2017**, *10*, 73. [CrossRef] [PubMed]

187. Li, W.; Zhang, X.; Wang, J.; Li, M.; Cao, C.; Tan, J.; Ma, D.; Gao, Q. TGFβ1 in fibroblasts-derived exosomes promotes epithelial-mesenchymal transition of ovarian cancer cells. *Oncotarget* **2017**, *8*, 96035–96047. [CrossRef] [PubMed]

188. Au Yeung, C.L.; Co, N.-N.; Tsuruga, T.; Yeung, T.-L.; Kwan, S.-Y.; Leung, C.S.; Li, Y.; Lu, E.S.; Kwan, K.; Wong, K.-K.; et al. Exosomal transfer of stroma-derived miR21 confers paclitaxel resistance in ovarian cancer cells through targeting APAF1. *Nat. Commun.* **2016**, *7*, 11150. [CrossRef] [PubMed]

189. Peng, P.; Yan, Y.; Keng, S. Exosomes in the ascites of ovarian cancer patients: Origin and effects on anti-tumor immunity. *Oncol. Rep.* **2011**, *25*, 749–762. [CrossRef] [PubMed]

190. Keerthikumar, S.; Chisanga, D.; Ariyaratne, D.; Al Saffar, H.; Anand, S.; Zhao, K.; Samuel, M.; Pathan, M.; Jois, M.; Chilamkurti, N.; et al. ExoCarta: A web-based compendium of exosomal cargo. *J. Mol. Biol.* **2016**, *428*, 688–692. [CrossRef] [PubMed]

191. Mathivanan, S.; Simpson, R.J. ExoCarta: A compendium of exosomal proteins and RNA. *Proteomics* **2009**, *9*, 4997–5000. [CrossRef] [PubMed]

192. Keller, S.; König, A.-K.; Marmé, F.; Runz, S.; Wolterink, S.; Koensgen, D.; Mustea, A.; Sehouli, J.; Altevogt, P. Systemic presence and tumor-growth promoting effect of ovarian carcinoma released exosomes. *Cancer Lett.* **2009**, *278*, 73–81. [CrossRef] [PubMed]

193. Valenti, R.; Huber, V.; Iero, M.; Filipazzi, P.; Parmiani, G.; Rivoltini, L. Tumor-released microvesicles as vehicles of immunosuppression. *Cancer Res.* **2007**, *67*, 2912–2915. [CrossRef] [PubMed]

194. Robbins, P.D.; Morelli, A.E. Regulation of immune responses by extracellular vesicles. *Nat. Rev. Immunol.* **2014**, *14*, 195–208. [CrossRef] [PubMed]

195. Cai, X.; Caballero-Benitez, A.; Gewe, M.M.; Jenkins, I.C.; Drescher, C.W.; Strong, R.K.; Spies, T.; Groh, V. Control of tumor initiation by NKG2D naturally expressed on ovarian cancer cells. *Neoplasia* **2017**, *19*, 471–482. [CrossRef] [PubMed]

196. Syn, N.L.; Wang, L.; Chow, E.K.-H.; Lim, C.T.; Goh, B.-C. Exosomes in cancer nanomedicine and immunotherapy: Prospects and challenges. *Trends Biotechnol.* **2017**, *35*, 665–676. [CrossRef] [PubMed]

197. Labiche, A.; Heutte, N.; Herlin, P.; Chasle, J.; Gauduchon, P.; Elie, N. Stromal compartment as a survival prognostic factor in advanced ovarian carcinoma. *Int. J. Gynecol. Cancer Off. J. Int. Gynecol. Cancer Soc.* **2010**, *20*, 28–33. [CrossRef] [PubMed]

198. Deying, W.; Feng, G.; Shumei, L.; Hui, Z.; Ming, L.; Hongqing, W. CAF-derived HGF promotes cell proliferation and drug resistance by up-regulating the c-Met/PI3K/Akt and GRP78 signalling in ovarian cancer cells. *Biosci. Rep.* **2017**, *37*. [CrossRef] [PubMed]

199. Kwon, Y.; Smith, B.D.; Zhou, Y.; Kaufman, M.D.; Godwin, A.K. Effective inhibition of c-MET-mediated signaling, growth and migration of ovarian cancer cells is influenced by the ovarian tissue microenvironment. *Oncogene* **2015**, *34*, 144–153. [CrossRef] [PubMed]

200. Erez, N.; Glanz, S.; Raz, Y.; Avivi, C.; Barshack, I. Cancer associated fibroblasts express pro-inflammatory factors in human breast and ovarian tumors. *Biochem. Biophys. Res. Commun.* **2013**, *437*, 397–402. [CrossRef] [PubMed]

201. Zhou, B.; Sun, C.; Li, N.; Shan, W.; Lu, H.; Guo, L.; Guo, E.; Xia, M.; Weng, D.; Meng, L.; et al. Cisplatin-induced CCL5 secretion from CAFs promotes cisplatin-resistance in ovarian cancer via regulation of the STAT3 and PI3K/Akt signaling pathways. *Int. J. Oncol.* **2016**, *48*, 2087–2097. [CrossRef] [PubMed]

202. Lau, T.-S.; Chung, T.K.-H.; Cheung, T.-H.; Chan, L.K.-Y.; Cheung, L.W.-H.; Yim, S.-F.; Siu, N.S.-S.; Lo, K.-W.; Yu, M.M.-Y.; Kulbe, H.; et al. Cancer cell-derived lymphotoxin mediates reciprocal tumour-stromal interactions in human ovarian cancer by inducing CXCL11 in fibroblasts. *J. Pathol.* **2014**, *232*, 43–56. [CrossRef] [PubMed]

203. Wang, L.; Zhang, F.; Cui, J.-Y.; Chen, L.; Chen, Y.-T.; Liu, B.-W. CAFs enhance paclitaxel resistance by inducing EMT through the IL-6/JAK2/STAT3 pathway. *Oncol. Rep.* **2018**, *39*, 2081–2090. [CrossRef] [PubMed]

204. Givel, A.-M.; Kieffer, Y.; Scholer-Dahirel, A.; Sirven, P.; Cardon, M.; Pelon, F.; Magagna, I.; Gentric, G.; Costa, A.; Bonneau, C.; et al. miR200-regulated CXCL12β promotes fibroblast heterogeneity and immunosuppression in ovarian cancers. *Nat. Commun.* **2018**, *9*, 1056. [CrossRef] [PubMed]

205. Schauer, I.G.; Zhang, J.; Xing, Z.; Guo, X.; Mercado-Uribe, I.; Sood, A.K.; Huang, P.; Liu, J. Interleukin-1β promotes ovarian tumorigenesis through a p53/NF-κB-mediated inflammatory response in stromal fibroblasts. *Neoplasia* **2013**, *15*, 409–420. [CrossRef] [PubMed]

206. Yeung, T.-L.; Leung, C.S.; Wong, K.-K.; Samimi, G.; Thompson, M.S.; Liu, J.; Zaid, T.M.; Ghosh, S.; Birrer, M.J.; Mok, S.C. TGF-β modulates ovarian cancer invasion by upregulating CAF-derived versican in the tumor microenvironment. *Cancer Res.* **2013**, *73*, 5016–5028. [CrossRef] [PubMed]

207. Giusti, I.; Francesco, M.D.; Ascenzo, S.D.; Palmerini, M.G.; Macchiarelli, G.; Carta, G.; Dolo, V. Ovarian cancer-derived extracellular vesicles affect normal human fibroblast behavior. *Cancer Biol. Ther.* **2018**, 1–44. [CrossRef] [PubMed]

208. Wei, R.; Lv, M.; Li, F.; Cheng, T.; Zhang, Z.; Jiang, G.; Zhou, Y.; Gao, R.; Wei, X.; Lou, J.; et al. Human CAFs promote lymphangiogenesis in ovarian cancer via the Hh-VEGF-C signaling axis. *Oncotarget* **2017**, *8*, 67315–67328. [CrossRef] [PubMed]

209. Leung, C.S.; Yeung, T.-L.; Yip, K.-P.; Wong, K.-K.; Ho, S.Y.; Mangala, L.S.; Sood, A.K.; Lopez-Berestein, G.; Sheng, J.; Wong, S.T.; et al. Cancer-associated fibroblasts regulate endothelial adhesion protein LPP to promote ovarian cancer chemoresistance. *J. Clin. Investig.* **2018**, *128*, 589–606. [CrossRef] [PubMed]

210. Lengyel, E. Ovarian Cancer Development and Metastasis. *Am. J. Pathol.* **2010**, *177*, 1053–1064. [CrossRef] [PubMed]

211. Lengyel, E.; Makowski, L.; DiGiovanni, J.; Kolonin, M.G. Cancer as a matter of fat: The crosstalk between adipose tissue and tumors. *Trends Cancer* **2018**, *4*, 374–384. [CrossRef] [PubMed]

212. Meza-Perez, S.; Randall, T.D. Immunological functions of the omentum. *Trends Immunol.* **2017**, *38*, 526–536. [CrossRef] [PubMed]

213. Clark, R.; Krishnan, V.; Schoof, M.; Rodriguez, I.; Theriault, B.; Chekmareva, M.; Rinker-Schaeffer, C. Milky spots promote ovarian cancer metastatic colonization of peritoneal adipose in experimental models. *Am. J. Pathol.* **2013**, *183*, 576–591. [CrossRef] [PubMed]

214. Gerber, S.A.; Rybalko, V.Y.; Bigelow, C.E.; Lugade, A.A.; Foster, T.H.; Frelinger, J.G.; Lord, E.M. Preferential attachment of peritoneal tumor metastases to omental immune aggregates and possible role of a unique vascular microenvironment in metastatic survival and growth. *Am. J. Pathol.* **2006**, *169*, 1739–1752. [CrossRef] [PubMed]

215. Krishnan, V.; Clark, R.; Chekmareva, M.; Johnson, A.; George, S.; Shaw, P.; Seewaldt, V.; Rinker-Schaeffer, C. In vivo and Ex vivo approaches to study ovarian cancer metastatic colonization of milky spot structures in peritoneal adipose. *J. Vis. Exp. JoVE* **2015**. [CrossRef] [PubMed]

216. Nieman, K.M.; Kenny, H.A.; Penicka, C.V.; Ladanyi, A.; Buell-Gutbrod, R.; Zillhardt, M.R.; Romero, I.L.; Carey, M.S.; Mills, G.B.; Hotamisligil, G.S.; et al. Adipocytes promote ovarian cancer metastasis and provide energy for rapid tumor growth. *Nat. Med.* **2011**, *17*, 1498–1503. [CrossRef] [PubMed]

217. Oosterling, S.J.; van der Bij, G.J.; Bögels, M.; van der Sijp, J.R.M.; Beelen, R.H.J.; Meijer, S.; van Egmond, M. Insufficient ability of omental milky spots to prevent peritoneal tumor outgrowth supports omentectomy in minimal residual disease. *Cancer Immunol. Immunother.* **2006**, *55*, 1043–1051. [CrossRef] [PubMed]

218. Ladanyi, A.; Mukherjee, A.; Kenny, H.A.; Johnson, A.; Mitra, A.K.; Sundaresan, S.; Nieman, K.M.; Pascual, G.; Benitah, S.A.; Montag, A.; et al. Adipocyte-induced CD36 expression drives ovarian cancer progression and metastasis. *Oncogene* **2018**, *37*, 2285–2301. [CrossRef] [PubMed]

219. Protani, M.M.; Nagle, C.M.; Webb, P.M. Obesity and ovarian cancer survival: A systematic review and meta-analysis. *Cancer Prev. Res.* **2012**, *5*, 901–910. [CrossRef] [PubMed]

220. Liu, Y.; Metzinger, M.N.; Lewellen, K.A.; Cripps, S.N.; Carey, K.D.; Harper, E.I.; Shi, Z.; Tarwater, L.; Grisoli, A.; Lee, E.; et al. Obesity contributes to ovarian cancer metastatic success through increased lipogenesis, enhanced vascularity, and decreased infiltration of M1 macrophages. *Cancer Res.* **2015**, *75*, 5046–5057. [CrossRef] [PubMed]

221. James, B.R.; Tomanek-Chalkley, A.; Askeland, E.J.; Kucaba, T.; Griffith, T.S.; Norian, L.A. Diet-induced obesity alters dendritic cell function in the presence and absence of tumor growth. *J. Immunol.* **2012**, *189*, 1311–1321. [CrossRef] [PubMed]

222. Macia, L.; Delacre, M.; Abboud, G.; Ouk, T.-S.; Delanoye, A.; Verwaerde, C.; Saule, P.; Wolowczuk, I. Impairment of dendritic cell functionality and steady-state number in obese mice. *J. Immunol.* **2006**, *177*, 5997–6006. [CrossRef] [PubMed]

223. Shirakawa, K.; Yan, X.; Shinmura, K.; Endo, J.; Kataoka, M.; Katsumata, Y.; Yamamoto, T.; Anzai, A.; Isobe, S.; Yoshida, N.; et al. Obesity accelerates T cell senescence in murine visceral adipose tissue. *J. Clin. Investig.* **2016**, *126*, 4626–4639. [CrossRef] [PubMed]

224. McCloskey, C.W.; Rodriguez, G.M.; Galpin, K.J.C.; Vanderhyden, B.C. Ovarian cancer immunotherapy: Preclinical models and emerging therapeutics. *Cancers* **2018**, in press.

The Role of Inflammation and Inflammatory Mediators in the Development, Progression, Metastasis and Chemoresistance of Epithelial Ovarian Cancer

Sudha S. Savant [1,†], Shruthi Sriramkumar [2,†] and Heather M. O'Hagan [1,3,*]

[1]   Medical Sciences, Indiana University School of Medicine, Bloomington, IN 47405, USA; ssavant@iu.edu
[2]   Cell, Molecular and Cancer Biology Graduate Program, Indiana University, Bloomington, IN 47405, USA; ssriramk@iu.edu
[3]   Indiana University Melvin and Bren Simon Cancer Center, Indianapolis, IN 46202, USA
*   Correspondence: hmohagan@indiana.edu
†   These authors contributed equally to this work.

Abstract: Inflammation plays a role in the initiation and development of many types of cancers, including epithelial ovarian cancer (EOC) and high grade serous ovarian cancer (HGSC), a type of EOC. There are connections between EOC and both peritoneal and ovulation-induced inflammation. Additionally, EOCs have an inflammatory component that contributes to their progression. At sites of inflammation, epithelial cells are exposed to increased levels of inflammatory mediators such as reactive oxygen species, cytokines, prostaglandins, and growth factors that contribute to increased cell division, and genetic and epigenetic changes. These exposure-induced changes promote excessive cell proliferation, increased survival, malignant transformation, and cancer development. Furthermore, the pro-inflammatory tumor microenvironment environment (TME) contributes to EOC metastasis and chemoresistance. In this review we will discuss the roles inflammation and inflammatory mediators play in the development, progression, metastasis, and chemoresistance of EOC.

Keywords: inflammation; epithelial ovarian cancer; cytokines; reactive oxygen species; growth factors

1. Inflammation and EOC

Inflammation is part of the immune response that protects against foreign pathogens and aids in healing. Inflammation is elicited in response to cellular damage either by infection, exposure to foreign particles (pollutants or irritants), or an increase in cellular stress [1]. The ultimate goal of the inflammatory response is to restore tissue homeostasis, either by destruction or healing of the damaged tissue. The acute or immediate inflammatory response involves modification of the vasculature surrounding the site of stress or damage to increase blood flow. This alteration is then followed by activation of innate immune cells already present in the tissue, including macrophages, dendritic cells (DC), and mast cells, and an increase in infiltration of additional innate immune cells into the affected tissue. At sites of inflammation there are high levels of reactive oxygen species (ROS), cytokines, chemokines, and growth factors that are produced by the immune cells and other cells in the tissue. Acute inflammation is essential for tissue homeostasis and to protect against normal exposure to pathogens. However, in certain cases the body is unable to resolve this response or is subjected to repeated stimulation resulting in chronic inflammation.

Ovarian cancer (OC) is the fifth leading cause of cancer-related deaths in women in the United States [2] and can originate in the germ cells, sex-cord stroma, the fallopian tube (FT), or ovary epithelium. Epithelial ovarian cancer (EOC) which originates from the ovary or fallopian tube epithelium, accounts for 85–90% of all OCs. Chronic inflammation is an important risk factor associated for EOC and high grade serous ovarian cancer (HGSC), the most malignant subtype of EOC. Chronic inflammation results in activation of signaling pathways, transcription factors, and the innate and adaptive immune responses [3,4]. In this review we primarily focus on inflammation as a risk factor for invasive EOC, but have also included supportive evidence from other OC subtypes, studies that do not define the subtype of OC, and other tumor types as indicated.

1.1. Signaling Pathways and Transcription Factors

Several signaling pathways and transcription factors involved in the inflammatory response also play critical roles in EOC. Here we briefly introduce relevant pathways that will be linked to OC formation in later sections. Cytokines produced during inflammation bind to and activate toll like receptors (TLRs) on cell surfaces, which results in activation of the signaling pathways involving mitogen-activated protein kinases (MAPKs) p38 and JNK (c-Jun N-terminal kinase) and transcription factors including nuclear factor kappa-light-chain-enhancer of activated B cells (NF-κB) and the signal transducer and activator of transcription (STATs). The MAPK pathway regulates cellular processes like proliferation, differentiation, growth, migration, and cell death by upregulating the expression of transcription factors like AP-1, c-Jun, FOS and by activating NF-κB and STATs, that either by themselves or along with AP-1 or c-Jun regulate expression of pro-survival and pro-growth genes. NF-κB and AP-1 also regulate production of cytokines like IL-6 [5–7].

During inflammation these transcription factors play an important role to maintain tissue homeostasis. However, in case of chronic inflammation, the signaling pathways are continuously stimulated, which can contribute to tumorigenesis.

1.2. Innate Immune Response

Inflammation activates the innate immune response, which signals macrophages and DCs to secrete chemoattractants like Interleukin-8 (IL-8), monocyte chemotactic protein-1 (MCP-1), and various other inflammatory mediators. These chemoattractants in turn result in recruitment of neutrophils, lymphocytes, and natural killer (NK) cells to the site of damage. All of these cells then secrete cytokines like IL-1, IL-3, IL-6, IL-8, tumor necrosis factor alpha (TNF-α), interferon (IFN) α, and colony-stimulating factors (CSF) like granulocyte macrophage CSF (GM-CSF). The cytokines bind to transmembrane receptors on the cell surfaces of other cells to activate transcription factors that regulate gene expression downstream of the cytokine activated pathway. This creates a pro-inflammatory environment resulting in recruitment of other immune cells, migration of endothelial cells, and proliferation of fibroblasts. Activation of macrophages and NK cells results in the production of high levels of ROS and reactive nitrogen species (RNS), which are used by these cells to kill foreign pathogens, but also end up damaging neighboring normal cells [8]. The lymphocytes also secrete growth factors like platelet derived growth factor (PDGF), transforming growth factor beta (TGF-β), and fibroblast growth factor (FGF), which facilitate wound healing. Overall the acute immune response is a rapid response that typically only lasts a few days. It results in removal of the pathogen, release of proteolytic enzymes to destroy damaged tissue, or stimulation of the proliferation of fibroblasts and epithelial cells to repair the tissue [1].

1.3. Adaptive Immune Response

If the infection is not resolved by the innate immune response, the adaptive immune response is activated, which is less inflammatory in nature. The adaptive immune response also provides longstanding protection against specific pathogens and/or antigens. B cells and T cells are the effector cells of the adaptive immune system that are derived from lymphocytes when they are presented with specific antigens by the antigen presenting cells (APC). T cells respond to the APCs by producing IL-2, which induces expression of transcription factors that facilitate T cells to differentiate into T regulatory (Tregs) and T effector (Teff) cells. There are two major classes of T effector cells;

CD8$^+$ cytotoxic T cells and CD4$^+$ T helper (Th) cells. Th cells are further differentiated into Th1, Th2, or Th17 depending on the ILs secreted and the transcription factors expressed. IFN-y activates STAT1 to induce formation of Th1 and IL-6, and TGF-β can induce Th17 cell formation. Th1 and Th17 secrete ILs and activate macrophages and B cells to create a pro-inflammatory microenvironment (ME) that can be protumorigenic depending on the context. Tregs are immunosuppressive cells that turn off the immune response [1,9,10].

2. Inflammation as a Risk Factor for EOC

Amongst other factors such as hereditary, environmental, and lifestyle, inflammation emerges as an important risk factor for EOC. EOC arises either in the epithelial layer surrounding the ovary or in the epithelium of the distal FT, which could then spread to the ovary. A significant portion of HGSC is thought to originate in the FT, in part because removal of the FT significantly reduces OC risk [11]. Interestingly, while surgical specimens from mutation carriers rarely had premalignant ovarian epithelial changes, early lesions called serous tubal intraepithelial carcinomas (STICs) were found in the FTs of 5–10% of the patients. Copy number and mutational analysis suggest that STICs shed cells with metastatic potential that then colonize the ovary to form HGSC. STICs are mostly found in the fimbriae, the distal end of the FT that shares a ME with the ovary. During a woman's lifetime, the repeated secretion of ROS, cytokines, and other growth factors by the ovaries and immune cells creates a chronic inflammatory ME in the peritoneum that in turn potentiates the initiation of normal cells to malignant ones in the FT and the ovary, supports tumor progression, metastasis, and development of resistance to chemotherapy.

During ovulation, infection and other causes of inflammation ovary and FT tissue is damaged and undergoes repair. We will briefly discuss how each of these processes evoke or involve an inflammatory response that can persist, leading to a cytokine and growth factor rich environment in the peritoneum and contribute to EOC.

2.1. Ovulation

The process of ovulation itself is comparable to that of inflammation as described in the early 20th century. The development of the follicle to its rupture and release of the egg results in recruitment of activated immune cells to the ovary and production of enormous amounts of chemokines, cytokines, and growth factors. Ovulation is initiated by a surge of Luteinizing hormones (LH) that results in increased blood flow to the ovarian follicles. Before release of the egg, the surge of LH hormone recruits neutrophils and macrophages to the graafian follicles [12–14]. Macrophages in the theca have been shown to support growth of follicles [15]. During ovulation macrophages secrete growth factors like hepatocyte growth factor (HGF), TGF-β, and epidermal growth factor (EGF), which stimulate cellular proliferation and follicle growth. Simultaneously the macrophages also secrete ROS, TNF-α, and IL1β, which stimulate local apoptosis resulting in rupture of the follicle, which bathes the ovarian surface and fimbriae with follicular fluid. Exposure of FT cells to follicular fluid results in altered expression of genes associated with inflammation, including increased expression of IL8 and cyclooxygenase-2 (COX-2) [16]. Quiescent fibroblasts are present in the thecal layer surrounding the follicles. Exposure to growth factors stimulates their proliferation and they then secrete prostaglandins, collagenases, and plasminogen activator. In the corpus luteum, after the follicle is released, the macrophages secrete prostaglandins, ROS, and TNF-α, which stimulate apoptosis of the corpus luteum cells. Therefore, ovulation results in the cyclic exposure of FT and ovarian epithelial cells to high levels of ROS, cytokines, and growth factors [17] Although the other causes of inflammation discussed below are important and result in increased overall risk for EOC, the process of ovulation itself occurs often in the lifetime of the majority of women and may be the most important inflammation-related risk factor for EOC. This hypothesis is corroborated by the laying hen model, which is commonly used to study ovarian cancer [18]. In this model, hens develop spontaneous EOC, likely due to their high ovulation rate, thus linking ovulation directly as an increased risk factor for EOC. Delayed onset of menarche and early onset of menopause have been shown to be inversely related to the risk of OC, likely due to the reduction in number of ovulation cycles in a woman's lifetime [19,20]. Further, ovulation has also been connected to EOC because contraceptive pills, pregnancy, and breastfeeding reduce the risk of OC. These factors reduce, halt, or delay overall ovulation cycles, respectively, which in turn reduces overall exposure to inflammation of the ovary and FT. The associations of parity and oral contraceptive use with invasive EOC were recently confirmed in a large, prospective study using the European Prospective Investigation into Cancer and Nutrition (EPIC) cohort that found only limited heterogeneity in the risk between reproductive factors and EOC subtypes [21]. Hysterectomy, tube ligation, and removal of ovaries are also protective against development of OC [22,23].

2.2. Infection

Pelvic inflammatory disorder (PID) is the infection of the female reproductive organs like cervix, uterus, FTs, and ovaries. It is a significant risk factor for OC and is caused by various bacteria and virus such as *Chlamydia trachomatis*, *Mycoplasma genitalium*, *Neisseria gonorrhoeae*, human papilloma virus, and cytomegalovirus [24,25]. Infection by these microbes results in DNA damage and production of ROS and induces a pro-inflammatory response, which involves secretion of cytokines and migration of immune cells [24]. PID is generally resolved with antibiotics within 48–72 hours of detection. However, repeated infection and unresolved inflammation can lead to chronic inflammation that is a risk factor for EOC.

2.3. Other Sources of Inflammation

The other causes of inflammation in the ovaries and/or FTs are endometriosis, obesity, Polycystic Ovarian Syndrome (PCOS), and talc exposure. Endometriosis is defined as presence of stroma and endometrial gland tissues in the pelvic peritoneum, rectovaginal septum, and ovaries [26]. Retrograde menstruation is the most commonly accepted theory for endometriosis. Retrograde menstruation results in aberrant accumulation of red blood cells (RBCs) and tissue, which can trigger an inflammatory response, activating the macrophages in the peritoneal cavity [27,28]. The macrophages lyse the RBCs, resulting in an increase in iron accumulation in the endometric implants and peritoneal fluid. The accumulated iron can catalyze formation of free radicals like RNS and ROS in the peritoneum and results in increased oxidative stress (OS). OS can activate NF-κB, in macrophages resulting in secretion of growth factors, cytokines, and IFNs. Around one third of women are affected by mild endometriosis, which resolves on its own over time. For the remaining cases, endometriosis results in chronic pain and inflammation, which can be resolved by excision of affected tissue or the outgrowth. However, in 45% of these cases, the endometriosis reoccurs resulting in repeated bouts of chronic inflammation [29,30].

Obese women have higher risks of EOC and HGSC and pro-inflammatory cytokines are associated with higher body mass index (BMI) levels. Adipose tissues secrete the cytokines TNF-α, IL-6, IL-8, and MCP-1, which can induce an inflammatory reaction in the peritoneum [31]. Continuous secretion of these cytokines leads to a state of chronic inflammation, which includes activation of macrophages and recruitment of NK cells and results in high levels of OS. Once the tumor has been initiated, the continuous secretion of cytokines by adipose tissue or omentum can facilitate migration of cancer cells to the omentum, promoting metastasis of the tumor into the peritoneum [30]. High levels (>10 mg/L) of C-reactive protein (CRP), a marker of global inflammation, are associated with an increased risk of EOC [32,33]. IL-6 itself is not a risk factor for EOC but in obese women IL-6 and CRP may be associated with increased EOC risk [33].

PCOS also contributes to inflammation in women and may increase risk of EOC [34]. PCOS is a hormonal disorder occurring in reproductive aged women during which ovaries may develop numerous small collections of fluid and fail to release eggs properly. Obesity, hyperandrogenism, and increased insulin resistance further characterize PCOS. Increased C-Reactive protein (CRP) and MCP-1 levels, indicative of low-level chronic inflammation, are elevated in women with PCOS [35–38].

Simultaneously chemokines like IL-18, IL-6, and TNF-α are also increased in circulation in women with PCOS [39–42]. The increase in inflammatory mediators correlates positively with BMI, suggesting that increased obesity in women with PCOS may be the source of inflammation. Increased DNA damage and OS is observed in women with PCOS, which may also increase risk for EOC [43]. Evidence linking PCOS directly to EOC is limited due to small study sizes, PCOS being associated with other EOC risk factors such as obesity, and PCOS possibly being only associated with one subtype of EOC, borderline serous [44].

Talc is a silicate mineral and exposure to it can cause inflammation of the ovaries and poses a risk hazard for development of EOC [45]. It has been proposed that talc from talcum powder used for dusting and from condoms and vaginal diaphragms can migrate up to the ovaries via retrograde flow of fluids and mucous and get lodged in the ovaries. Tubal ligation, which is protective for EOC, is thought to block the transport off talc from the lower genital tract. Talc behaves as a foreign particle, triggering an inflammatory response [46,47]. The talc attracts macrophages, which try to phagocytose it. The macrophages then send chemotactic signals to other immune response mediators and initiate a wound healing process. Since talc is not degradable by the body, it inhibits the wound healing process, resulting in chronic inflammation.

2.4. NSAIDS and Reduced Risk of EOC

Further connecting inflammation to EOC are several studies that demonstrate that intake of non-steroidal anti-inflammatory drugs (NSAIDs), specifically of aspirin, correlates inversely with risk of OC and endometrial cancer [48–52]. In vitro studies with OC cell lines and NSAIDS show that NSAIDs and COX-2 inhibitors facilitate apoptosis, however this effect is not dependent on COX-2 and may be due to upregulation of p21, a protein important for cell cycle arrest [53]. Another study by Arango et al., demonstrates that acetylsalicylic acid or aspirin resulted in increased apoptosis via downregulation of Bcl2 in an endometrial cancer cell line [54]. A third study has shown that a selective COX-2 inhibitor, JTE-522, can inhibit proliferation and increase apoptosis of endometrial cancer cells by increasing levels of p53 and p21 and decreasing phosphorylation of retinoblastoma (Rb) protein, which results in its activation; all of which results in cell cycle arrest [55,56]. Simultaneously, there was an increase in caspase-3 activity, which is indicative of increased apoptosis. Another mechanism by which aspirin could facilitate its chemopreventive nature is by inhibiting oxidative induced DNA damage [57]. COX-1 is also expressed in normal ovaries of the laying hen, with expression increasing in post-ovulatory follicles suggesting its importance for or a role in ovulation. With the onset of OC, COX-1 expression is increased [58] and COX-1 inhibition and NSAIDs have shown to decrease proliferation of ascites in the laying hen OC model [59]. Further, when 0.1% aspirin was included in their diet for one year, although the onset of OC was not different, the progression of cancer was slower when compared to hens fed with regular diet [60].

As discussed, inflammation results in secretion of ROS, growth factors, cytokines, and chemokines into the shared environment surrounding the ovary and distal FT. Exposure of normal tissue to these inflammatory mediators results in activation of downstream signaling that can promote the transformation of normal cells or survival of already transformed cells. Once EOC has already formed further exposure of cancer cells to these inflammatory mediators also results in activation of downstream signaling within the cancer cell and in the surrounding tissue, creating an inflammatory environment that can further promote EOC (Figure 1). We will discuss in more detail how key inflammatory mediators contribute to EOC initiation, progression, metastasis, and chemoresistance.

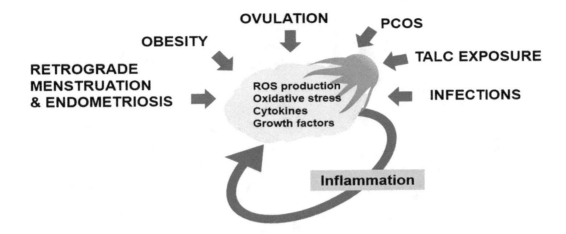

Figure 1. Sources of inflammation in the ovary and fimbriae. Ovulation, retrograde menstruation, endometriosis, infections, exposure to talc, Polycystic Ovarian Syndrome (PCOS), and obesity result in exposure of the ovary and fimbriae to reactive oxygen species (ROS), oxidative stress, cytokines, and growth factors, generating an inflammatory response that leads to additional production of ROS and cytokines in the ovary. Unresolved, chronic inflammation is a critical risk factor for tumor initiation.

3. Inflammation and EOC Initiation and Progression

Tumorigenesis is a multistep process that requires cells to gain the ability to evade apoptosis and antigrowth signals, proliferate independently of stimuli, develop a support system (angiogenesis), and have the capacity to invade and metastasize. Tumorigenesis is initiated by the transformation of a normal cell to a malignant one. The deregulation of the above mentioned processes in the malignant cell could potentiate its progression to cancer.

One mechanism of cancer initiation is genomic instability due to DNA damage [61] and EOCs exhibit a high number of chromosomal aberrations and genomic instability [62]. The most common gene mutations in HGSCs include *BRCA*, *TP53*, and genes in involved in mismatch repair and the DNA damage response [63]. A pro-inflammatory ME can also contribute to genetic instability and therefore play a role in EOC cancer initiation. A pro-inflammatory ME, which is continuously supplemented by ROS, cytokines, and growth factors, can cause DNA damage in epithelial ovarian and FT cells, switch on antiapoptotic pathways, and initiate transformation of normal cells. When cells transformed either by oncogenic alterations or by exposure to inflammation are in a pro-inflammatory ME they are able to turn on pro-survival signaling pathways rather than the senescence pathways that are normally induced by oncogene expression in normal cells. For example, disruption of the RAS pathway results in activated NF-κB signaling and upregulation of its downstream targets including cytokines like IL-1β, IL-6, and IL-8. These cytokines are upregulated in EOC patients and their increased levels correlate with decreased survival [64–71]. The inflammatory mediators like cytokines, chemokines, growth factors, and prostaglandins secreted by the transformed epithelial cells further promote a pro-inflammatory environment, which can reprogram the surrounding cells to form the TME. The TME is mainly composed of endothelial cells, cancer associated fibroblasts (CAFs), adipocytes, tumor associated macrophages (TAMs), regulatory T-cells, pericytes, infiltrated immune cells such as neutrophils, lymphocytes, and various other cells that further secrete growth factors and cytokines which potentiate tumor progression (Figure 2, Table 1). Furthermore, OC-initiating cells (OCICs) have been identified in tumors and ascites that exhibit stem cell like properties and are capable of forming tumors [65,66,72]. Cytokines can promote self-renewal of CD133$^+$ OCICs to potentiate tumor progression [73].

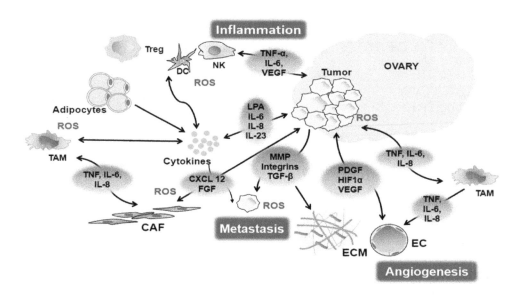

Figure 2. Inflammatory mediators contributing to EOC progression, metastasis, and angiogenesis. EOC cells produce ROS, chemokines, cytokines, and growth factors that can: (1) Lead to recruitment of immune cells like Dentric cells (DC), Natural killer cells (NK), Tumor associated macrophages (TAMs), and T-regulatory (Treg) cells into the TME, which generate additional cytokines, ROS, and growth factors, resulting in chronic inflammation. (2) Stimulate the tumor cells themselves, the TAMs, and the surrounding fibroblasts (also known as cancer associated fibroblasts or CAFs) to proliferate and secrete growth factors like TGF-β and FGF that stimulate production of integrins and Matrix Metalloproteins (MMPs), resulting in migration of the tumor cell via degradation of the extra cellular matrix (ECM). (3) Stimulate endothelial cells (EC) to produce growth factors like PDGF and EGF and factors like VEGF that stimulate angiogenesis. The double arrows indicate that the cells are a source of the factor as well as stimulated by it.

The innate immune response can prevent tumorigenesis by recognizing and eliminating transformed cells. However, chronic inflammation can contribute to the ability of premalignant cells to evade apoptosis, escape the immune surveillance, and continue to grow, resulting in tumor formation. As mentioned, EOC can originate from either distal FT or ovarian epithelial cells. Since both the ovary and fimbria are exposed to the same ME, exposures reviewed here are relevant to initiation in either tissue. [74]. In this section we will review the role of OS and some specific pro-inflammatory mediators and signaling pathways in the initiation and progression of EOC.

3.1. ROS and Oxidative Stress

ROS plays an important role in the normal female reproductive cycle, from affecting maturation of the oocyte to ovulation, apoptosis of cells in corpus luteum, and embryo development [75]. Ovulation results in increased levels of DNA damage in the FT epithelium that is likely a result of the ROS generated during ovulation or the ovulation-associated increase in numbers of infiltrating macrophages in the FT [17]. Additionally, during infection and inflammatory responses immune and damaged cells produce ROS resulting in continuous exposure of the ovaries, FTs, and peritoneal cavity to ROS [76–78]. ROS exposure could potentially lead to epithelial cells in the ovary and FT undergoing transformative changes, as has been demonstrated for ovarian surface epithelium cells grown in 3D culture [79]. Elevated ROS and RNS levels beyond the level that cells can neutralize results in OS. Increased OS results in DNA damage, activation of signaling cascades, and epigenetic alterations.

DNA damage in a cell results in stimulation of DNA damage repair pathways. These repair pathways can be inactivated or be erroneous, which results in increased genotoxic stress and mutated DNA. Secretory tubal epithelial cells in the FT, a cell of origin for HGSC, are particularly susceptible to genotoxic injury with persistent DNA damage that could lead to mutation and STIC formation [80].

Mutations in tumor oncogenes and suppressors result in overexpression, constitutive activation of the protein, loss of expression, or expression of nonfunctional proteins, resulting in a transformed cell. Follicular fluid may have transformative properties as it has been demonstrated that bathing fimbriae with follicular fluid containing high levels of ROS results in increased levels of DNA damage. Bathing fimbriae that have loss of p53 and Rb with this follicular fluid results in evasion of apoptosis and cells with persistent DNA damage [81].

ROS can activate pro-survival intracellular tyrosine phosphorylation signaling cascades, mainly regulated by the MAPKs and redox sensitive kinases. Activation of c-Jun, JNK, ERK (extracellular signal-regulated kinase), and p38-MAPK signaling cascades results in upregulation of cell cycle proteins that enhances proliferation. Activation of JNK can also activate NF-κB, which can suppress apoptosis. The MAPK pathway inhibits apoptosis and regulates differentiation. When activated in transformed cells these pathways are important for tumor initiation. ROS affects redox sensitive factors like thioreoxin, which is also found elevated in OC cell lines [82]. Thioredoxin is involved in redox regulation of transcription factors such as NF-κB, NRF2, forkhead box class O (FOXO) proteins, reducing factor-1 (ref-1), and hypoxia inducible factor (HIF-1α), thereby increasing their binding to the DNA. Most of these transcription factors promote tumor growth and progression by regulating expression of genes that affect cell survival and growth [83,84]. For example, FOXO, NRF2, and ref-1 transcription factors upregulate transcription of anti-oxidant proteins that scavenge free radicals and allow survival of damaged or transformed cells [85]. HIF-1α upregulates the antiapoptotic factor, bcl-2 as well as vascular endothelial growth factor (VEGF), a factor important for angiogenesis.

OS has also been shown to facilitate epigenetic mechanisms in many cancers, including EOC [86]. Innate immune-mediated inflammation drives epigenetic silencing of tumor suppressor genes (TSGs) [87]. At sites of inflammation high levels of OS result in oxidative DNA damage that is recognized by the mismatch repair proteins mutS homolog MSH2 and MSH6. MSH2 and MSH6 then recruit epigenetic silencing proteins, including DNA methyltransferase 1 (DNMT1) to the sites of damage [88]. In an in vivo model of inflammation-driven colon tumorigenesis this early recruitment to sites of oxidative DNA damage results in permanent methylation of TSGs in tumors that form at the sites of inflammation [89]. While such a mechanism has not been directly proven in EOC models, Sapoznik et al. have demonstrated that exposure to follicular fluid or inflammation can induce Activation-Induced Cytidine Deaminase (AIDS) in fallopian tube epithelial cells, which results in epigenetic and genetic changes, increase in DNA damage and genotoxic stress and may be a contributing factor to EOC [90].

3.2. TNF-α

The cytokine TNF-α plays an important role in the process of ovulation and in removal of damaged corpus luteum. TNF-α ligand and its receptors, TNFRI and TNFRII are upregulated in ovarian tumors compared to normal ovarian tissue and high levels of TNF-α are found in ascites from OC patients [91–93]. OC cells have also been shown to secrete high levels of TNF-α as compared to normal ovarian epithelial cells resulting in autocrine upregulation of TNF-α mRNA and in expression of other pro-inflammatory cytokines, chemokines, and angiogenic factors like IL-6, M-CSF, CXCL2, CCL2, and VEGF [93,94]. Kellie et al. have shown using mouse models that TNF-α stimulates IL-17 production via TNFRI resulting in myeloid cell recruitment to the ovarian TME and increased tumor growth [95]. TNF-α, also upregulates AIDS transcript levels which can contribute to genotoxic stress [90].

3.3. IL-6

The cytokine IL-6 has been associated with poor survival in OC and is emerging as a potential therapeutic target for EOC [67,68,96,97]. IL-6 is normally produced by ovarian epithelial and OC cells. Macrophage migration inhibitory factor (MIF), EGF, and Transglutaminase secreted by OC cells can stimulate IL-6 production via activation of NF-κB [98–100]. IL-6 increases proliferation of OC cells by facilitating their exit from G1 into S phase of the cell cycle and by activation of the MAPK-ERK-Akt (protein kinase B) growth promoting signaling pathway [101]. ERK activation can promote formation of ascites by increasing the migration of tumor cells [70]. IL-6 production by M2 macrophages present in ascites in later stages of EOC can also stimulate cancer cell proliferation via STAT3 activation [102]. High levels of IL-6 can result in immune suppression by downregulation of IL-2, which stimulates Teff cell production [103]. IL-6 also stimulates production of Metallomatrix proteins (MMPs) in OC cells, which increases their invasive properties and promotes tumorigenesis [101,104].

3.4. IL-8

IL-8 a member of C-X-C chemokine family is present in the preovulatory follicle [105] where it may play a role in increasing leukocyte infiltration [106]. It is also elevated in ovarian cysts and in OC patients compared to healthy controls [107,108]. IL-8 has been found to be present in significantly higher levels in the ascites of patients with OC in comparison to patients with benign gynecological disorders [109]. Increased IL-8 expression has been associated with poor prognosis in OC patients [107]. Treatment of EOC cells with IL-8 results in their increased proliferation, which is accompanied by an increase in cyclins B1 and D1 and is dependent on phosphorylation of Akt and ERK [110]. Cyclins B1 and D1 are important for cell cycle progression, and an increase in their expression leads to increased cell growth. On the other hand, two independent studies have demonstrated that IL-8 inhibits EOC growth by increasing neutrophil infiltration [111,112].

3.5. Lyophosphotidic Acid (LPA)

LPA is a phospholipid that binds to and activates the endothelial differentiation gene (Edg) family of receptors. LPA is present in ovarian follicular fluid and it stimulates IL-6 and IL-8 production in the corpus luteum [113,114]. OC cells have been shown to produce LPA, which functions like a growth factor [115–119]. Plasma and ascites of OC patients have elevated levels of LPA that contribute to OC progression via upregulation of COX-2 and MMP2 [115,120,121]. LPA can bind to LPA_2 receptor and induce expression of IL-6 and IL-8 via activation of NF-κB and AP-1 in OC cell lines [122]. It can induce ROS dependent Akt and ERK phosphorylation and inhibition of LPA can increase apoptosis of EOC cells [123]. ERK phosphorylation can induce phosphorylation of HIF-1α, which then can upregulate VEGF and promote tumorigenesis. Another group demonstrated that stimulating EOC cells with ether-linked LPA resulted in their increased proliferation and survival by increased synthesis of DNA and activation of Akt via PI3K, which contributes to tumor progression [124].

3.6. Prostaglandins and COX-1 and COX-2

Prostaglandins are secreted in the ovary, FT, and uterus. They are important for maturation of the oocyte and facilitate the movement of the FT so that the mature oocyte can move from the ovary to the uterus. In the uterus prostaglandins help regulate and maintain uterine blood flow. COX-1 and COX-2 are enzymes that catalyze the production of prostaglandins from arachidonic acid and are overexpressed in OC patients [22,125,126]. High COX levels positively correlate with increased cell proliferation, angiogenesis, and malignancy in ovarian tumors [126,127]. COX-1 and COX-2 are normally involved in the acute inflammatory response but can become dysregulated in chronic inflammatory or TMEs. Obermajer et al. have demonstrated that prostaglandins produced by COX-2 can stimulate production of CXCR4 and its ligand Stromal cell derived factor 1 (SDF1) CXCL12 in myeloid derived suppressor cells (MDSC), which stimulates them to migrate towards OC ascites [128]. MDSCs inhibit the proliferation and differentiation of T cells, resulting in overall immune suppression, which allows the tumor cells to escape immune surveillance and continue to grow. Genetically engineered mouse models of EOC; one harboring the *p53* and *Rb* deletion and other the *KRAS*^{G12D} mutation and *Pten* deletion, demonstrate increased COX-1 levels, thus suggestive that COX-1 could be used as a potential biomarker and therapeutic target for EOC [129]. Further when

COX-1 was inhibited in EOC cells, it led to reduction in prostacyclin (a type of prostaglandin) synthesis and reduced tumor growth by enhanced apoptosis [130].

4. Inflammation and EOC Angiogenesis

Angiogenesis is required for the growth of both primary and metastatic tumors [131]. The process of angiogenesis is a complex multi-step process reviewed previously [132]. It is regulated by a balance between pro-angiogenic and antiangiogenic factors. Hypoxic and ischemic areas are present at sites of inflammation and also in tumors mainly due to obstruction of local blood vessels, differences in pace of growth of blood vessels and growth of the tumor and/or infiltration of immune cells. Macrophages accumulate at hypoxic sites and alter their gene expression profiles in response to the hypoxic conditions. One of the important genes for angiogenesis that is upregulated by hypoxia is VEGF [133,134]. The rate-limiting step in angiogenesis is VEGF signaling in endothelial cells (ECs) [135]. VEGF functions via tyrosine kinase receptors VEGF-1 and VEGF-2 and promotes migration, survival, proliferation of ECs, and formation of new blood vessels [136–138]. Many of the inflammatory mediators discussed so far are also involved in promoting angiogenesis in EOC as detailed below (Figure 2, Table 1).

4.1. TNF-α

TNF-α creates a pro-inflammatory TME and has also been associated with promoting angiogenesis. It has been hypothesized that TNF-α induces the production of soluble factors that promote tumor angiogenesis. Culture supernatants from TNF-α expressing cells induce the growth of mouse lung endothelial cells in vitro while culture supernatants from TNF-α lacking cells do not exert the same effect [94]. In pituitary adenomas TNF-α is known to induce VEGF that in turn induces CXCL12 [139,140]. VEGF and CXCL12 synergistically induce angiogenesis in EOC [141]. Mice injected with OC cells lacking TNF-α have reduced vascular density in their tumors and reduced formation of blood vessels in the peritoneal deposits. These mice also did not have accumulation of ascetic fluid suggesting the importance of TNF-α in angiogenesis and EOC progression [94].

4.2. IL-6

In physiological conditions, IL-6 is involved in angiogenesis in the ovary during the development of ovarian follicles [142]. IL-6 induces the phosphorylation of STAT3 and MAPK in ovarian endothelial cells thereby enhancing their migratory ability, a key step in angiogenesis [143]. As explained before, OC cells also secrete increased amounts of IL-6. Some OC cells also secrete an alternative splice variant of IL-6Rα, the soluble form sIL-6R, which consists of only the ectodomain of the transmembrane receptor. By a process called trans-signaling, the sIL-6R-IL-6 complex initiates signaling in cells in the ME that do not express the transmembrane receptor facilitating angiogenesis [144].

4.3. IL-8

Several studies have clearly established the role of IL-8 in promoting angiogenesis. Hu et al., demonstrated that IL-8 plays a role in angiogenesis using a rat sponge model [145]. IL-8 was also able to induce angiogenesis in the rat cornea, which is normally avascular [146]. As explained in the previous section, there are several sources of IL-8 in ovarian TME. Overexpression of IL-8 in A2780 (non-IL-8 expressing) OC cells has been shown to increase the expression of VEGF, MMP-2, and MMP-9; while depletion of IL-8 in SKOV3 (IL-8 expressing) cells has been shown to reduce VEGF, MMP-2, and MMP-9 [110]. The process of angiogenesis involves degradation of extracellular matrix components and proliferation and migration of endothelial cells. MMPs are a family of endopeptidases that breakdown components of extracellular matrix and have been implicated in angiogenesis [147]. Because of the importance of VEGF and MMPs in angiogenesis these findings suggest that IL-8 in the ovarian TME will promote the formation of new blood vessels in EOC. Targeting IL-8 using mouse models reduces EOC growth and decreases angiogenesis [112].

Table 1. Role of inflammatory mediators in different stages of tumor progression.

Inflammatory Mediators	Secreting Cell Type	Stages in Tumor Progression			
		Initiation and Progression	Angiogenesis	Metastasis	Chemoresistance
TNF-α ligands, TNFRI, TNFRII	OC cells, infiltrating monocytes, macrophages	↑ autocrine production of TNF-α and IL-6, M-CSF, CXCL2, CCL2 [93,94] and AIDS mRNA level [90]	↑VEGF, VEGF↑ CXCL12 and promotes angiogenesis [139–141]	↑TGF-α secretion by stromal fibroblasts which promote peritoneal metastasis [148] Enhances migration of OC cells towards CXCL12 [149,150]	
IL-6	Ovarian epithelial cells, OC cells, M2 macrophages, mesothelial cells, TAMS, ascites	↑Proliferation by promoting G1 to S transition and MAPK-ERK- Akt activation and STAT3 activation [101,102] ↓IL-2, resulting in immune suppression [103]	Induces STAT3 and MAPK phosphorylation which enhances migration of endothelial cells [143] sIL-6R–IL-6 facilitates angiogenesis in cells lacking IL-6 receptor [144]	Stimulates production of MMPs in OCs which ↑ invasion and migration [101,104] ↑ IL-6 in ascites enhances invasion via JAK-STAT signaling [151]	↓ Caspase- 3 cleavage and makes OC cells resistant to cisplatin and paclitaxel [152] ↑Expression of MDR1, GSTpi, Bcl-2, Bcl-xL, and XIAP [152]
IL-8	Pre-ovulatory follicles, OC cells, ascites	↑ Proliferation by ↑ cyclin B1 and cyclin D1 via pAkt [110]	↑ Expression of VEGF, MMP-2, MMP-9 promoting angiogenesis [110]	Activates TAK1/ NF-κB via CXCR2 [153]	Blocks TRAIL induced apoptosis to promote resistance [154]
LPA	Follicular fluid, corpus luteum, OC cells, ascites	↑IL-6 and IL-8 via NF-κB and AP-1 [113,114,122] ↑COX-2 AND MMP2 [115,120,121] ↑ phosphorylation of Akt and ERK resulting in increased cell cycle [123,124]	↑ Expression of VEGF via Myc and Sp-1 [155]	↑ urokinase, which results in degradation of basemembrane protein to promote metastasis [156,157]	
Prostaglandins, COX-1 and COX-2	Ovary, FT, uterus, MDSCs	↑CXCR4 and SDF1 in MDSCs resulting in immune suppression [128]	↑ Bcl-2 and blood vessel formation [158,159]		↑ Bcl-2, thus inhibiting apoptosis in lung, colon, breast and prostate cancers [158,159]
TGF-β and EGF	OC cells, CAFs			TGF-β ↑ VCAN, which activates NF-κB and ↑MM-9 [160]	↑ EGF protects cells from cisplatin-induced apoptosis [161]. Inhibiting TGF-β sensitizes resistant cells [162]

4.4. LPA

In addition to playing a role in initiation, and progression, LPA has also been implicated in angiogenesis in OC. LPA has been shown to induce transcriptional activation of VEGF in EOC cell lines [163]. Transcriptional activation of VEGF primarily occurs through HIF-1α under oxygen limiting conditions in Hep3B hepatocellular carcinoma cells [164]. LPA mediated induction of VEGF expression has been shown to be independent of HIF-1α in EOC cell lines. Transition metal cobalt treatment also leads to stabilization of HIF1α similar to hypoxia. Combination treatment of EOC cells with cobalt and LPA additively increased VEGF production suggesting the effect of two different pathways [155]. LPA activates c-Myc and Sp-1, which induce VEGF expression through consensus binding sites in the VEGF promoter that have been implicated in HIFα independent induction of VEGF [155].

5. Inflammation and EOC Metastasis

Tumor metastasis is the major cause of mortality in most cancers, including EOC. Most EOC patients are diagnosed at an advanced stage when the cancer has already metastasized [165]. Dissemination of cancer cells to distant sites is a complex multi-step process called the invasion-metastasis cascade and is reviewed in detail in previous papers [166–168]. Briefly, some major steps in metastasis are—invasion through the basement membrane, intravasation into the lymphatics and circulation, survival of disseminating cancer cells in circulation, extravasation into surrounding tissues, colonization, and finally, formation of micro and macro metastases. However, unlike other epithelial malignancies, EOC has a different pattern of metastasis. EOC cells directly shed from the primary tumor into the peritoneal space and disseminate to organs in the peritoneal cavity. One of the prerequisites for cancer cells to metastasize is to undergo a process called epithelial to mesenchymal transition (EMT) where they lose their ability to attach to the basement membrane and acquire a mesenchymal phenotype and characteristics. Several recent evidences have indicated that the TME aids tumor cells to acquire these properties facilitating the metastatic cascade. An example of the ME promoting metastasis is the presence of STICs in the distal part of the FT, which shares its ME with ovary. Yang-Hartwich et al. have demonstrated that granulosa cells in the ovary secrete SDF-1 (stromal cell-derived factor 1) [169]. SDF-1 functions as a chemoattractant and recruits malignant FT cells to the ovary suggesting that the ovary is a primary site of metastasis, not the primary tumor site. Russo et al. demonstrated that loss of PTEN (phosphatase and tensin homolog) by the malignant FT cells and upregulation of WNT4 (wingless-related MMTV integration site 4) is crucial for initial metastasis to the ovary thereby supporting the tubal origin of EOC and the ovary as the primary site of metastasis [170]. The cells that make up the TME also secrete various inflammatory mediators, which facilitate progression and metastasis of OC cells (Figure 2, Table 1). These factors enable tumor metastasis by deregulating signal transduction pathways. Examples include the PI3-Akt and RAS-ERK pathways, which control migration and invasion through downstream effectors like Rho family GTPases, extracellular proteases, integrins, matrix associated proteins like focal adhesion kinases (FAK), and transcription factors like ETS2 and AP-1 [171–173]. Robinson-Smith et al. demonstrated that peritoneal inflammation correlated with dissemination of cancer cells from the ovaries in SCID mice. Augmenting the inflammatory response using thioglycolate accelerated ascites formation and metastasis while suppressing the inflammation using acetyl salicyclic acid impeded ascites formation and reduced metastasis. This inflammation-induced metastasis of OC cells was found to be primarily mediated by macrophages and not neutrophils or NK cells [174]. As explained in one of the previous sections a pro-inflammatory environment can be created in the peritoneum due to secretion of cytokines like IL-6 and TNF-α by adipose cells [31]. Omentum, the primary site of metastasis of OC, is largely composed of adipose cells. In addition to adipocytes, omentum also consists of blood and lymph vessels, immune cells, and stromal cells [175]. Adipocytes have been shown to increase migration, invasion, and proliferation of EOC cells. Upregulation of SUSD2 a secreted tumor suppressor by adipocytes by guadecitabine treatment reduced EOC migration and invasion. This finding suggests that epigenetic changes in the stromal cells in addition to EOC cells can facilitate EOC metastasis [176]. Omentum has aggregates of immune cells around the vasculature commonly referred to as milky spots [177]. Melanoma, lung carcinoma, ovarian carcinoma, and mammary carcinoma cell lines have been shown to specifically metastasize to the immune cell aggregates in the omentum when injected intraperitonealy into C57BL/6 mice [178]. These milky spots in the omentum have also been shown to facilitate metastatic colonization of the OC cells. Clark et al. have suggested that both adipocytes and milky spots have specific and important roles in metastatic colonization of OC cells [179]. These evidences imply that omentum potentially provides a good niche for the growth of ovarian cancer cells. Here we will specifically discuss how inflammatory mediators promote tumor metastasis in EOC.

5.1. ROS

EOC cells produce a large amount of ROS [180]. Loss of E-cadherin is one of the characteristic features of tumor cells with increased ability to migrate and invade. Wang et al. demonstrated that ROS leads to HIFα mediated activation of lysl oxidase. Lysl oxidase was shown to inversely correlate with E-cadherin expression promoting migration and invasion in EOC cells [181]. Tumor cells treated with sub-lethal doses of H_2O_2 failed to attach to the extracellular matrix components fibronectin and laminin and had increased metastatic colonization of lung, thereby establishing a role for ROS in tumor cell metastasis [182].

5.2. TNF-α

TNF-α provides a good example of how interactions between cancer and stroma aid in OC metastasis. Ascitic fluid and OCs contain a large number infiltrating macrophages in part because OCs constitutively produce M-CSF, which functions as a chemoattractant for monocytes [183]. These infiltrating monocytes produce many cytokines one of which is TNF-α [184,185]. OC cells also have elevated TNF-α expression that is regulated by DNA hypomethylation and chromatin remodeling of the TNF-α promoter. Increased TNF-α produced by OC cells and macrophages stimulates increased expression of TGF-α in stromal fibroblasts. TGF-α secreting stromal fibroblasts promote peritoneal metastasis of OC via EGF receptor signaling [148].

Furthermore, in EOC cells and clinical biopsies TNF-α expression correlates with one of the most commonly expressed cytokine receptors CXCR4. TNF-α stimulation of EOC cells enhanced their migration toward the only CXCR4 ligand, CXCL12. Stimulation of EOC cells by CXCL12 induced mRNA and protein expression of TNF-α. Therefore, a positive feedback loop has been suggested where in CXCL12 induced TNF-α potentially acts on the cancer cells and induces CXCR4 expression thereby enhancing tumor cell migration [149,150].

5.3. IL-6

IL-6 has also been implicated in metastasis of OC. Elevated levels of IL-6 found in serum and peritoneal fluid of EOC and OC patients have many sources [186–188]. Mesothelial cells in the peritoneum, TAMs, and EOC cells all secrete IL-6 [67]. M2 polarized macrophages in the ovarian TME induce proliferation and invasion of EOC cells by secretion of IL-6 [189]. Increased IL-6 present in ascites from OC patients enhanced the invasive ability of OC cells via the JAK-STAT signaling pathway. Canonically IL-6 signaling occurs by binding of the ligand to its transmembrane receptor IL-6Rα. The effect of IL-6 on invasion of OC cells correlated with their IL-6R expression [151]. Because through trans-signaling, the sIL-6R–IL-6 complex initiates signaling in cells that do not express the transmembrane receptor [144], we hypothesize that IL-6 produced by macrophages could also promote invasion of OC cells similar to the mechanism of induction of angiogenesis.

5.4. IL-8

Increased proliferation, anchorage independent growth, and angiogenic potential are some prerequisites for cells to metastasize. IL-8 increases the proliferation of OC cells and upregulates VEGF and MMP2 and 9 via activation of NF-κB, which results in enhanced invasive phenotype of OC cells. IL-8 has been shown to activate TAK1/NF-κB signaling via CXCR2, thereby facilitating the seeding and growth of OC cells in the peritoneal cavity during metastasis [153].

5.5. LPA

LPA promotes proliferation, survival, and metastasis of EOC cells by inducing the expression of c-Myc, VEGF, IL-8, MMPs and COX-2 [163,190–193]. LPA acts through its receptors LPAR1-3, which are members of G-protein coupled receptor superfamily. Invasive EOC cells have significantly higher expression of LPAR1 in comparison to non-invasive cell lines and LPA induces EOC cell invasion specifically through LPAR1 and not through LPAR2 or LPAR3 [194]. It can also induce secretion of urokinase in EOC cells, which has been shown to play a role in metastasis and its high levels correlate with advanced OC and poor survival in patients. LPA has been shown to increase promoter activity, mRNA levels, protein levels, and enzyme activity of Urokinase plasminogen activator (uPA) possibly via the edg-4 LPA receptor [156]. uPA is involved in converting plasminogen to plasmin, which facilitates the degradation of basement membrane and extracellular membrane proteins like fibronection aiding in metastasis [157].

5.6. TGF-β

TGF-β initiates signaling by dimerization of serine/threonine kinase receptors. The dimerization of receptors results in their phosphorylation, which then relays signals downstream via SMAD dependent and SMAD independent pathways. Phosphorylation by the TGF-β receptor causes R-SMADs to bind to Co-SMAD and translocate to the nucleus, where they activate transcription of genes that promote invasion, migration. Bone morphogenic proteins (BMPs) are cytokines that belong to TGF-β family and have been associated with progression of many different cancer types. Their mechanism of promoting tumor progression depends on the TME in which the cancer grows and their mode of metastatic spread [195]. Specifically, BMP-2 overexpression has been associated with poor prognosis in OC [196]. Additionally, TGF-β could potentially modify the TME to promote tumorigenesis. Veriscan (VCAN), an extracellular matrix associated protein, was upregulated by TGF-β through TGF-β receptor II (TGFBR2) and SMAD signaling making the EOC cells more aggressive. Increased VCAN expression enhanced motility and invasion of EOC cells by activating NF-κB signaling, increased expression of MMP-9, and hyaluronidase mediated motility receptor [160]. CAFs have higher expression of TGF-β receptors in comparison to normal ovarian fibroblasts and EOC cells suggesting that CAFs within the TME are more responsive to TGF-β then the other cell types [160].

6. Inflammation and EOC Chemoresistance

The standard treatment for EOC patients is cytoreductive surgery followed by platinum/taxane-based chemotherapy [197]. The main obstacle in treatment of EOC patients is development of chemoresistance. Resistance to chemotherapy can be either intrinsic or acquired. Inherent gene expression patterns harbored by chemo-naïve tumor cells contribute to intrinsic resistance. Acquired resistance is a consequence of different alterations induced after exposure to chemotherapeutic agents [198]. Different mechanisms, including increased drug efflux, decreased uptake of the drug, inactivation of the drug, increased DNA repair, and reduced apoptotic response, have been implicated in development of platinum resistance [199]. Several recent studies have demonstrated that the TME contributes to both intrinsic and acquired resistance. One type of intrinsic drug resistance influenced by the TME is referred to as environment mediated drug resistance (EMDR). In EMDR, factors and cells present in the TME activate diverse signaling events, transiently protecting the tumor cells from undergoing apoptosis in response to chemotherapeutic agents [200,201]. Another type of drug resistance induced by cytokines, chemokines, and growth factors secreted by fibroblast cells in the tumor stroma is called soluble factor mediated drug resistance (SFM-DR). A good example of SFM-DR is IL-6 mediated drug resistance in multiple myeloma. IL-6 is important for growth of multiple myeloma cells. IL-6 activates STAT3 signaling in these cells and protects them from Fas mediated apoptosis by upregulating antiapoptotic protein Bcl-X_L [202]. Myeloma cells that produced IL-6 in an autocrine manner were found to be resistant to dexamethasone induced apoptosis while non-IL-6 producing cells were sensitive [203]. Cell adhesion mediated drug resistance (CAM-DR) occurs due to adhesion of tumor cells to extracellular matrix components like laminin, collagen, and fibronectin or due to fibroblasts present in the tumor stroma [204]. An example of this type of resistance is when drug sensitive myeloma cells were adhered to an extracellular matrix component fibronectin, they exhibited a reversible drug resistant phenotype which was not due reduced drug accumulation or increase in antiapoptotic proteins like Bcl-X_L [201]. Here we will discuss specific inflammatory mediators and their role in OC chemoresistance (Figure 3).

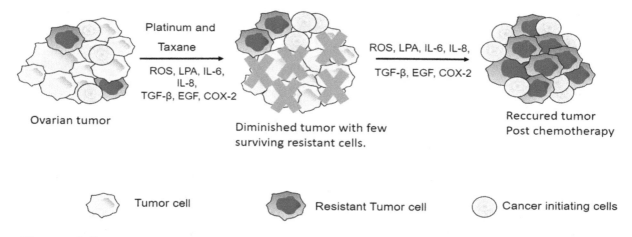

Figure 3. Inflammatory mediators contribute to chemoresistance of EOC. A combination of platinum and taxane drugs is currently used as chemotherapy for OC. ROS, Lyophosphotidic Acid (LPA), cytokines, and growth factors like TGF-β and EGF increase tumor cell survival by upregulating antiapoptotic genes, by stimulating stemness and proliferation of cancer initiating cells, by increasing repair of damaged DNA, or by increasing efflux of the drug. The resistant tumor cells and the cancer initiating cells can then proliferate under the influence of growth factors and cytokines resulting in a recurrent chemoresistant tumor.

6.1. ROS

ROS are abundant in the pro-inflammatory TME. Malignant EOC tissues have been shown to have 96% higher ROS levels than normal controls [205]. OC stem like cells or OCICs are more drug resistant and responsible for relapse of chemoresistant tumors [66]. OCICs produce ROS and superoxide. This ROS induces the expression of peroxisome proliferator-activated receptor-gamma coactivator (PCG)-1α, which regulates mitochondrial biogenesis and is required for expression of detoxifying enzymes [206,207]. PCG1α increases the aldehyde dehydrogenase (ALDH) activity and expression of multidrug resistance gene (MDR1). MDR1 is an ATP dependent transporter that has been associated with efflux of platinum based drugs from OC cells contributing to platinum resistance. Scavenging ROS reduced expression of PCG1α and drug resistant related genes thereby linking ROS to development of chemoresistance [207].

6.2. IL-6

IL-6 in the OC TME is associated with increased chemoresistance. Wang et al. demonstrated that autocrine production of IL-6 by EOC cells makes them resistant to cisplatin and paclitaxel by causing decreased proteolytic cleavage of capase-3. Paclitaxel resistant EOC cells have increased expression of IL-6 and one of its downstream effectors STAT3 [208,209]. IL-6 producing OC cells also had increased expression of multidrug resistant genes MDR1 and GSTpi and anti-apoptotic genes

Bcl-2, Bcl-xL, and XIAP, suggesting that IL6 promotes drug resistance by increasing drug efflux and reducing apoptosis [152].

6.3. IL-8

IL-8 blocks TRAIL-induced apoptosis and reduces caspase cleavage in EOC cell lines by decreasing the expression of death receptor (DR) 4 [210]. TRAIL is a cell death inducing ligand that belongs to the TNF superfamily and has been shown to induce apoptosis specifically in tumor cells and not in nontransformed cells [211,212]. Combination of TRAIL and the chemotherapeutic drugs—cisplatin, doxorubicin, and paclitaxel has been shown to induce apoptosis in chemoresistant EOC cell lines by causing increased caspase and PARP cleavage [154]. This finding suggests that IL8 may contribute to chemoresistance by blocking TRAIL.

6.4. LPA

LPA has been shown to contribute to platinum resistance by preventing cells from undergoing cisplatin-induced apoptosis without affecting their proliferation rate. The mechanism of how LPA inhibits apoptosis in EOC cells in response to cisplatin is not yet clearly understood [161].

6.5. TGF-β and EGF

Recurrent OC show significantly higher expression of TGF-β1 and TGF-β3 in comparison to primary tumors and normal ovary tissue [213]. Inhibition of TGF-β by the inhibitor LY2109761 sensitizes resistant SKOV3 cells to cisplatin suggesting that TGF-β contributes to the development of platinum resistance in EOC cells [162]. Cisplatin resistant A2780P cells had hypomethylation and upregulation of TGFBR2 confirming the involvement of the pathway in acquisition of platinum resistance [214]. An elevated level of EGF receptor (EGFR) has also been associated with poor prognosis in OC patients [215]. EGF has been shown to stimulate the growth of EOC cells expressing EGFR and alters their cell cycle distribution [216]. EGF similar to LPA has been shown to protect EOC cells from undergoing cisplatin induced apoptosis [161].

6.6. COX-2

In addition to being associated with tumor initiation and progression, COX-2 has also been associated with chemoresistance. Ferrandina et al. reported that a statistically significant higher percentage of primary OC patients unresponsive to platinum-containing chemotherapy were positive for COX-2 than responsive patients (84.6% versus 34.6%, respectively) [217]. The percentage of positive COX-2 staining per tumor area in COX-2 positive patients ranged from 15 to 45%. The results from this study suggest that COX-2 levels may influence the response of patients to different chemotherapy regimens, but the sample size of this study was small and the results need to be confirmed in a larger group of patients. Furthermore, this association needs to be corroborated biochemically [217]. In both patients groups undergoing cytoreductive surgery and explorative laparotomy, COX-2 expression was higher in nonresponders [218]. Using lung, colon, and prostate cancer models, COX-2 has been shown to induce Bcl-2 and promote tumor growth by facilitating the formation of new blood vessels [158,159]. These findings suggest that COX-2 may contribute to chemoresistance by inhibiting apoptosis and promoting angiogenesis in OC as well.

7. Treatment Strategies Targeting Inflammatory Mediators in EOC

As discussed, development of resistance to available chemotherapeutic drugs remains the major obstacle in management of OC patients. While several immunotherapies have been developed to improve the antitumor response of T-cells and/or modulate the immune response, here we will discuss EOC treatment strategies that specifically target the inflammatory mediators that have been reviewed above.

A monoclonal antibody directed at VEGF, bevacizumab, has been widely studied and is a promising target in EOC [219]. Bevacizumab is a recombinant humanized monoclonal antibody and has been approved by the FDA for treatment of metastatic breast, non-small cell lung, and colorectal cancer. Phase II clinical studies have shown that it is active in treatment of recurrent OC patients [220]. OCEANS trial was a randomized phase III clinical trial that evaluated the safety and efficacy of bevacizumab in combination with gemcitabine and carboplatin (GC) in comparison with GC alone in recurrent platinum sensitive ovarian, primary peritoneal, or FT cancer. This trial demonstrated that bevacizumab was able to prolong the PFS in platinum-sensitive recurrent EOC patients [221]. In addition to OCEANS, GOG218, and ICON7 have also shown that bevacizumab prolongs the PFS in OC patients confirming the promise this therapeutic target holds for management of OC [222,223].

We have discussed some mechanisms by which the pro-inflammatory cytokine TNF-α promotes OC metastasis and angiogenesis making it a good target for development of therapeutic agents. The safety profile and biological activity of a monoclonal anti-TNF-α antibody, Infliximab was assessed in a clinical study consisting of patients with advanced solid tumors, including OC. Infliximab did not have any toxic effects and was well tolerated by these patients. Reduced plasma levels of IL-6 and CCL12 in these patients was observed 24 h and 48 h after administration of Infliximab, while neutralization of TNF-α was detected after an hour indicating some biological activity [224]. This response warrants further study of Infliximab as a therapeutic agent for treatment of OC.

IL-6/STAT3 signaling has been implicated at different stages of OC progression and is a promising target although most agents are still in preclinical or early clinical trial stages. Siltuximab, an anti-IL-6 antibody, suppresses IL-6-induced STAT3 phosphorylation and nuclear translocation in OC cell lines. Siltuximab treatment also reduced the level of pro-survival proteins like Bcl-X_L and Survivin, which are downstream of STAT3. Siltuximab was able to sensitize paclitaxel resistant OC cell lines, but did not show the same effect in vivo [225]. sc144 is a novel small molecule inhibitor has shown significant promise in preclinical studies. sc144 binds gp130, which is a signal transducer in STAT3 signaling. It causes phosphorylation of gp130 leading to its deglycosylation. This abrogates downstream STAT3 phosphorylation and nuclear translocation inhibiting transcription of downstream genes. sc144 has increased potency in EOC cells in comparison to normal epithelial cells and slows down the growth of tumors in xenograft models of EOC [226]. A phase I clinical trial combining carboplatin, the monoclonal antibody Tocilizumab, which blocks IL-6R, and immune enhancer INF-α showed good promise. The EOC patients who received the highest dose of Tocilizumab had increased serum levels of IL-6 and sIL-6R and also showed longer median overall survival [227].

We have discussed the role of TGF-β in EOC tumor progression substantiating it as a good therapeutic target. A preclinical study of LY2109761 (TGFβRI and TGFβRII kinase inhibitor) in combination with cisplatin was conducted by Gao et al. This inhibitor significantly increased apoptosis in cisplatin resistant cells. Combining LY2109761 with cisplatin had antiproliferative effects and increased the rate of apoptosis in parental and cisplatin resistant xenograft models [162]. In triple negative breast cancer, LY2157299 a TGF-β1 receptor kinase inhibitor, prevented recurrence of tumors in xenograft models after treatment with paclitaxel [228]. Early phase clinical trials of LY2157299 in patients with advanced or metastasized pancreatic cancer have been completed. Early phase trials in triple negative metastatic breast cancer, unresectable hepatocellular carcinoma, and metastatic castration resistant prostate cancer are underway [229].

EGF has also been associated with chemoresistance in EOC. Cetuximab, a chimerized monoclonal antibody that targets EGFR, was tested in combination with carboplatin in patients with recurrent platinum sensitive OC. Cetuximab showed modest activity in these patients [230]. Panitumumab, a human monoclonal antibody specific to EGFR, in combination with carboplatin did not improve efficacy or progression free survival in platinum sensitive EOC patients [231].

8. Conclusions and Future Perspectives

Several studies in the last decade have associated increased inflammation and inflammatory mediators with increased EOC risk and reduced survival in EOC patients. We have presented published evidence suggesting that inflammation and inflammatory mediators promote ovarian tumorigenesis. However the mechanisms by which the process of inflammation culminates in ovarian tumor initiation need to be further understood. Such links have been established in colon and pancreatic cancer. Understanding these mechanisms is important for developing ways to target inflammatory mediators and reduce OC risk. Furthermore, epidemiological studies of NSAIDs and early clinical trials targeting IL-6 and TNF-α have shown significant promise, thus suggesting that targeting inflammatory mediators as treatment for OC warrants future research.

Author Contributions: S.S.S. and S.S wrote the manuscript. S.S.S., S.S. and H.M.O. edited the manuscript.

Acknowledgments: We acknowledge the Leo and Anne Albert Charitable Trust for its ongoing support of ovarian cancer research.

References

1. Maiuri, A.R.; O'Hagan, H.M. Interplay Between Inflammation and Epigenetic Changes in Cancer. *Prog. Mol. Biol. Transl. Sci.* **2016**, *144*, 69–117. [PubMed]

2. Siegel, R.L.; Miller, K.D.; Jemal, A. Cancer statistics, 2018. *CA Cancer J. Clin.* **2018**, *68*, 7–30. [CrossRef] [PubMed]

3. Grivennikov, S.I.; Greten, F.R.; Karin, M. Immunity, inflammation, and cancer. *Cell* **2010**, *140*, 883–899. [CrossRef] [PubMed]

4. Clendenen, T.V.; Lundin, E.; Zeleniuch-Jacquotte, A.; Koenig, K.L.; Berrino, F.; Lukanova, A.; Lokshin, A.E.; Idahl, A.; Ohlson, N.; Hallmans, G.; et al. Circulating inflammation markers and risk of epithelial ovarian cancer. *Cancer Epidemiol. Biomark. Prev.* **2011**, *20*, 799–810. [CrossRef] [PubMed]

5. Chou, C.H.; Wei, L.H.; Kuo, M.L.; Huang, Y.J.; Lai, K.P.; Chen, C.A.; Hsieh, C.Y. Up-regulation of interleukin-6 in human ovarian cancer cell via a Gi/PI3K-Akt/NF-κB pathway by lysophosphatidic acid, an ovarian cancer-activating factor. *Carcinogenesis* **2005**, *26*, 45–52. [CrossRef] [PubMed]

6. Dhillon, A.S.; Hagan, S.; Rath, O.; Kolch, W. MAP kinase signalling pathways in cancer. *Oncogene* **2007**, *26*, 3279–3290. [CrossRef] [PubMed]

7. Schulze-Osthoff, K.; Ferrari, D.; Riehemann, K.; Wesselborg, S. Regulation of NF-κ B activation by MAP kinase cascades. *Immunobiology* **1997**, *198*, 35–49. [CrossRef]

8. Coussens, L.M.; Werb, Z. Inflammation and cancer. *Nature* **2002**, *420*, 860–867. [CrossRef] [PubMed]

9. Gajewski, T.F.; Schreiber, H.; Fu, Y.X. Innate and adaptive immune cells in the tumor microenvironment. *Nat. Immunol.* **2013**, *14*, 1014–1022. [CrossRef] [PubMed]

10. Wilson, C.B.; Rowell, E.; Sekimata, M. Epigenetic control of T-helper-cell differentiation. *Nat. Rev. Immunol.* **2009**, *9*, 91–105. [CrossRef] [PubMed]

11. Tone, A.A.; Salvador, S.; Finlayson, S.J.; Tinker, A.V.; Kwon, J.S.; Lee, C.H.; Cohen, T.; Ehlen, T.; Lee, M.; Carey, M.S.; et al. The role of the fallopian tube in ovarian cancer. *Clin. Adv. Hematol. Oncol.* **2012**, *10*, 296–306. [PubMed]

12. Petrovska, M.; Dimitrov, D.G.; Michael, S.D. Quantitative changes in macrophage distribution in normal mouse ovary over the course of the estrous cycle examined with an image analysis system. *Am. J. Reprod. Immunol.* **1996**, *36*, 175–183. [CrossRef] [PubMed]

13. Takaya, R.; Fukaya, T.; Sasano, H.; Suzuki, T.; Tamura, M.; Yajima, A. Macrophages in normal cycling human ovaries; immunohistochemical localization and characterization. *Hum. Reprod.* **1997**, *12*, 1508–1512. [CrossRef] [PubMed]

14. Wu, R.; Van der Hoek, K.H.; Ryan, N.K.; Norman, R.J.; Robker, R.L. Macrophage contributions to ovarian function. *Hum. Reprod. Update* **2004**, *10*, 119–133. [CrossRef] [PubMed]

15. Tingen, C.M.; Kiesewetter, S.E.; Jozefik, J.; Thomas, C.; Tagler, D.; Shea, L.; Woodruff, T.K. A macrophage and theca cell-enriched stromal cell population influences growth and survival of immature murine follicles in vitro. *Reproduction* **2011**, *141*, 809–820. [CrossRef] [PubMed]

16. Lau, A.; Kollara, A.; St John, E.; Tone, A.A.; Virtanen, C.; Greenblatt, E.M.; King, W.A.; Brown, T.J. Altered expression of inflammation-associated genes in oviductal cells following follicular fluid exposure: Implications for ovarian carcinogenesis. *Exp. Biol. Med.* **2014**, *239*, 24–32. [CrossRef] [PubMed]

17. King, S.M.; Hilliard, T.S.; Wu, L.Y.; Jaffe, R.C.; Fazleabas, A.T.; Burdette, J.E. The impact of ovulation on fallopian tube epithelial cells: Evaluating three hypotheses connecting ovulation and serous ovarian cancer. *Endocr. Relat. Cancer* **2011**, *18*, 627–642. [CrossRef] [PubMed]

18. Johnson, P.A.; Giles, J.R. The hen as a model of ovarian cancer. *Nat. Rev. Cancer* **2013**, *13*, 432–436. [CrossRef] [PubMed]

19. Gong, T.T.; Wu, Q.J.; Vogtmann, E.; Lin, B.; Wang, Y.L. Age at menarche and risk of ovarian cancer: A meta-analysis of epidemiological studies. *Int. J. Cancer* **2013**, *132*, 2894–2900. [CrossRef] [PubMed]

20. Chiaffarino, F.; Pelucchi, C.; Parazzini, F.; Negri, E.; Franceschi, S.; Talamini, R.; Conti, E.; Montella, M.; La Vecchia, C. Reproductive and hormonal factors and ovarian cancer. *Ann. Oncol.* **2001**, *12*, 337–341. [CrossRef] [PubMed]

21. Fortner, R.T.; Ose, J.; Merritt, M.A.; Schock, H.; Tjonneland, A.; Hansen, L.; Overvad, K.; Dossus, L.; Clavel-Chapelon, F.; Baglietto, L.; et al. Reproductive and hormone-related risk factors for epithelial ovarian cancer by histologic pathways, invasiveness and histologic subtypes: Results from the EPIC cohort. *Int. J. Cancer* **2015**, *137*, 1196–1208. [CrossRef] [PubMed]

22. Espey, L.L. Ovulation as an inflammatory reaction—A hypothesis. *Biol. Reprod.* **1980**, *22*, 73–106. [CrossRef] [PubMed]

23. Machelon, V.; Emilie, D. Production of ovarian cytokines and their role in ovulation in the mammalian ovary. *Eur. Cytokine Netw.* **1997**, *8*, 137–143. [PubMed]

24. Chumduri, C.; Gurumurthy, R.K.; Zadora, P.K.; Mi, Y.; Meyer, T.F. Chlamydia infection promotes host DNA damage and proliferation but impairs the DNA damage response. *Cell. Host Microbe* **2013**, *13*, 746–758. [CrossRef] [PubMed]

25. Ingerslev, K.; Hogdall, E.; Schnack, T.H.; Skovrider-Ruminski, W.; Hogdall, C.; Blaakaer, J. The potential role of infectious agents and pelvic inflammatory disease in ovarian carcinogenesis. *Infect. Agent Cancer* **2017**, *12*, 25. [CrossRef] [PubMed]

26. Burney, R.O.; Giudice, L.C. Pathogenesis and pathophysiology of endometriosis. *Fertil. Steril.* **2012**, *98*, 511–519. [CrossRef] [PubMed]

27. Vercellini, P.; Crosignani, P.; Somigliana, E.; Viganò, P.; Buggio, L.; Bolis, G.; Fedele, L. The 'incessant menstruation' hypothesis: A mechanistic ovarian cancer model with implications for prevention. *Hum. Reprod.* **2011**, *26*, 2262–2273. [CrossRef] [PubMed]

28. Burghaus, S.; Haberle, L.; Schrauder, M.G.; Heusinger, K.; Thiel, F.C.; Hein, A.; Wachter, D.; Strehl, J.; Hartmann, A.; Ekici, A.B.; et al. Endometriosis as a risk factor for ovarian or endometrial cancer—Results of a hospital-based case-control study. *BMC Cancer* **2015**, *15*, 751. [CrossRef] [PubMed]

29. Sayasneh, A.; Tsivos, D.; Crawford, R. Endometriosis and ovarian cancer: A systematic review. *ISRN Obstet. Gynecol.* **2011**, *2011*, 140310. [CrossRef] [PubMed]

30. Rizi, B.S.; Nagrath, D. Linking omentum and ovarian cancer: NO. *Oncoscience* **2015**, *2*, 797–798. [PubMed]

31. Gunderson, C.C.; Ding, K.; Dvorak, J.; Moore, K.N.; McMeekin, D.S.; Benbrook, D.M. The pro-inflammatory effect of obesity on high grade serous ovarian cancer. *Gynecol. Oncol.* **2016**, *143*, 40–45. [CrossRef] [PubMed]

32. Poole, E.M.; Lee, I.M.; Ridker, P.M.; Buring, J.E.; Hankinson, S.E.; Tworoger, S.S. A prospective study of circulating C-reactive protein, interleukin-6, and tumor necrosis factor alpha receptor 2 levels and risk of ovarian cancer. *Am. J. Epidemiol.* **2013**, *178*, 1256–1264. [CrossRef] [PubMed]

33. Ose, J.; Schock, H.; Tjonneland, A.; Hansen, L.; Overvad, K.; Dossus, L.; Clavel-Chapelon, F.; Baglietto, L.; Boeing, H.; Trichopolou, A.; et al. Inflammatory Markers and Risk of Epithelial Ovarian Cancer by Tumor Subtypes: The EPIC Cohort. *Cancer Epidemiol. Biomark. Prev.* **2015**, *24*, 951–961. [CrossRef] [PubMed]

34. Duleba, A.J.; Dokras, A. Is PCOS an inflammatory process? *Fertil. Steril.* **2012**, *97*, 7–12. [CrossRef] [PubMed]

35. Kelly, C.C.; Lyall, H.; Petrie, J.R.; Gould, G.W.; Connell, J.M.; Sattar, N. Low grade chronic inflammation in women with polycystic ovarian syndrome. *J. Clin. Endocrinol. Metab.* **2001**, *86*, 2453–2455. [CrossRef] [PubMed]

36. Escobar-Morreale, H.F.; Luque-Ramirez, M.; Gonzalez, F. Circulating inflammatory markers in polycystic ovary syndrome: A systematic review and metaanalysis. *Fertil. Steril.* **2011**, *95*, 1048–1058.e1041-1042. [CrossRef] [PubMed]

37. Gonzalez, F.; Rote, N.S.; Minium, J.; Kirwan, J.P. Evidence of proatherogenic inflammation in polycystic ovary syndrome. *Metabolism* **2009**, *58*, 954–962. [CrossRef] [PubMed]

38. Glintborg, D.; Andersen, M.; Richelsen, B.; Bruun, J.M. Plasma monocyte chemoattractant protein-1 (MCP-1) and macrophage inflammatory protein-1α are increased in patients with polycystic ovary syndrome (PCOS) and associated with adiposity, but unaffected by pioglitazone treatment. *Clin. Endocrinol.* **2009**, *71*, 652–658. [CrossRef] [PubMed]

39. Escobar-Morreale, H.F.; Botella-Carretero, J.I.; Villuendas, G.; Sancho, J.; San Millan, J.L. Serum interleukin-18 concentrations are increased in the polycystic ovary syndrome: Relationship to insulin resistance and to obesity. *J. Clin. Endocrinol. Metab.* **2004**, *89*, 806–811. [CrossRef] [PubMed]

40. Yang, Y.; Qiao, J.; Li, R.; Li, M.Z. Is interleukin-18 associated with polycystic ovary syndrome? *Reprod. Biol. Endocrinol.* **2011**, *9*, 7. [CrossRef] [PubMed]

41. Tarkun, I.; Cetinarslan, B.; Turemen, E.; Canturk, Z.; Biyikli, M. Association between Circulating Tumor Necrosis Factor-α, Interleukin-6, and Insulin Resistance in Normal-Weight Women with Polycystic Ovary Syndrome. *Metab. Syndr. Relat. Disord.* **2006**, *4*, 122–128. [CrossRef] [PubMed]

42. Vgontzas, A.N.; Trakada, G.; Bixler, E.O.; Lin, H.M.; Pejovic, S.; Zoumakis, E.; Chrousos, G.P.; Legro, R.S. Plasma interleukin 6 levels are elevated in polycystic ovary syndrome independently of obesity or sleep apnea. *Metabolism* **2006**, *55*, 1076–1082. [CrossRef] [PubMed]

43. Dinger, Y.; Akcay, T.; Erdem, T.; Ilker Saygili, E.; Gundogdu, S. DNA damage, DNA susceptibility to oxidation and glutathione level in women with polycystic ovary syndrome. *Scand. J. Clin Lab. Investig.* **2005**, *65*, 721–728.

44. Harris, H.R.; Terry, K.L. Polycystic ovary syndrome and risk of endometrial, ovarian, and breast cancer: A systematic review. *Fertil. Res. Pract.* **2016**, *2*, 14. [CrossRef] [PubMed]

45. Heller, D.S.; Westhoff, C.; Gordon, R.E.; Katz, N. The relationship between perineal cosmetic talc usage and ovarian talc particle burden. *Am. J. Obstet. Gynecol.* **1996**, *174*, 1507–1510. [CrossRef]

46. Henderson, W.J.; Hamilton, T.C.; Griffiths, K. Talc in normal and malignant ovarian tissue. *Lancet* **1979**, *1*, 499. [CrossRef]

47. Muscat, J.E.; Huncharek, M.S. Perineal talc use and ovarian cancer: A critical review. *Eur J. Cancer Prev.* **2008**, *17*, 139–146. [CrossRef] [PubMed]

48. Brasky, T.M.; Moysich, K.B.; Cohn, D.E.; White, E. Non-steroidal anti-inflammatory drugs and endometrial cancer risk in the VITamins And Lifestyle (VITAL) cohort. *Gynecol. Oncol.* **2013**, *128*, 113–119. [CrossRef] [PubMed]

49. Prizment, A.E.; Folsom, A.R.; Anderson, K.E. Nonsteroidal anti-inflammatory drugs and risk for ovarian and endometrial cancers in the Iowa Women's Health Study. *Cancer Epidemiol. Biomark. Prev.* **2010**, *19*, 435–442. [CrossRef] [PubMed]

50. Fairfield, K.M.; Hunter, D.J.; Fuchs, C.S.; Colditz, G.A.; Hankinson, S.E. Aspirin, other NSAIDs, and ovarian cancer risk (United States). *Cancer Causes Control.* **2002**, *13*, 535–542. [CrossRef] [PubMed]

51. Trabert, B.; Poole, E.M.; White, E.; Visvanathan, K.; Adami, H.O.; Anderson, G.L.; Brasky, T.M.; Brinton, L.A.; Fortner, R.T.; Gaudet, M.; et al. Analgesic Use and Ovarian Cancer Risk: An Analysis in the Ovarian Cancer Cohort Consortium. *J. Natl. Cancer Inst.* **2018**. [CrossRef] [PubMed]

52. Peres, L.C.; Camacho, F.; Abbott, S.E.; Alberg, A.J.; Bandera, E.V.; Barnholtz-Sloan, J.; Bondy, M.; Cote, M.L.; Crankshaw, S.; Funkhouser, E.; et al. Analgesic medication use and risk of epithelial ovarian cancer in African American women. *Br. J. Cancer* **2016**, *114*, 819–825. [CrossRef] [PubMed]

53. Rodriguez-Burford, C.; Barnes, M.N.; Oelschlager, D.K.; Myers, R.B.; Talley, L.I.; Partridge, E.E.; Grizzle, W.E. Effects of nonsteroidal anti-inflammatory agents (NSAIDs) on ovarian carcinoma cell lines: Preclinical evaluation of NSAIDs as chemopreventive agents. *Clin. Cancer Res.* **2002**, *8*, 202–209. [PubMed]

54. Arango, H.A.; Icely, S.; Roberts, W.S.; Cavanagh, D.; Becker, J.L. Aspirin effects on endometrial cancer cell growth. *Obstet. Gynecol.* **2001**, *97*, 423–427. [PubMed]

55. Gao, J.; Niwa, K.; Sun, W.; Takemura, M.; Lian, Z.; Onogi, K.; Seishima, M.; Mori, H.; Tamaya, T. Non-steroidal anti-inflammatory drugs inhibit cellular proliferation and upregulate cyclooxygenase-2 protein expression in endometrial cancer cells. *Cancer Sci.* **2004**, *95*, 901–907. [CrossRef] [PubMed]

56. Li, H.L.; Zhang, H.W.; Chen, D.D.; Zhong, L.; Ren, X.D.; St-Tu, R. JTE-522, a selective COX-2 inhibitor, inhibits cell proliferation and induces apoptosis in RL95-2 cells. *Acta Pharmacol Sin.* **2002**, *23*, 631–637. [PubMed]

57. Hsu, C.S.; Li, Y. Aspirin potently inhibits oxidative DNA strand breaks: Implications for cancer chemoprevention. *Biochem. Biophys. Res. Commun.* **2002**, *293*, 705–709. [PubMed]

58. Hales, D.B.; Zhuge, Y.; Lagman, J.A.; Ansenberger, K.; Mahon, C.; Barua, A.; Luborsky, J.L.; Bahr, J.M. Cyclooxygenases expression and distribution in the normal ovary and their role in ovarian cancer in the domestic hen (Gallus domesticus). *Endocrine* **2008**, *33*, 235–244. [CrossRef] [PubMed]

59. Urick, M.E.; Giles, J.R.; Johnson, P.A. VEGF expression and the effect of NSAIDs on ascites cell proliferation in the hen model of ovarian cancer. *Gynecol. Oncol.* **2008**, *110*, 418–424. [CrossRef] [PubMed]

60. Urick, M.E.; Giles, J.R.; Johnson, P.A. Dietary aspirin decreases the stage of ovarian cancer in the hen. *Gynecol. Oncol.* **2009**, *112*, 166–170. [CrossRef] [PubMed]

61. Hanahan, D.; Weinberg, R.A. Hallmarks of cancer: The next generation. *Cell* **2011**, *144*, 646–674. [CrossRef] [PubMed]

62. Cancer Genome Atlas Research, N. Integrated genomic analyses of ovarian carcinoma. *Nature* **2011**, *474*, 609–615.

63. Toss, A.; Tomasello, C.; Razzaboni, E.; Contu, G.; Grandi, G.; Cagnacci, A.; Schilder, R.J.; Cortesi, L. Hereditary ovarian cancer: Not only BRCA 1 and 2 genes. *Biomed. Res. Int.* **2015**, *2015*, 341723. [CrossRef] [PubMed]

64. Liu, J.; Yang, G.; Thompson-Lanza, J.A.; Glassman, A.; Hayes, K.; Patterson, A.; Marquez, R.T.; Auersperg, N.; Yu, Y.; Hahn, W.C.; et al. A genetically defined model for human ovarian cancer. *Cancer Res.* **2004**, *64*, 1655–1663. [CrossRef] [PubMed]

65. Szotek, P.P.; Pieretti-Vanmarcke, R.; Masiakos, P.T.; Dinulescu, D.M.; Connolly, D.; Foster, R.; Dombkowski, D.; Preffer, F.; Maclaughlin, D.T.; Donahoe, P.K. Ovarian cancer side population defines cells with stem cell-like characteristics and Mullerian Inhibiting Substance responsiveness. *Proc. Natl. Acad. Sci. USA* **2006**, *103*, 11154–11159. [CrossRef] [PubMed]

66. Zhang, S.; Balch, C.; Chan, M.W.; Lai, H.C.; Matei, D.; Schilder, J.M.; Yan, P.S.; Huang, T.H.; Nephew, K.P. Identification and characterization of ovarian cancer-initiating cells from primary human tumors. *Cancer Res.* **2008**, *68*, 4311–4320. [CrossRef] [PubMed]

67. Lane, D.; Matte, I.; Rancourt, C.; Piche, A. Prognostic significance of IL-6 and IL-8 ascites levels in ovarian cancer patients. *BMC Cancer* **2011**, *11*, 210. [CrossRef] [PubMed]

68. Masoumi-Moghaddam, S.; Amini, A.; Wei, A.Q.; Robertson, G.; Morris, D.L. Intratumoral interleukin-6 predicts ascites formation in patients with epithelial ovarian cancer: A potential tool for close monitoring. *J. Ovarian Res.* **2015**, *8*, 58. [CrossRef] [PubMed]

69. Rath, K.S.; Funk, H.M.; Bowling, M.C.; Richards, W.E.; Drew, A.F. Expression of soluble interleukin-6 receptor in malignant ovarian tissue. *Am. J. Obstet. Gynecol.* **2010**, *203*, 230.e1–230.e8. [CrossRef] [PubMed]

70. Lo, C.W.; Chen, M.W.; Hsiao, M.; Wang, S.; Chen, C.A.; Hsiao, S.M.; Chang, J.S.; Lai, T.C.; Rose-John, S.; Kuo, M.L.; et al. IL-6 trans-signaling in formation and progression of malignant ascites in ovarian cancer. *Cancer Res.* **2011**, *71*, 424–434. [CrossRef] [PubMed]

71. Dalal, V.; Kumar, R.; Kumar, S.; Sharma, A.; Kumar, L.; Sharma, J.B.; Roy, K.K.; Singh, N.; Vanamail, P. Biomarker potential of IL-6 and VEGF-A in ascitic fluid of epithelial ovarian cancer patients. *Clin. Chim. Acta* **2018**, *482*, 27–32. [CrossRef] [PubMed]

72. Bapat, S.A.; Mali, A.M.; Koppikar, C.B.; Kurrey, N.K. Stem and progenitor-like cells contribute to the aggressive behavior of human epithelial ovarian cancer. *Cancer Res.* **2005**, *65*, 3025–3029. [CrossRef] [PubMed]

73. Wang, D.; Xiang, T.; Zhao, Z.; Lin, K.; Yin, P.; Jiang, L.; Liang, Z.; Zhu, B. Autocrine interleukin-23 promotes self-renewal of CD133+ ovarian cancer stem-like cells. *Oncotarget* **2016**, *7*, 76006–76020. [CrossRef] [PubMed]

74. Maccio, A.; Madeddu, C. Inflammation and ovarian cancer. *Cytokine* **2012**, *58*, 133–147. [CrossRef] [PubMed]

75. Agarwal, A.; Gupta, S.; Sharma, R.K. Role of oxidative stress in female reproduction. *Reprod. Biol. Endocrinol.* **2005**, *3*, 28. [CrossRef] [PubMed]

76. Shkolnik, K.; Tadmor, A.; Ben-Dor, S.; Nevo, N.; Galiani, D.; Dekel, N. Reactive oxygen species are indispensable in ovulation. *Proc. Natl. Acad. Sci. USA* **2011**, *108*, 1462–1467. [CrossRef] [PubMed]

77. Waris, G.; Ahsan, H. Reactive oxygen species: Role in the development of cancer and various chronic conditions. *J. Carcinog.* **2006**, *5*, 14. [CrossRef] [PubMed]

78. Liou, G.Y.; Storz, P. Reactive oxygen species in cancer. *Free Radic. Res.* **2010**, *44*, 479–496. [CrossRef] [PubMed]

79. King, S.M.; Quartuccio, S.M.; Vanderhyden, B.C.; Burdette, J.E. Early transformative changes in normal ovarian surface epithelium induced by oxidative stress require Akt upregulation, DNA damage and epithelial-stromal interaction. *Carcinogenesis* **2013**, *34*, 1125–1133. [CrossRef] [PubMed]

80. Levanon, K.; Ng, V.; Piao, H.Y.; Zhang, Y.; Chang, M.C.; Roh, M.H.; Kindelberger, D.W.; Hirsch, M.S.; Crum, C.P.; Marto, J.A.; et al. Primary ex vivo cultures of human fallopian tube epithelium as a model for serous ovarian carcinogenesis. *Oncogene* **2010**, *29*, 1103–1113. [CrossRef] [PubMed]

81. Huang, H.S.; Chu, S.C.; Hsu, C.F.; Chen, P.C.; Ding, D.C.; Chang, M.Y.; Chu, T.Y. Mutagenic, surviving and tumorigenic effects of follicular fluid in the context of p53 loss: Initiation of fimbria carcinogenesis. *Carcinogenesis* **2015**, *36*, 1419–1428. [CrossRef] [PubMed]

82. Kalinina, E.V.; Chernov, N.N.; Saprin, A.N.; Kotova, Y.N.; Gavrilova, Y.A.; Chermnykh, N.S.; Shcherbak, N.P. Expression of genes for thioredoxin 1 and thioredoxin 2 in multidrug resistance ovarian carcinoma cells SKVLB. *Bull. Exp. Biol. Med.* **2007**, *144*, 301–303. [CrossRef] [PubMed]

83. Ohno, T.; Hirota, K.; Nakamura, H.; Masutani, H.; Sasada, T.; Yodoi, J. Thioredoxin and Its Involvement in the Redox Regulation of Transcription Factors, NF-κB and AP-1. In *Oxygen Homeostasis and Its Dynamics*; Springer: Tokyo, Japan, 1998; pp. 450–456.

84. Van der Wijst, M.G.; Huisman, C.; Mposhi, A.; Roelfes, G.; Rots, M.G. Targeting Nrf2 in healthy and malignant ovarian epithelial cells: Protection versus promotion. *Mol. Oncol.* **2015**, *9*, 1259–1273. [CrossRef] [PubMed]

85. Klotz, L.O.; Sanchez-Ramos, C.; Prieto-Arroyo, I.; Urbanek, P.; Steinbrenner, H.; Monsalve, M. Redox regulation of FoxO transcription factors. *Redox Biol* **2015**, *6*, 51–72. [CrossRef] [PubMed]

86. Ozdemir, F.; Altinisik, J.; Karateke, A.; Coksuer, H.; Buyru, N. Methylation of tumor suppressor genes in ovarian cancer. *Exp. Ther. Med.* **2012**, *4*, 1092–1096. [CrossRef] [PubMed]

87. Niwa, T.; Tsukamoto, T.; Toyoda, T.; Mori, A.; Tanaka, H.; Maekita, T.; Ichinose, M.; Tatematsu, M.; Ushijima, T. Inflammatory processes triggered by Helicobacter pylori infection cause aberrant DNA methylation in gastric epithelial cells. *Cancer Res.* **2010**, *70*, 1430–1440. [CrossRef] [PubMed]

88. Ding, N.; Bonham, E.M.; Hannon, B.E.; Amick, T.R.; Baylin, S.B.; O'Hagan, H.M. Mismatch repair proteins recruit DNA methyltransferase 1 to sites of oxidative DNA damage. *J. Mol. Cell. Biol.* **2016**, *8*, 244–254. [CrossRef] [PubMed]

89. Maiuri, A.R.; Peng, M.; Sriramkumar, S.; Kamplain, C.M.; DeStefano Shields, C.E.; Sears, C.L.; O'Hagan, H.M. Mismatch Repair Proteins Initiate Epigenetic Alterations during Inflammation-Driven Tumorigenesis. *Cancer Res.* **2017**, *77*, 3467–3478. [CrossRef] [PubMed]

90. Sapoznik, S.; Bahar-Shany, K.; Brand, H.; Pinto, Y.; Gabay, O.; Glick-Saar, E.; Dor, C.; Zadok, O.; Barshack, I.; Zundelevich, A.; et al. Activation-Induced Cytidine Deaminase Links Ovulation-Induced Inflammation and Serous Carcinogenesis. *Neoplasia* **2016**, *18*, 90–99. [CrossRef] [PubMed]

91. Gupta, M.; Babic, A.; Beck, A.H.; Terry, K. TNF-α expression, risk factors, and inflammatory exposures in ovarian cancer: Evidence for an inflammatory pathway of ovarian carcinogenesis? *Hum. Pathol.* **2016**, *54*, 82–91. [CrossRef] [PubMed]

92. Moradi, M.M.; Carson, L.F.; Weinberg, B.; Haney, A.F.; Twiggs, L.B.; Ramakrishnan, S. Serum and ascitic fluid levels of interleukin-1, interleukin-6, and tumor necrosis factor-α in patients with ovarian epithelial cancer. *Cancer* **1993**, *72*, 2433–2440. [CrossRef]

93. Szlosarek, P.W.; Grimshaw, M.J.; Kulbe, H.; Wilson, J.L.; Wilbanks, G.D.; Burke, F.; Balkwill, F.R. Expression and regulation of tumor necrosis factor alpha in normal and malignant ovarian epithelium. *Mol. Cancer Ther.* **2006**, *5*, 382–390. [CrossRef] [PubMed]

94. Kulbe, H.; Thompson, R.; Wilson, J.L.; Robinson, S.; Hagemann, T.; Fatah, R.; Gould, D.; Ayhan, A.; Balkwill, F. The inflammatory cytokine tumor necrosis factor-α generates an autocrine tumor-promoting network in epithelial ovarian cancer cells. *Cancer Res.* **2007**, *67*, 585–592. [CrossRef] [PubMed]

95. Charles, K.A.; Kulbe, H.; Soper, R.; Escorcio-Correia, M.; Lawrence, T.; Schultheis, A.; Chakravarty, P.; Thompson, R.G.; Kollias, G.; Smyth, J.F.; et al. The tumor-promoting actions of TNF-α involve TNFR1 and IL-17 in ovarian cancer in mice and humans. *J. Clin. Investig.* **2009**, *119*, 3011–3023. [CrossRef] [PubMed]

96. Berek, J.S.; Chung, C.; Kaldi, K.; Watson, J.M.; Knox, R.M.; Martinez-Maza, O. Serum interleukin-6 levels correlate with disease status in patients with epithelial ovarian cancer. *Am. J. Obstet. Gynecol.* **1991**, *164*, 1038–1042; discussion 1042–1033. [CrossRef]

97.   Scambia, G.; Testa, U.; Benedetti Panici, P.; Foti, E.; Martucci, R.; Gadducci, A.; Perillo, A.; Facchini, V.;
       Peschle, C.; Mancuso, S. Prognostic significance of interleukin 6 serum levels in patients with ovarian cancer.
       Br. J. Cancer **1995**, *71*, 354. [CrossRef] [PubMed]
98.   Alberti, C.; Pinciroli, P.; Valeri, B.; Ferri, R.; Ditto, A.; Umezawa, K.; Sensi, M.; Canevari, S.; Tomassetti, A.
       Ligand-dependent EGFR activation induces the co-expression of IL-6 and PAI-1 via the NFkB pathway in
       advanced-stage epithelial ovarian cancer. *Oncogene* **2012**, *31*, 4139–4149. [CrossRef] [PubMed]
99.   Hagemann, T.; Robinson, S.C.; Thompson, R.G.; Charles, K.; Kulbe, H.; Balkwill, F.R. Ovarian
       cancer cell-derived migration inhibitory factor enhances tumor growth, progression, and angiogenesis.
       Mol. Cancer Ther. **2007**, *6*, 1993–2002. [CrossRef] [PubMed]
100.   Oh, K.; Moon, H.G.; Lee, D.S.; Yoo, Y.B. Tissue transglutaminase-interleukin-6 axis facilitates peritoneal
       tumor spreading and metastasis of human ovarian cancer cells. *Lab. Anim. Res.* **2015**, *31*, 188–197. [CrossRef]
       [PubMed]
101.   Wang, Y.; Li, L.; Guo, X.; Jin, X.; Sun, W.; Zhang, X.; Xu, R.C. Interleukin-6 signaling regulates
       anchorage-independent growth, proliferation, adhesion and invasion in human ovarian cancer cells. *Cytokine*
       2012, *59*, 228–236. [CrossRef] [PubMed]
102.   Takaishi, K.; Komohara, Y.; Tashiro, H.; Ohtake, H.; Nakagawa, T.; Katabuchi, H.; Takeya, M. Involvement of
       M2-polarized macrophages in the ascites from advanced epithelial ovarian carcinoma in tumor progression
       via Stat3 activation. *Cancer Sci.* **2010**, *101*, 2128–2136. [CrossRef] [PubMed]
103.   Maccio, A.; Lai, P.; Santona, M.C.; Pagliara, L.; Melis, G.B.; Mantovani, G. High serum levels of soluble IL-2
       receptor, cytokines, and C reactive protein correlate with impairment of T cell response in patients with
       advanced epithelial ovarian cancer. *Gynecol. Oncol.* **1998**, *69*, 248–252. [CrossRef] [PubMed]
104.   Rabinovich, A.; Medina, L.; Piura, B.; Segal, S.; Huleihel, M. Regulation of ovarian carcinoma SKOV-3 cell
       proliferation and secretion of MMPs by autocrine IL-6. *Anticancer Res.* **2007**, *27*, 267–272. [PubMed]
105.   Runesson, E.; Bostrom, E.K.; Janson, P.O.; Brannstrom, M. The human preovulatory follicle is a source of the
       chemotactic cytokine interleukin-8. *Mol. Hum. Reprod* **1996**, *2*, 245–250. [CrossRef] [PubMed]
106.   Brannstrom, M.; Mayrhofer, G.; Robertson, S.A. Localization of leukocyte subsets in the rat ovary during the
       periovulatory period. *Biol. Reprod.* **1993**, *48*, 277–286. [CrossRef] [PubMed]
107.   Kassim, S.K.; El-Salahy, E.M.; Fayed, S.T.; Helal, S.A.; Helal, T.; Azzam Eel, D.; Khalifa, A. Vascular endothelial
       growth factor and interleukin-8 are associated with poor prognosis in epithelial ovarian cancer patients.
       Clin. Biochem. **2004**, *37*, 363–369. [CrossRef] [PubMed]
108.   Ivarsson, K.; Runesson, E.; Sundfeldt, K.; Haeger, M.; Hedin, L.; Janson, P.O.; Brannstrom, M. The chemotactic
       cytokine interleukin-8—A cyst fluid marker for malignant epithelial ovarian cancer? *Gynecol. Oncol.* **1998**,
       71, 420–423. [CrossRef] [PubMed]
109.   Radke, J.; Schmidt, D.; Bohme, M.; Schmidt, U.; Weise, W.; Morenz, J. Cytokine level in malignant ascites and
       peripheral blood of patients with advanced ovarian carcinoma. *Geburtshilfe Frauenheilkd.* **1996**, *56*, 83–87.
       [CrossRef] [PubMed]
110.   Wang, Y.; Xu, R.C.; Zhang, X.L.; Niu, X.L.; Qu, Y.; Li, L.Z.; Meng, X.Y. Interleukin-8 secretion by ovarian cancer
       cells increases anchorage-independent growth, proliferation, angiogenic potential, adhesion and invasion.
       Cytokine **2012**, *59*, 145–155. [CrossRef] [PubMed]
111.   Hirose, K.; Hakozaki, M.; Nyunoya, Y.; Kobayashi, Y.; Matsushita, K.; Takenouchi, T.; Mikata, A.; Mukaida, N.;
       Matsushima, K. Chemokine gene transfection into tumour cells reduced tumorigenicity in nude mice in
       association with neutrophilic infiltration. *Br. J. Cancer* **1995**, *72*, 708–714. [CrossRef] [PubMed]
112.   Lee, L.F.; Hellendall, R.P.; Wang, Y.; Haskill, J.S.; Mukaida, N.; Matsushima, K.; Ting, J.P. IL-8 reduced
       tumorigenicity of human ovarian cancer in vivo due to neutrophil infiltration. *J. Immunol.* **2000**, *164*, 2769–2775.
       [CrossRef] [PubMed]
113.   Tokumura, A.; Miyake, M.; Nishioka, Y.; Yamano, S.; Aono, T.; Fukuzawa, K. Production of lysophosphatidic
       acids by lysophospholipase D in human follicular fluids of In vitro fertilization patients. *Biol. Reprod.* **1999**,
       61, 195–199. [CrossRef] [PubMed]
114.   Chen, S.U.; Chou, C.H.; Lee, H.; Ho, C.H.; Lin, C.W.; Yang, Y.S. Lysophosphatidic acid
       up-regulates expression of interleukin-8 and -6 in granulosa-lutein cells through its receptors and
       nuclear factor-κB dependent pathways: Implications for angiogenesis of corpus luteum and ovarian
       hyperstimulation syndrome. *J. Clin. Endocrinol. Metab.* **2008**, *93*, 935–943. [CrossRef] [PubMed]

115. Fang, X.; Gaudette, D.; Furui, T.; Mao, M.; Estrella, V.; Eder, A.; Pustilnik, T.; Sasagawa, T.; Lapushin, R.; Yu, S.; et al. Lysophospholipid growth factors in the initiation, progression, metastases, and management of ovarian cancer. *Ann. N. Y. Acad. Sci.* **2000**, *905*, 188–208. [CrossRef] [PubMed]

116. Xu, Y.; Shen, Z.; Wiper, D.W.; Wu, M.; Morton, R.E.; Elson, P.; Kennedy, A.W.; Belinson, J.; Markman, M.; Casey, G. Lysophosphatidic acid as a potential biomarker for ovarian and other gynecologic cancers. *JAMA* **1998**, *280*, 719–723. [CrossRef] [PubMed]

117. Xiao, Y.J.; Schwartz, B.; Washington, M.; Kennedy, A.; Webster, K.; Belinson, J.; Xu, Y. Electrospray ionization mass spectrometry analysis of lysophospholipids in human ascitic fluids: Comparison of the lysophospholipid contents in malignant vs nonmalignant ascitic fluids. *Anal. Biochem.* **2001**, *290*, 302–313. [CrossRef] [PubMed]

118. Mills, G.B.; Eder, A.; Fang, X.; Hasegawa, Y.; Mao, M.; Lu, Y.; Tanyi, J.; Tabassam, F.H.; Wiener, J.; Lapushin, R.; et al. Critical role of lysophospholipids in the pathophysiology, diagnosis, and management of ovarian cancer. *Cancer Treat. Res.* **2002**, *107*, 259–283. [PubMed]

119. Westermann, A.M.; Havik, E.; Postma, F.R.; Beijnen, J.H.; Dalesio, O.; Moolenaar, W.H.; Rodenhuis, S. Malignant effusions contain lysophosphatidic acid (LPA)-like activity. *Ann. Oncol.* **1998**, *9*, 437–442. [CrossRef] [PubMed]

120. Xu, Y.; Gaudette, D.C.; Boynton, J.D.; Frankel, A.; Fang, X.J.; Sharma, A.; Hurteau, J.; Casey, G.; Goodbody, A.; Mellors, A.; et al. Characterization of an ovarian cancer activating factor in ascites from ovarian cancer patients. *Clin. Cancer Res.* **1995**, *1*, 1223–1232. [PubMed]

121. Symowicz, J.; Adley, B.P.; Woo, M.M.; Auersperg, N.; Hudson, L.G.; Stack, M.S. Cyclooxygenase-2 functions as a downstream mediator of lysophosphatidic acid to promote aggressive behavior in ovarian carcinoma cells. *Cancer Res.* **2005**, *65*, 2234–2242. [CrossRef] [PubMed]

122. Fang, X.; Yu, S.; Bast, R.C.; Liu, S.; Xu, H.J.; Hu, S.X.; LaPushin, R.; Claret, F.X.; Aggarwal, B.B.; Lu, Y.; et al. Mechanisms for lysophosphatidic acid-induced cytokine production in ovarian cancer cells. *J. Biol. Chem.* **2004**, *279*, 9653–9661. [CrossRef] [PubMed]

123. Saunders, J.A.; Rogers, L.C.; Klomsiri, C.; Poole, L.B.; Daniel, L.W. Reactive oxygen species mediate lysophosphatidic acid induced signaling in ovarian cancer cells. *Free Radic. Biol. Med.* **2010**, *49*, 2058–2067. [CrossRef] [PubMed]

124. Lu, J.; Xiao Yj, Y.J.; Baudhuin, L.M.; Hong, G.; Xu, Y. Role of ether-linked lysophosphatidic acids in ovarian cancer cells. *J. Lipid Res.* **2002**, *43*, 463–476. [PubMed]

125. Ali-Fehmi, R.; Morris, R.T.; Bandyopadhyay, S.; Che, M.; Schimp, V.; Malone, J.M., Jr.; Munkarah, A.R. Expression of cyclooxygenase-2 in advanced stage ovarian serous carcinoma: Correlation with tumor cell proliferation, apoptosis, angiogenesis, and survival. *Am. J. Obstet. Gynecol.* **2005**, *192*, 819–825. [CrossRef] [PubMed]

126. Rask, K.; Zhu, Y.; Wang, W.; Hedin, L.; Sundfeldt, K. Ovarian epithelial cancer: A role for PGE2-synthesis and signalling in malignant transformation and progression. *Mol. Cancer* **2006**, *5*, 62. [CrossRef] [PubMed]

127. Heinonen, P.K.; Metsa-Ketela, T. Prostaglandin and thromboxane production in ovarian cancer tissue. *Gynecol. Obstet. Investig.* **1984**, *18*, 225–229. [CrossRef] [PubMed]

128. Obermajer, N.; Muthuswamy, R.; Odunsi, K.; Edwards, R.P.; Kalinski, P. PGE(2)-induced CXCL12 production and CXCR4 expression controls the accumulation of human MDSCs in ovarian cancer environment. *Cancer Res.* **2011**, *71*, 7463–7470. [CrossRef] [PubMed]

129. Daikoku, T.; Tranguch, S.; Trofimova, I.N.; Dinulescu, D.M.; Jacks, T.; Nikitin, A.Y.; Connolly, D.C.; Dey, S.K. Cyclooxygenase-1 is overexpressed in multiple genetically engineered mouse models of epithelial ovarian cancer. *Cancer Res.* **2006**, *66*, 2527–2531. [CrossRef] [PubMed]

130. Li, W.; Cai, J.H.; Zhang, J.; Tang, Y.X.; Wan, L. Effects of cyclooxygenase inhibitors in combination with taxol on expression of cyclin D1 and Ki-67 in a xenograft model of ovarian carcinoma. *Int. J. Mol. Sci.* **2012**, *13*, 9741–9753. [CrossRef] [PubMed]

131. Paweletz, N.; Knierim, M. Tumor-related angiogenesis. *Crit. Rev. Oncol. Hematol.* **1989**, *9*, 197–242. [CrossRef]

132. Potente, M.; Gerhardt, H.; Carmeliet, P. Basic and therapeutic aspects of angiogenesis. *Cell* **2011**, *146*, 873–887. [CrossRef] [PubMed]

133. Burke, B.; Giannoudis, A.; Corke, K.P.; Gill, D.; Wells, M.; Ziegler-Heitbrock, L.; Lewis, C.E. Hypoxia-induced gene expression in human macrophages: Implications for ischemic tissues and hypoxia-regulated gene therapy. *Am. J. Pathol.* **2003**, *163*, 1233–1243. [CrossRef]

134. Murdoch, C.; Muthana, M.; Lewis, C.E. Hypoxia regulates macrophage functions in inflammation. *J. Immunol.* **2005**, *175*, 6257–6263. [CrossRef] [PubMed]

135. Ferrara, N.; Gerber, H.P.; LeCouter, J. The biology of VEGF and its receptors. *Nat. Med.* **2003**, *9*, 669–676. [CrossRef] [PubMed]

136. Wheeler-Jones, C.; Abu-Ghazaleh, R.; Cospedal, R.; Houliston, R.A.; Martin, J.; Zachary, I. Vascular endothelial growth factor stimulates prostacyclin production and activation of cytosolic phospholipase A2 in endothelial cells via p42/p44 mitogen-activated protein kinase. *FEBS Lett.* **1997**, *420*, 28–32. [CrossRef]

137. Gerber, H.P.; McMurtrey, A.; Kowalski, J.; Yan, M.; Keyt, B.A.; Dixit, V.; Ferrara, N. Vascular endothelial growth factor regulates endothelial cell survival through the phosphatidylinositol 3'-kinase/Akt signal transduction pathway. Requirement for Flk-1/KDR activation. *J. Biol. Chem.* **1998**, *273*, 30336–30343. [CrossRef] [PubMed]

138. Gerber, H.P.; Dixit, V.; Ferrara, N. Vascular endothelial growth factor induces expression of the antiapoptotic proteins Bcl-2 and A1 in vascular endothelial cells. *J. Biol. Chem.* **1998**, *273*, 13313–13316. [CrossRef] [PubMed]

139. Xiao, Z.; Liu, Q.; Mao, F.; Wu, J.; Lei, T. TNF-α-induced VEGF and MMP-9 expression promotes hemorrhagic transformation in pituitary adenomas. *Int. J. Mol. Sci.* **2011**, *12*, 4165–4179. [CrossRef] [PubMed]

140. Liang, Z.; Brooks, J.; Willard, M.; Liang, K.; Yoon, Y.; Kang, S.; Shim, H. CXCR4/CXCL12 axis promotes VEGF-mediated tumor angiogenesis through Akt signaling pathway. *Biochem. Biophys. Res. Commun.* **2007**, *359*, 716–722. [CrossRef] [PubMed]

141. Kryczek, I.; Lange, A.; Mottram, P.; Alvarez, X.; Cheng, P.; Hogan, M.; Moons, L.; Wei, S.; Zou, L.; Machelon, V.; et al. CXCL12 and vascular endothelial growth factor synergistically induce neoangiogenesis in human ovarian cancers. *Cancer Res.* **2005**, *65*, 465–472. [PubMed]

142. Motro, B.; Itin, A.; Sachs, L.; Keshet, E. Pattern of interleukin 6 gene expression in vivo suggests a role for this cytokine in angiogenesis. *Proc. Natl. Acad. Sci. USA* **1990**, *87*, 3092–3096. [CrossRef] [PubMed]

143. Nilsson, M.B.; Langley, R.R.; Fidler, I.J. Interleukin-6, secreted by human ovarian carcinoma cells, is a potent proangiogenic cytokine. *Cancer Res.* **2005**, *65*, 10794–10800. [CrossRef] [PubMed]

144. Rose-John, S.; Scheller, J.; Elson, G.; Jones, S.A. Interleukin-6 biology is coordinated by membrane-bound and soluble receptors: Role in inflammation and cancer. *J. Leukocyte Biol.* **2006**, *80*, 227–236. [CrossRef] [PubMed]

145. Hu, D.E.; Hori, Y.; Fan, T.P. Interleukin-8 stimulates angiogenesis in rats. *Inflammation* **1993**, *17*, 135–143. [CrossRef] [PubMed]

146. Koch, A.E.; Polverini, P.J.; Kunkel, S.L.; Harlow, L.A.; DiPietro, L.A.; Elner, V.M.; Elner, S.G.; Strieter, R.M. Interleukin-8 as a macrophage-derived mediator of angiogenesis. *Science* **1992**, *258*, 1798–1801. [CrossRef] [PubMed]

147. Stetler-Stevenson, W.G. Matrix metalloproteinases in angiogenesis: A moving target for therapeutic intervention. *J. Clin. Investig.* **1999**, *103*, 1237–1241. [CrossRef] [PubMed]

148. Lau, T.S.; Chan, L.K.; Wong, E.C.; Hui, C.W.; Sneddon, K.; Cheung, T.H.; Yim, S.F.; Lee, J.H.; Yeung, C.S.; Chung, T.K.; et al. A loop of cancer-stroma-cancer interaction promotes peritoneal metastasis of ovarian cancer via TNFα-TGFα-EGFR. *Oncogene* **2017**, *36*, 3576–3587. [CrossRef] [PubMed]

149. Scotton, C.J.; Wilson, J.L.; Scott, K.; Stamp, G.; Wilbanks, G.D.; Fricker, S.; Bridger, G.; Balkwill, F.R. Multiple actions of the chemokine CXCL12 on epithelial tumor cells in human ovarian cancer. *Cancer Res.* **2002**, *62*, 5930–5938. [PubMed]

150. Kulbe, H.; Hagemann, T.; Szlosarek, P.W.; Balkwill, F.R.; Wilson, J.L. The inflammatory cytokine tumor necrosis factor-α regulates chemokine receptor expression on ovarian cancer cells. *Cancer Res.* **2005**, *65*, 10355–10362. [CrossRef] [PubMed]

151. Kim, S.; Gwak, H.; Kim, H.S.; Kim, B.; Dhanasekaran, D.N.; Song, Y.S. Malignant ascites enhances migratory and invasive properties of ovarian cancer cells with membrane bound IL-6R in vitro. *Oncotarget* **2016**, *7*, 83148–83159. [CrossRef] [PubMed]

152. Wang, Y.; Niu, X.L.; Qu, Y.; Wu, J.; Zhu, Y.Q.; Sun, W.J.; Li, L.Z. Autocrine production of interleukin-6 confers cisplatin and paclitaxel resistance in ovarian cancer cells. *Cancer Lett.* **2010**, *295*, 110–123. [CrossRef] [PubMed]

153. Yung, M.M.; Tang, H.W.; Cai, P.C.; Leung, T.H.; Ngu, S.F.; Chan, K.K.; Xu, D.; Yang, H.; Ngan, H.Y.; Chan, D.W. GRO-α and IL-8 enhance ovarian cancer metastatic potential via the CXCR2-mediated TAK1/NFκB signaling cascade. *Theranostics* **2018**, *8*, 1270–1285. [CrossRef] [PubMed]

154. Cuello, M.; Ettenberg, S.A.; Nau, M.M.; Lipkowitz, S. Synergistic induction of apoptosis by the combination of trail and chemotherapy in chemoresistant ovarian cancer cells. *Gynecol. Oncol.* **2001**, *81*, 380–390. [CrossRef] [PubMed]

155. Song, Y.; Wu, J.; Oyesanya, R.A.; Lee, Z.; Mukherjee, A.; Fang, X. Sp-1 and c-Myc mediate lysophosphatidic acid-induced expression of vascular endothelial growth factor in ovarian cancer cells via a hypoxia-inducible factor-1-independent mechanism. *Clin. Cancer Res.* **2009**, *15*, 492–501. [CrossRef] [PubMed]

156. Pustilnik, T.B.; Estrella, V.; Wiener, J.R.; Mao, M.; Eder, A.; Watt, M.A.; Bast, R.C., Jr.; Mills, G.B. Lysophosphatidic acid induces urokinase secretion by ovarian cancer cells. *Clin. Cancer Res.* **1999**, *5*, 3704–3710. [PubMed]

157. Duffy, M.J. Proteases as prognostic markers in cancer. *Clin. Cancer Res.* **1996**, *2*, 613–618. [PubMed]

158. Masferrer, J.L.; Leahy, K.M.; Koki, A.T.; Zweifel, B.S.; Settle, S.L.; Woerner, B.M.; Edwards, D.A.; Flickinger, A.G.; Moore, R.J.; Seibert, K. Antiangiogenic and antitumor activities of cyclooxygenase-2 inhibitors. *Cancer Res.* **2000**, *60*, 1306–1311. [PubMed]

159. Liu, X.H.; Yao, S.; Kirschenbaum, A.; Levine, A.C. NS398, a selective cyclooxygenase-2 inhibitor, induces apoptosis and down-regulates bcl-2 expression in LNCaP cells. *Cancer Res.* **1998**, *58*, 4245–4249. [PubMed]

160. Yeung, T.L.; Leung, C.S.; Wong, K.K.; Samimi, G.; Thompson, M.S.; Liu, J.; Zaid, T.M.; Ghosh, S.; Birrer, M.J.; Mok, S.C. TGF-beta modulates ovarian cancer invasion by upregulating CAF-derived versican in the tumor microenvironment. *Cancer Res.* **2013**, *73*, 5016–5028. [CrossRef] [PubMed]

161. Frankel, A.; Mills, G.B. Peptide and lipid growth factors decrease cis-diamminedichloroplatinum-induced cell death in human ovarian cancer cells. *Clin. Cancer Res.* **1996**, *2*, 1307–1313. [PubMed]

162. Gao, Y.; Shan, N.; Zhao, C.; Wang, Y.; Xu, F.; Li, J.; Yu, X.; Gao, L.; Yi, Z. LY2109761 enhances cisplatin antitumor activity in ovarian cancer cells. *Int J. Clin. Exp. Pathol.* **2015**, *8*, 4923–4932. [PubMed]

163. Hu, Y.L.; Tee, M.K.; Goetzl, E.J.; Auersperg, N.; Mills, G.B.; Ferrara, N.; Jaffe, R.B. Lysophosphatidic acid induction of vascular endothelial growth factor expression in human ovarian cancer cells. *J. Natl. Cancer Inst.* **2001**, *93*, 762–768. [CrossRef] [PubMed]

164. Forsythe, J.A.; Jiang, B.H.; Iyer, N.V.; Agani, F.; Leung, S.W.; Koos, R.D.; Semenza, G.L. Activation of vascular endothelial growth factor gene transcription by hypoxia-inducible factor 1. *Mol. Cell. Biol.* **1996**, *16*, 4604–4613. [CrossRef] [PubMed]

165. Tan, D.S.; Agarwal, R.; Kaye, S.B. Mechanisms of transcoelomic metastasis in ovarian cancer. *Lancet Oncol.* **2006**, *7*, 925–934. [CrossRef]

166. Fidler, I.J. The pathogenesis of cancer metastasis: The 'seed and soil' hypothesis revisited. *Nat. Rev. Cancer* **2003**, *3*, 453–458. [CrossRef] [PubMed]

167. Gupta, G.P.; Massague, J. Cancer metastasis: Building a framework. *Cell* **2006**, *127*, 679–695. [CrossRef] [PubMed]

168. Talmadge, J.E.; Fidler, I.J. AACR centennial series: The biology of cancer metastasis: Historical perspective. *Cancer Res.* **2010**, *70*, 5649–5669. [CrossRef] [PubMed]

169. Yang-Hartwich, Y.; Gurrea-Soteras, M.; Sumi, N.; Joo, W.D.; Holmberg, J.C.; Craveiro, V.; Alvero, A.B.; Mor, G. Ovulation and extra-ovarian origin of ovarian cancer. *Sci. Rep.* **2014**, *4*, 6116. [CrossRef] [PubMed]

170. Russo, A.; Czarnecki, A.A.; Dean, M.; Modi, D.A.; Lantvit, D.D.; Hardy, L.; Baligod, S.; Davis, D.A.; Wei, J.J.; Burdette, J.E. PTEN loss in the fallopian tube induces hyperplasia and ovarian tumor formation. *Oncogene* **2018**, *37*, 1976–1990. [CrossRef] [PubMed]

171. Cain, R.J.; Ridley, A.J. Phosphoinositide 3-kinases in cell migration. *Biol. Cell* **2009**, *101*, 13–29. [CrossRef] [PubMed]

172. Raftopoulou, M.; Hall, A. Cell migration: Rho GTPases lead the way. *Dev. Biol.* **2004**, *265*, 23–32. [CrossRef] [PubMed]

173. Devreotes, P.; Horwitz, A.R. Signaling networks that regulate cell migration. *Cold Spring Harb Perspect. Biol.* **2015**, *7*, a005959. [CrossRef] [PubMed]

174. Robinson-Smith, T.M.; Isaacsohn, I.; Mercer, C.A.; Zhou, M.; Van Rooijen, N.; Husseinzadeh, N.; McFarland-Mancini, M.M.; Drew, A.F. Macrophages mediate inflammation-enhanced metastasis of ovarian tumors in mice. *Cancer Res.* **2007**, *67*, 5708–5716. [CrossRef] [PubMed]

175. Wilkosz, S.; Ireland, G.; Khwaja, N.; Walker, M.; Butt, R.; de Giorgio-Miller, A.; Herrick, S.E. A comparative study of the structure of human and murine greater omentum. *Anat. Embryol.* **2005**, *209*, 251–261. [CrossRef] [PubMed]

176. Tang, J.; Pulliam, N.; Ozes, A.; Buechlein, A.; Ding, N.; Keer, H.; Rusch, D.; O'Hagan, H.; Stack, M.S.; Nephew, K.P. Epigenetic Targeting of Adipocytes Inhibits High-Grade Serous Ovarian Cancer Cell Migration and Invasion. *Mol. Cancer Res.* **2018**. [CrossRef] [PubMed]

177. Meza-Perez, S.; Randall, T.D. Immunological Functions of the Omentum. *Trends Immunol.* **2017**, *38*, 526–536. [CrossRef] [PubMed]

178. Gerber, S.A.; Rybalko, V.Y.; Bigelow, C.E.; Lugade, A.A.; Foster, T.H.; Frelinger, J.G.; Lord, E.M. Preferential attachment of peritoneal tumor metastases to omental immune aggregates and possible role of a unique vascular microenvironment in metastatic survival and growth. *Am. J. Pathol.* **2006**, *169*, 1739–1752. [CrossRef] [PubMed]

179. Clark, R.; Krishnan, V.; Schoof, M.; Rodriguez, I.; Theriault, B.; Chekmareva, M.; Rinker-Schaeffer, C. Milky spots promote ovarian cancer metastatic colonization of peritoneal adipose in experimental models. *Am. J. Pathol.* **2013**, *183*, 576–591. [CrossRef] [PubMed]

180. Szatrowski, T.P.; Nathan, C.F. Production of large amounts of hydrogen peroxide by human tumor cells. *Cancer Res.* **1991**, *51*, 794–798. [PubMed]

181. Wang, Y.; Ma, J.; Shen, H.; Wang, C.; Sun, Y.; Howell, S.B.; Lin, X. Reactive oxygen species promote ovarian cancer progression via the HIF-1α/LOX/E-cadherin pathway. *Oncol. Rep.* **2014**, *32*, 2150–2158. [CrossRef] [PubMed]

182. Kundu, N.; Zhang, S.; Fulton, A.M. Sublethal oxidative stress inhibits tumor cell adhesion and enhances experimental metastasis of murine mammary carcinoma. *Clin. Exp. Metast.* **1995**, *13*, 16–22. [CrossRef]

183. Haskill, S.; Becker, S.; Fowler, W.; Walton, L. Mononuclear-cell infiltration in ovarian cancer. I. Inflammatory-cell infiltrates from tumour and ascites material. *Br. J. Cancer* **1982**, *45*, 728–736. [CrossRef] [PubMed]

184. Wang, J.M.; Griffin, J.D.; Rambaldi, A.; Chen, Z.G.; Mantovani, A. Induction of monocyte migration by recombinant macrophage colony-stimulating factor. *J. Immunol.* **1988**, *141*, 575–579. [PubMed]

185. Ramakrishnan, S.; Xu, F.J.; Brandt, S.J.; Niedel, J.E.; Bast, R.C., Jr.; Brown, E.L. Constitutive production of macrophage colony-stimulating factor by human ovarian and breast cancer cell lines. *J. Clin. Investig.* **1989**, *83*, 921–926. [CrossRef] [PubMed]

186. Plante, M.; Rubin, S.C.; Wong, G.Y.; Federici, M.G.; Finstad, C.L.; Gastl, G.A. Interleukin-6 level in serum and ascites as a prognostic factor in patients with epithelial ovarian cancer. *Cancer* **1994**, *73*, 1882–1888. [CrossRef]

187. Scambia, G.; Testa, U.; Panici, P.B.; Martucci, R.; Foti, E.; Petrini, M.; Amoroso, M.; Masciullo, V.; Peschle, C.; Mancuso, S. Interleukin-6 serum levels in patients with gynecological tumors. *Int. J. Cancer* **1994**, *57*, 318–323. [CrossRef] [PubMed]

188. Tempfer, C.; Zeisler, H.; Sliutz, G.; Haeusler, G.; Hanzal, E.; Kainz, C. Serum evaluation of interleukin 6 in ovarian cancer patients. *Gynecol. Oncol.* **1997**, *66*, 27–30. [CrossRef] [PubMed]

189. Isobe, A.; Sawada, K.; Kinose, Y.; Ohyagi-Hara, C.; Nakatsuka, E.; Makino, H.; Ogura, T.; Mizuno, T.; Suzuki, N.; Morii, E.; et al. Interleukin 6 receptor is an independent prognostic factor and a potential therapeutic target of ovarian cancer. *PLoS ONE* **2015**, *10*, e0118080. [CrossRef] [PubMed]

190. Fishman, D.A.; Liu, Y.; Ellerbroek, S.M.; Stack, M.S. Lysophosphatidic acid promotes matrix metalloproteinase (MMP) activation and MMP-dependent invasion in ovarian cancer cells. *Cancer Res.* **2001**, *61*, 3194–3199. [PubMed]

191. Reiser, C.O.; Lanz, T.; Hofmann, F.; Hofer, G.; Rupprecht, H.D.; Goppelt-Struebe, M. Lysophosphatidic acid-mediated signal-transduction pathways involved in the induction of the early-response genes prostaglandin G/H synthase-2 and Egr-1: A critical role for the mitogen-activated protein kinase p38 and for Rho proteins. *Biochem. J.* **1998**, *330 (Pt 3)*, 1107–1114. [CrossRef] [PubMed]

192. Moolenaar, W.H.; Kruijer, W.; Tilly, B.C.; Verlaan, I.; Bierman, A.J.; de Laat, S.W. Growth factor-like action of phosphatidic acid. *Nature* **1986**, *323*, 171–173. [CrossRef] [PubMed]

193. Schwartz, B.M.; Hong, G.; Morrison, B.H.; Wu, W.; Baudhuin, L.M.; Xiao, Y.J.; Mok, S.C.; Xu, Y. Lysophospholipids increase interleukin-8 expression in ovarian cancer cells. *Gynecol. Oncol.* **2001**, *81*, 291–300. [CrossRef] [PubMed]

194. Yu, X.; Zhang, Y.; Chen, H. LPA receptor 1 mediates LPA-induced ovarian cancer metastasis: An in vitro and in vivo study. *BMC Cancer* **2016**, *16*, 846. [CrossRef] [PubMed]

195. Loizzi, V.; Del Vecchio, V.; Gargano, G.; De Liso, M.; Kardashi, A.; Naglieri, E.; Resta, L.; Cicinelli, E.; Cormio, G. Biological Pathways Involved in Tumor Angiogenesis and Bevacizumab Based Anti-Angiogenic Therapy with Special References to Ovarian Cancer. *Int. J. Mol. Sci.* **2017**, *18*, 1967. [CrossRef] [PubMed]

196. Le Page, C.; Puiffe, M.L.; Meunier, L.; Zietarska, M.; de Ladurantaye, M.; Tonin, P.N.; Provencher, D.; Mes-Masson, A.M. BMP-2 signaling in ovarian cancer and its association with poor prognosis. *J. Ovarian Res.* **2009**, *2*, 4. [CrossRef] [PubMed]

197. Ozols, R.F. Treatment goals in ovarian cancer. *Int. J. Gynecol. Cancer* **2005**, *15* (Suppl. 1), 3–11. [CrossRef] [PubMed]

198. Koti, M.; Siu, A.; Clement, I.; Bidarimath, M.; Turashvili, G.; Edwards, A.; Rahimi, K.; Mes-Masson, A.M.; Squire, J.A. A distinct pre-existing inflammatory tumour microenvironment is associated with chemotherapy resistance in high-grade serous epithelial ovarian cancer. *Br. J. Cancer* **2015**, *112*, 1215–1222. [CrossRef] [PubMed]

199. Stewart, D.J. Mechanisms of resistance to cisplatin and carboplatin. *Crit Rev. Oncol Hematol* **2007**, *63*, 12–31. [CrossRef] [PubMed]

200. Damiano, J.S.; Cress, A.E.; Hazlehurst, L.A.; Shtil, A.A.; Dalton, W.S. Cell adhesion mediated drug resistance (CAM-DR): Role of integrins and resistance to apoptosis in human myeloma cell lines. *Blood* **1999**, *93*, 1658–1667. [PubMed]

201. Meads, M.B.; Hazlehurst, L.A.; Dalton, W.S. The bone marrow microenvironment as a tumor sanctuary and contributor to drug resistance. *Clin. Cancer Res.* **2008**, *14*, 2519–2526. [CrossRef] [PubMed]

202. Catlett-Falcone, R.; Landowski, T.H.; Oshiro, M.M.; Turkson, J.; Levitzki, A.; Savino, R.; Ciliberto, G.; Moscinski, L.; Fernandez-Luna, J.L.; Nunez, G.; et al. Constitutive activation of Stat3 signaling confers resistance to apoptosis in human U266 myeloma cells. *Immunity* **1999**, *10*, 105–115. [CrossRef]

203. Frassanito, M.A.; Cusmai, A.; Iodice, G.; Dammacco, F. Autocrine interleukin-6 production and highly malignant multiple myeloma: Relation with resistance to drug-induced apoptosis. *Blood* **2001**, *97*, 483–489. [CrossRef] [PubMed]

204. Meads, M.B.; Gatenby, R.A.; Dalton, W.S. Environment-mediated drug resistance: A major contributor to minimal residual disease. *Nat. Rev. Cancer* **2009**, *9*, 665–674. [CrossRef] [PubMed]

205. Cohen, S.; Mehrabi, S.; Yao, X.; Millingen, S.; Aikhionbare, F.O. Reactive Oxygen Species and Serous Epithelial Ovarian Adenocarcinoma. *Cancer Res. J.* **2016**, *4*, 106–114. [CrossRef] [PubMed]

206. St-Pierre, J.; Drori, S.; Uldry, M.; Silvaggi, J.M.; Rhee, J.; Jager, S.; Handschin, C.; Zheng, K.; Lin, J.; Yang, W.; et al. Suppression of reactive oxygen species and neurodegeneration by the PGC-1 transcriptional coactivators. *Cell* **2006**, *127*, 397–408. [CrossRef] [PubMed]

207. Kim, B.; Jung, J.W.; Jung, J.; Han, Y.; Suh, D.H.; Kim, H.S.; Dhanasekaran, D.N.; Song, Y.S. PGC1α induced by reactive oxygen species contributes to chemoresistance of ovarian cancer cells. *Oncotarget* **2017**, *8*, 60299–60311. [PubMed]

208. Duan, Z.; Feller, A.J.; Penson, R.T.; Chabner, B.A.; Seiden, M.V. Discovery of differentially expressed genes associated with paclitaxel resistance using cDNA array technology: Analysis of interleukin (IL) 6, IL-8, and monocyte chemotactic protein 1 in the paclitaxel-resistant phenotype. *Clin. Cancer Res.* **1999**, *5*, 3445–3453. [PubMed]

209. Duan, Z.; Foster, R.; Bell, D.A.; Mahoney, J.; Wolak, K.; Vaidya, A.; Hampel, C.; Lee, H.; Seiden, M.V. Signal transducers and activators of transcription 3 pathway activation in drug-resistant ovarian cancer. *Clin. Cancer Res.* **2006**, *12*, 5055–5063. [CrossRef] [PubMed]

210. Abdollahi, T.; Robertson, N.M.; Abdollahi, A.; Litwack, G. Identification of interleukin 8 as an inhibitor of tumor necrosis factor-related apoptosis-inducing ligand-induced apoptosis in the ovarian carcinoma cell line OVCAR3. *Cancer Res.* **2003**, *63*, 4521–4526. [PubMed]

211. Wiley, S.R.; Schooley, K.; Smolak, P.J.; Din, W.S.; Huang, C.P.; Nicholl, J.K.; Sutherland, G.R.; Smith, T.D.; Rauch, C.; Smith, C.A.; et al. Identification and characterization of a new member of the TNF family that induces apoptosis. *Immunity* **1995**, *3*, 673–682. [CrossRef]

212. Walczak, H.; Miller, R.E.; Ariail, K.; Gliniak, B.; Griffith, T.S.; Kubin, M.; Chin, W.; Jones, J.; Woodward, A.; Le, T.; et al. Tumoricidal activity of tumor necrosis factor-related apoptosis-inducing ligand in vivo. *Nat. Med.* **1999**, *5*, 157–163. [CrossRef] [PubMed]

213. Bristow, R.E.; Baldwin, R.L.; Yamada, S.D.; Korc, M.; Karlan, B.Y. Altered expression of transforming growth factor-beta ligands and receptors in primary and recurrent ovarian carcinoma. *Cancer* **1999**, *85*, 658–668. [CrossRef]

214. Li, M.; Balch, C.; Montgomery, J.S.; Jeong, M.; Chung, J.H.; Yan, P.; Huang, T.H.; Kim, S.; Nephew, K.P. Integrated analysis of DNA methylation and gene expression reveals specific signaling pathways associated with platinum resistance in ovarian cancer. *BMC Med. Genom.* **2009**, *2*, 34. [CrossRef] [PubMed]

215. Psyrri, A.; Kassar, M.; Yu, Z.; Bamias, A.; Weinberger, P.M.; Markakis, S.; Kowalski, D.; Camp, R.L.; Rimm, D.L.; Dimopoulos, M.A. Effect of epidermal growth factor receptor expression level on survival in patients with epithelial ovarian cancer. *Clin. Cancer Res.* **2005**, *11*, 8637–8643. [CrossRef] [PubMed]

216. Crew, A.J.; Langdon, S.P.; Miller, E.P.; Miller, W.R. Mitogenic effects of epidermal growth factor and transforming growth factor-α on EGF-receptor positive human ovarian carcinoma cell lines. *Eur. J. Cancer* **1992**, *28*, 337–341. [CrossRef]

217. Ferrandina, G.; Ranelletti, F.O.; Martinelli, E.; Paglia, A.; Zannoni, G.F.; Scambia, G. Cyclo-oxygenase-2 (Cox-2) expression and resistance to platinum versus platinum/paclitaxel containing chemotherapy in advanced ovarian cancer. *BMC Cancer* **2006**, *6*, 182. [CrossRef] [PubMed]

218. Ferrandina, G.; Lauriola, L.; Zannoni, G.F.; Fagotti, A.; Fanfani, F.; Legge, F.; Maggiano, N.; Gessi, M.; Mancuso, S.; Ranelletti, F.O.; et al. Increased cyclooxygenase-2 (COX-2) expression is associated with chemotherapy resistance and outcome in ovarian cancer patients. *Ann. Oncol.* **2002**, *13*, 1205–1211. [CrossRef] [PubMed]

219. Kim, A.; Ueda, Y.; Naka, T.; Enomoto, T. Therapeutic strategies in epithelial ovarian cancer. *J. Exp. Clin. Cancer Res.* **2012**, *31*, 14. [CrossRef] [PubMed]

220. Ellis, L.M.; Hicklin, D.J. VEGF-targeted therapy: Mechanisms of anti-tumour activity. *Nat. Rev. Cancer* **2008**, *8*, 579–591. [CrossRef] [PubMed]

221. Aghajanian, C.; Blank, S.V.; Goff, B.A.; Judson, P.L.; Teneriello, M.G.; Husain, A.; Sovak, M.A.; Yi, J.; Nycum, L.R. OCEANS: A randomized, double-blind, placebo-controlled phase III trial of chemotherapy with or without bevacizumab in patients with platinum-sensitive recurrent epithelial ovarian, primary peritoneal, or fallopian tube cancer. *J. Clin. Oncol.* **2012**, *30*, 2039–2045. [CrossRef] [PubMed]

222. Burger, R.A.; Brady, M.F.; Bookman, M.A.; Fleming, G.F.; Monk, B.J.; Huang, H.; Mannel, R.S.; Homesley, H.D.; Fowler, J.; Greer, B.E.; et al. Incorporation of bevacizumab in the primary treatment of ovarian cancer. *N. Engl. J. Med.* **2011**, *365*, 2473–2483. [CrossRef] [PubMed]

223. Perren, T.J.; Swart, A.M.; Pfisterer, J.; Ledermann, J.A.; Pujade-Lauraine, E.; Kristensen, G.; Carey, M.S.; Beale, P.; Cervantes, A.; Kurzeder, C.; et al. A phase 3 trial of bevacizumab in ovarian cancer. *N. Engl. J. Med.* **2011**, *365*, 2484–2496. [CrossRef] [PubMed]

224. Brown, E.R.; Charles, K.A.; Hoare, S.A.; Rye, R.L.; Jodrell, D.I.; Aird, R.E.; Vora, R.; Prabhakar, U.; Nakada, M.; Corringham, R.E.; et al. A clinical study assessing the tolerability and biological effects of infliximab, a TNF-α inhibitor, in patients with advanced cancer. *Ann. Oncol.* **2008**, *19*, 1340–1346. [CrossRef] [PubMed]

225. Guo, Y.; Nemeth, J.; O'Brien, C.; Susa, M.; Liu, X.; Zhang, Z.; Choy, E.; Mankin, H.; Hornicek, F.; Duan, Z. Effects of siltuximab on the IL-6-induced signaling pathway in ovarian cancer. *Clin. Cancer Res.* **2010**, *16*, 5759–5769. [CrossRef] [PubMed]

226. Xu, S.; Grande, F.; Garofalo, A.; Neamati, N. Discovery of a novel orally active small-molecule gp130 inhibitor for the treatment of ovarian cancer. *Mol. Cancer Ther.* **2013**, *12*, 937–949. [CrossRef] [PubMed]

227. Dijkgraaf, E.M.; Santegoets, S.J.; Reyners, A.K.; Goedemans, R.; Wouters, M.C.; Kenter, G.G.; van Erkel, A.R.; van Poelgeest, M.I.; Nijman, H.W.; van der Hoeven, J.J.; et al. A phase I trial combining carboplatin/doxorubicin with tocilizumab, an anti-IL-6R monoclonal antibody, and interferon-α2b in patients with recurrent epithelial ovarian cancer. *Ann. Oncol.* **2015**, *26*, 2141–2149. [CrossRef] [PubMed]

228. Bhola, N.E.; Balko, J.M.; Dugger, T.C.; Kuba, M.G.; Sanchez, V.; Sanders, M.; Stanford, J.; Cook, R.S.; Arteaga, C.L. TGF-beta inhibition enhances chemotherapy action against triple-negative breast cancer. *J. Clin. Investig.* **2013**, *123*, 1348–1358. [CrossRef] [PubMed]

229. Alsina-Sanchis, E.; Figueras, A.; Lahiguera, A.; Gil-Martin, M.; Pardo, B.; Piulats, J.M.; Marti, L.; Ponce, J.; Matias-Guiu, X.; Vidal, A.; et al. TGFbeta Controls Ovarian Cancer Cell Proliferation. *Int. J. Mol. Sci.* **2017**, *18*, 1658. [CrossRef] [PubMed]

230. Secord, A.A.; Blessing, J.A.; Armstrong, D.K.; Rodgers, W.H.; Miner, Z.; Barnes, M.N.; Lewandowski, G.; Mannel, R.S.; Gynecologic Oncology, G. Phase II trial of cetuximab and carboplatin in relapsed

platinum-sensitive ovarian cancer and evaluation of epidermal growth factor receptor expression: A Gynecologic Oncology Group study. *Gynecol. Oncol.* **2008**, *108*, 493–499. [CrossRef] [PubMed]

231. Chekerov, R.; Klare, P.; Krabisch, P.; Potenberg, J.; Heinrich, G.; Mueller, L.; Kurbacher, C.M.; Grischke, E.-M.; Braicu, E.I.; Wimberger, P.; et al. Panitumumab in platinum-sensitive epithelial ovarian cancer patients with KRAS wild-type: The PROVE-study, a phase II randomized multicenter study of the North-Eastern German Society of Gynaecologic Oncology. *J. Clin. Oncol.* **2017**, *35* (Suppl. 1), 5558.

5

Ovarian Tumor Microenvironment Signaling: Convergence on the Rac1 GTPase

Laurie G. Hudson [1,2,*,†], Jennifer M. Gillette [2,3,†], Huining Kang [2,4], Melanie R. Rivera [2,3] and Angela Wandinger-Ness [2,3,†]

[1] Department of Pharmaceutical Sciences, University of New Mexico Health Sciences Center, Albuquerque, NM 87131, USA

[2] Comprehensive Cancer Center, University of New Mexico Health Sciences Center, Albuquerque, NM 87131, USA; jgillette@salud.unm.edu (J.M.G.); HuKang@salud.unm.edu (H.K.); MelRivera@salud.unm.edu (M.R.R.); awandinger-ness@salud.unm.edu (A.W.-N.)

[3] Department of Pathology, University of New Mexico Health Sciences Center, Albuquerque, NM 87131, USA

[4] Department of Medicine, University of New Mexico Health Sciences Center, Albuquerque, NM 87131, USA

* Correspondence: lhudson@salud.unm.edu

† These authors contributed equally to this manuscript.

Abstract: The tumor microenvironment for epithelial ovarian cancer is complex and rich in bioactive molecules that modulate cell-cell interactions and stimulate numerous signal transduction cascades. These signals ultimately modulate all aspects of tumor behavior including progression, metastasis and therapeutic response. Many of the signaling pathways converge on the small GTPase Ras-related C3 botulinum toxin substrate (Rac)1. In addition to regulating actin cytoskeleton remodeling necessary for tumor cell adhesion, migration and invasion, Rac1 through its downstream effectors, regulates cancer cell survival, tumor angiogenesis, phenotypic plasticity, quiescence, and resistance to therapeutics. In this review we discuss evidence for Rac1 activation within the ovarian tumor microenvironment, mechanisms of Rac1 dysregulation as they apply to ovarian cancer, and the potential benefits of targeting aberrant Rac1 activity in this disease. The potential for Rac1 contribution to extraperitoneal dissemination of ovarian cancer is addressed.

Keywords: Rho-GTPase; Rac1; guanine nucleotide exchange factors (GEFs); GTPase activating proteins (GAPs); oncogene; oncoprotein; ovarian cancer; tumor microenvironment; bone niche; therapeutic targeting

1. Introduction

Despite advances in treatment, long-term outcomes for epithelial ovarian cancer (EOC) patients remain discouraging. Challenges to effective treatment include factors such as diagnosis after tumor dissemination, presence of residual disease after treatment, a limited number of identified targets for maintenance therapy, and acquired chemoresistance leading to relapse after initial clinical remission [1,2]. EOC displays a high degree of genomic heterogeneity [3,4] and it has been proposed that tumor microenvironmental factors may also contribute to tumor heterogeneity [5].

EOC dissemination occurs predominantly through tumor cell exfoliation into the peritoneal cavity thereby providing a unique environment for tumor growth and metastasis when compared to the majority of solid tumors [6–10]. There is heterogeneity of sites within the peritoneal cavity leading to diverse localized environments. For example, the omentum is rich in adipocytes and provides a distinct niche when compared to the mesothelium of the peritoneal wall [10–18]. Furthermore, the tissue underlying the mesothelial lining at various locations differs in architecture and local production of chemotactic factors thus promoting different adhesive and invasive behaviors [11]. It may be more accurate to consider the peritoneal cavity as home to multiple tumor microenvironments (TMEs) presenting additional challenges to effective treatment.

Tumor cells within the ovarian cancer TME are exposed to a variety of regulatory signals. Tumor cells interact with mesothelium, fibroblasts, endothelium, immune cells and other cells in the TME [6–10,19,20]. Invasive cells come into contact with the extracellular matrix (ECM) underlying the mesothelium. This leads to intracellular signaling due to integrin engagement and exposure to ECM-associated growth factors. Each cell type in the TME, as well as the tumor cells themselves, secrete bioactive molecules that accumulate in the peritoneal fluids and drive adverse tumor cell behaviors such as proliferation, invasion, and phenotypes promoting chemoresistance. These cell-cell interactions between tumor cells or other cells in the TME, cell-matrix interactions, and exposure to growth factors and cytokines present in peritoneal fluids all stimulate signaling cascades that dictate aspects of tumor cell function. Many of these diverse signals converge upon, and are integrated through, the small GTPase Ras-related C3 botulinum toxin substrate (Rac) 1 (Figure 1) [21–26].

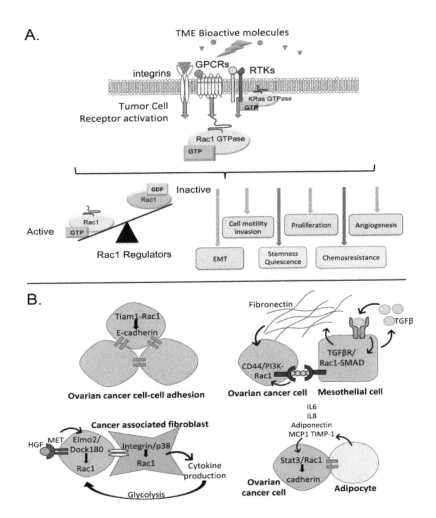

Figure 1. Bioactive molecules in the tumor microenvironment (TME) activate multiple receptors that converge on Rac1. (**A**) Examples of receptors that activate Rac1 in response to bioactive molecules in the TME are shown (GPCR = G protein-coupled receptor; RTK = receptor tyrosine kinase). Rac1 activity is balanced through multiple regulatory mechanisms discussed in this review that serve to control diverse physiological outcomes. (**B**) Cell-cell interactions between tumor cells themselves or with cells in the TME (adipocytes, cancer-associated fibroblasts, mesothelia) can also cause Rac1 activation and further modulate the TME. See Section 3.3 for further detail.

The Rac subfamily of Rho family small GTPases has three members. Rac1 is the best-characterized member of this subfamily with strong evidence for Rac1 dysregulation in cancer [21,23–25,27,28]. Rac2 expression is confined to hematopoietic cells [29] and Rac3 has not been studied in the context of ovarian cancer so these two proteins will not be discussed further in this review. Rac1 acts as a molecular switch by cycling between active and inactive states that depend upon nucleotide binding (Figure 1A) and other regulatory mechanisms discussed below. As a focal point for multiple signaling pathways, Rac1 is capable of shunting cells between proliferation, apoptosis or quiescence, altering cell differentiation and transcription, and modulating cell-environment interactions. Based on the known activities of Rac1, this protein can play important roles in multiple steps of tumor development, dissemination and disease recurrence.

2. Consequences of Rac1 Activation in Cancer

Rac1 cycles between an active GTP-bound state and an inactive GDP-bound conformation (Figure 1A) regulated by guanine nucleotide exchange factors (GEFs), GTPase-activating proteins (GAPs) and guanine nucleotide dissociation inhibitors (GDIs) [24]. Aberrant activation of Rac1 is implicated in numerous aspects of tumor development and progression and is the subject of several recent reviews [25,26,30,31]. Rac1 is best recognized for translating extracellular signaling into downstream changes in actin remodeling, cell adhesion, motility and invasion [23,26,32]. There is strong emerging evidence that Rac1 also contributes to the tumor stem cell phenotype, epithelial to mesenchymal transition (EMT), angiogenesis, and chemoresistance [33–38]. Elevated Rac1 activity is associated with enhanced stem cell characteristics in multiple cancers and its inhibition attenuates the stem cell phenotype [34,36,39]. Although the relationship between Rac1 expression and/or elevated activity and cancer stem cells has been reported for several cancer types, there is little information for ovarian cancer. However, a splice variant of Vav3, a GEF and enhancer of Rac1 activity, is overexpressed in multi-drug resistant stem cell-like fractions of ovarian cancer cells [40]. This finding suggests that elevated Rac1 activity may promote stem cell characteristics in ovarian cancer similar to the reports for other tumor types.

Ovarian cancer cells display phenotypic plasticity with gains and losses of epithelial characteristics during tumor development and peritoneal metastasis [41–43]. EMT is viewed as a critical aspect of tumor invasion and metastasis [44,45] and Rac1 is implicated in promoting EMT in a number of cancers [25]. Experimental evidence demonstrates that elevated Rac1 activity is sufficient to drive aspects of EMT in ovarian tumor cells. When a mutationally activated form of Rac1 (Rac1G12V) was introduced into ovarian tumor cells with an epithelial phenotype, cells displayed morphologic characteristics of EMT including down-regulation of the epithelial marker E-cadherin, up-regulation of the mesenchymal marker vimentin, and increased invasive capacity [46]. Inhibition of Rac1 activity or knockdown of Rac1 expression restored epithelial characteristics to ovarian tumor cells [13,46,47] and inhibited migration and invasion [47–49]. The significance of EMT in ovarian cancer is demonstrated by the presence of ovarian cancer cells in extraperitoneal sites [50–52] and the circulation [50,53–55] where the circulating tumor cells display mesenchymal characteristics [54,56]

Tumor angiogenesis supplies necessary nutrients and fosters tumor growth [22]. Angiogenesis is a critical aspect of ovarian cancer and this process is targeted by therapeutics in current care [57–59]. Rac1 is involved in angiogenesis and required for vascular integrity and blood vessel sprouting as demonstrated in a conditional Rac1 knockout mouse model [60]. In humans, Rac1 expression correlated with blood vessel invasion in a meta-analysis of multiple cancer studies [38]. Rac1 is activated by the angiogenic factors vascular endothelial growth factor (VEGF)-A, angiopoietin 1, basic fibroblast growth factor (FGF) and others [61]. Activation of Rac1 in endothelial cells regulates adhesion, filopodia, morphogenesis, cell proliferation and migration [33,62–65]. Two different Rac1 inhibitors displayed anti-angiogenic activity in breast cancer models in vivo [66,67] supporting a potential benefit of Rac1 inhibition as an alternate anti-angiogenic strategy in cancer, including ovarian cancer.

Lymphangiogenesis is driven by the VEGF-C ligand and its high affinity receptor VEGFR3 [68,69]. The well-established omental niche site has vessels that express high levels of the neoangiogenic VEGFR3, which serve to recruit ovarian tumor cells and offer a supportive environment for neovascularization [70]. High VEGF-C expression is associated with worse overall survival in ovarian cancer patients and tumor cell expression of VEGF-C is critical for lymphatic invasion and lymphangiogenesis [71,72]. Mechanistic studies show VEGF-C signaling to Rac1 requires VEGFR3 endocytosis mediated by EphrinB2 [73]. In colorectal and lung cancers, lymph node metastasis mediated by VEGF-C is linked to high expression of the Rac1 activating GEF Tiam1 [74,75]. Conversely, a chemical library screen identified statins as potent inhibitors of lymphangiogenesis by blocking Rac1 prenylation and plasma membrane recruitment [69]. In this regard it is worth noting that inhibition of VEGFR3 signaling in OVCAR8 cells, via Maz51, induced chemosensitization through downregulation of BRCA gene expression. This finding suggests that combined targeting of VEGFR3 and Rac1 may have benefit for dually blocking metastasis and enhancing tumor cell killing [76].

Rac1 is gaining substantial attention as a mediator of chemoresistance [37,77,78]. Rac1 is implicated in treatment resistance in multiple cancers [37] and Rac1 inhibition increases sensitivity to doxorubicin for squamous cell carcinoma cells, 5-fluorouracil and cisplatin in gastric adenocarcinoma spheroids, and fludarabine for chronic lymphocytic leukemia (reviewed in [37]). In addition to these conventional chemotherapies, Rac1 is suspected in resistance to a number of targeted therapies through regulation of compensatory mechanisms. These include therapies directed against the epidermal growth factor (EGF) receptor and human epidermal growth factor receptor (HER)-2 for lung and breast cancers, B-RAF protein inhibitors in melanoma, estrogen targeted therapies in breast cancer and VEGF/VEGFR targeted therapies in prostate cancer (reviewed in [30]). In many cases sensitivity to the targeted therapeutic is restored upon Rac1 inhibition. The contributions of Rac1 activation to chemoresistance is likely multifaceted based on specific mechanisms along distinct drug action pathways, as well as non-specific mechanisms related to Rac1 promotion of EMT and stem cell characteristics [42,79–81].

3. Pathways for Rac1 Activation by the Ovarian Tumor Microenvironment

Extracellular signals mediated by various cell surface receptors such as integrins, cadherins, cytokine receptors, G-protein-coupled receptors (GPCRs) and receptor tyrosine kinases (RTKs) activate GEFs and recruit Rac1 (sequestered with GDIs) from the cytosol to the plasma membrane or other cellular locations (Figure 3A [21,30,82,83]). Rac1 then activates effector molecules including proteins involved in actin remodeling, kinases, and adapter proteins that are responsible for propagating Rac1-dependent signals and subsequent biological responses. The specific stimulus can dictate distinct responses to Rac1 activation based on post-translational modifications of Rac1, GEFs or other Rac1 modulatory molecules or effectors [21]. Because Rac1 is responsive to an array of signals, Rac1 is capable of driving multiple steps of tumor development, dissemination and recurrence. A few examples of Rac1 activation by common components of ascitic fluids are described in more detail below.

3.1. Activators of G-Protein Coupled Receptors and Rac1 Activity

The bioactive lipids lysophosphatidic acid (LPA) and sphingosine-1-phosphate (S1P) are present in ascitic fluid of ovarian cancer patients and activate GPCRs upstream of Rac1. Elevated levels of LPA and S1P are both associated with ovarian tumor cell migration, invasion and metastasis [6,84] and these processes require Rac1-dependent actin remodeling. Pharmacologic inhibition of Rac1 decreased S1P-dependent ovarian tumor cell invasion [85]. When multiple ovarian tumor cell lines were studied, the ability of LPA to stimulate migration was highly correlated with LPA-dependent Rac1 activation [86]. Expression of a dominant negative form of Rac1 ablated LPA-stimulated cell migration and in vivo metastatic colonization in responsive cell lines. Conversely, expression of a constitutively active form of Rac1 conferred migration and in vivo implantation to cell lines non-responsive to LPA [86]. Knock-down strategies determined that a Rac1-activating SOS1/EPS8/ABI1 complex unique to metastatic cells was responsible for the LPA stimulated migration and invasive implantation in mice [86]. LPA activation of Rac1 has also been reported to be dependent on a Src/p130Cas pathway for ovarian cell migration [87] and the Rac1 GEF βPIX was necessary for LPA-induced invadopodia formation [88] although βPIX knock-down did not disrupt LPA-stimulated migration in certain ovarian tumor cell lines [86]. The reported observations indicate that distinct Rac1 regulatory mechanisms are responsible for different functional outputs and there may be cell-specific differences based on the expression or activity of Rac1 regulators.

3.2. Activators of Tyrosine Kinases and Rac1 Activity

Ligands for RTKs such as the EGF receptor and VEGF receptor are prevalent in ovarian cancer ascites and regulate Rac1 activation through multiple mechanisms. Signaling through RTKs activate phosphatidylinositol-3 kinase and phospholipase C-γ to modulate targeting of Rac1 regulatory proteins such as GEFs and GAPs and recruit GEFs to signaling complexes through post-translational modifications (reviewed in [21,89]). In certain cases, signaling receptors can modify Rac1 activity directly. For example, EGF receptor-stimulated ERK phosphorylation of Rac1 on T108 targets Rac1 for nuclear translocation [21]. Rac1 has been shown to be an essential component of EGF receptor signaling in different tumor types [90,91] and implicated in EGF receptor driven tumorigenesis [91]. Ligands present in the ovarian TME are likely to activate Rac1 by impinging on ErbB3, ErbB4 and MET receptors, which are expressed in 76–98% of ovarian tumors [92]. For example, heregulin stimulation of ErbB3 and ErbB4 causes upregulation of C-X-C chemokine receptor type 4 (CXCR4) and increases Rac1 activation through a stromal cell-derived factor (SDF)-1-CXCR4 mediated PREX1 GEF mechanism in breast cancer cells [93]. Hepatocyte growth factor (HGF) induces a MET-AXL-ELMO2-DOCK180 complex that activates Rac1-dependent cancer cell migration and invasion [94]. Pharmacologic inhibition of Rac1 inhibited EGF-stimulated p21-activating kinase (PAK) phosphorylation, filopodia formation and invadopodia [48,95] in ovarian tumor cell lines indicating contributions of Rac1 in cancer-relevant functions. Although specific mechanisms of Rac1 activation by VEGF have not been explored in ovarian cancer models, there is abundant evidence that Rac1 is a component of VEGF signaling to angiogenesis. Ablation of Rac1 in endothelial cells in development is embryonic lethal due to lack of neovascularization [96]. Studies show that Rac1 activation is critical for normal in vivo angiogenesis in adult mice due to junctional stabilization required for mature vessels [97]. More recent work indicates that lumen formation and stable cell:cell contacts are mediated through the GEF DOCK4 activation of Rac1 [62]. The combined data indicate that further study of Rac1 activation in ovarian cancer by tyrosine kinase receptors and their interfaces with G-protein coupled receptors is warranted.

3.3. Cell Interactions Leading to Rac1 Activation

An article in the present series and other recent reviews provide an in depth analysis of cell-cell interactions in the ovarian tumor microenvironment that drive ovarian cancer progression [9,57,98]. Here, we briefly highlight how some of these interactions may promote ovarian cancer metastasis through Rac1-dependent mechanisms (Figure 1B).

3.3.1. Tumor Cell-Cell Adhesion

Rac1 signaling is important for cell-cell adhesion. Ovarian cancer cells in the ascites fluid form multicellular aggregates (spheroids) that facilitate angiogenesis and invasion of various peritoneal organs [11]. Tumor cell-cell adhesions are mediated by E-cadherin maintenance of cell-cell junctions that depend on a Rac1-Tiam1 GEF-IQGAP1 effector complex and promote an anti-migratory phenotype [99]. Ovarian cancer spheroids with high E-cadherin expression are less sensitive to cisplatin treatment suggesting an important role for cell-cell adhesions in spheroid chemoresistance [100].

3.3.2. Mesothelial Cells

Ovarian cancer frequently metastasizes to the peritoneal wall, which is lined with mesothelial cells. Ovarian cancer cell interactions with mesothelial cells can stimulate mesothelial cell production of fibronectin through the autocrine secretion of transforming growth factor (TGF)-β1. This activates a TGF-βR1/Rac1/SMAD-dependent signaling pathway in mesothelial cells. The activated mesothelial cells and production of fibronectin contributes to metastasis by supporting tumor cell adhesion, invasion, and proliferation [13,57]. Co-culture of ovarian cancer cell lines with mesothelial cells led to upregulated expression of the hyaluronan receptor and stem cell marker CD44 and promoted tumorigenesis in a xenograft model [101]. CD44 promotes ovarian tumor cell-peritoneal cell adhesion through binding of its ligand hyaluronan in complex with versican [102] and is generally known to signal through multiple pathways downstream of Rac1 to promote tumor cell invasion [103].

3.3.3. Fibroblasts

Ovarian tumor cell-fibroblast interactions cause conversion of normal fibroblasts to cancer-associated fibroblasts (CAFs, distinguished by smooth muscle actin expression) and lead to increased tumor cell adhesion and overexpression of HGF and matrix metalloproteinase (MMP) [104]. MET receptor activation by HGF induced recruitment of the bipartite Rac1 GEF Elmo2/Dock180 and promoted Rac1-dependent migration and invasion of multiple cancer cell lines in vitro, though ovarian cell lines were not specifically tested [94]. Interactions between human omental CAF and ovarian tumor cells also result in an integrin/p38/Rac1-dependent activation of cytokine secretion by CAFs, which in turn promotes tumor cell proliferation and metastasis through activated glycogen breakdown and glycolysis [105].

3.3.4. Adipocytes

The omentum is a favored ovarian tumor cell niche based on initial chemoattraction by adipocyte secreted factors that can stimulate Stat3-mediated Rac1 activation [106]. In turn, the activation of these pathways can strengthen cadherin-dependent binding of tumor cells, provide tumor cells with an energy source through mutual changes in lipid metabolism, and promote invasion [14,106].

The selected illustrations do not capture the entire scope of potential ovarian cancer TME regulation of Rac1 activity. Inflammatory cytokines such as interleukins 6 and 8, tumor necrosis factor (TNF) α, and TGFβ are among the additional soluble factors in ascites fluids that are associated with worse prognosis and variously associated with proliferation, metastatic spread, angiogenesis, EMT and treatment resistance [6,107]. Each of these bioactive molecules is capable of stimulating signaling cascades leading to Rac1 activation through direct or indirect mechanisms [24]. In addition, integrin engagement and focal adhesion kinase activation recruits Rac1 to regulate spreading and adhesion on the extracellular matrix [26,89,108]. Immune cells are an integral part of the ovarian cancer TME and perform immune suppressive and activating functions that are pivotal in disease pathology [109,110] and these cells serve as important therapeutic targets [111,112]. The best-studied example of immune cell coupling to Rac1 activation in ovarian cancer is through cytokine activation of CXCR4 as detailed in Sections 4.2 and 6. A more complete understanding of the complexities of Rac1 regulation by the ovarian cancer TME will require further study.

4. Mechanisms of Rac1 Dysregulation and Evidence in Ovarian Cancer

We reported that Rac1 protein is overexpressed and hyperactivated in ovarian cancer patient samples [113]. Addressing the function of Rac1 hyperactivation in ovarian cancer is an important research area because of the known roles of Rac1 in cancer metastasis and recurrence. In cancer, Rac1 is frequently released from normal control mechanisms through mutation [114–118], aberrant regulation of nucleotide binding and hydrolysis [26,30,119], and altered splicing [120–130]. Insight into possible mechanisms leading to Rac1 overexpression and hyperactivation in ovarian cancer is garnered from analyses of the Catalogue of Somatic Mutations in Cancer (COSMIC) and The Cancer Genome Atlas (TCGA) databases as detailed below.

4.1. Rac1 Overexpression and Somatic Mutation

There are 239 pathogenic missense mutations across diverse cancer types affecting 46 of the 192 amino acids in RAC1 (COSMIC v86 database updated in August 2018, https://cancer.sanger.ac.uk/ cosmic/download). The mutants are clustered in conserved residues relevant to GTPase activity or affect residues close in 3D space that are important to Rac1 function (Figure 2A,B [117,118,131–133]). Select point mutants are the primary cause of constitutive Rac1 activation in some cancer types (melanoma, lung and germ cell cancers) (Figure 2A [114–118,132,134]). The highest prevalence (9%) of the constitutively active, fast cycling P29S mutant is found in melanoma [115]. To date, the functionally characterized Rac1 missense mutants (P29S, A159V, C18S and G15) all increase Rac1 activation and possibly expression [118,135]. Rac1 is not found mutant in the 315 serous ovarian cancer patient samples in the TCGA. However, given the low frequency of Rac1 missense mutants (0.01–0.02% for G15, C18 [118]) such rare mutations would be undetectable in the sample size and should not be taken as lack of evidence for the importance of Rac1 in ovarian cancer. For example, an shRNA essentiality screen of 29 ovarian cancer cell lines showed SKOV3, COV362, JHM + OM1 and SNU840 to have significantly decreased growth fitness with the loss of Rac1 (Harmonizome Achilles [136,137]. As another case in point, Rac1 is overexpressed due to gene amplification or mRNA upregulation in 21% (66/316) of the primary tumors in TCGA [138]. Despite the low frequency of RAC1 gene mutations, RAC1 is similar to well-known oncogenes and tumor suppressors in being categorized as a Tier 1 cancer-causing gene in the COSMIC cancer gene census. Therefore, further systematic study of the 239 Rac1 missense mutations is warranted. In contrast to tumor suppressor genes, where truncating mutations are prevalent and cause loss of function, the Rac1 mutations are like those in the oncoprotein Ras. The mutations appear in hotspots and tend to be activating mutations [139]. Thus, RAC1 is a Tier 1 cancer-causing gene and the mutational patterns in Rac1 are similar to many well-known oncogenes which are positive drivers of cancer.

4.2. Rac1 Regulators

The activity of Rac1 is tightly controlled through a large network of GEF and GAP regulatory factors (Figure 3A,B [30,131,140–143]). This network is much greater than most other Ras-related GTPases. Rac1 GEF and GAP regulatory factors are mutant or exhibit altered expression in ovarian serous adenocarcinoma with a frequency of 0.3–1.6% based on our analyses of 28 relevant regulatory proteins in COSMIC v86 [144] and the cBioPortal platform for TCGA data viewing [19,131] (Figure 4 [20,83,118,138,144–147]).

Notably, the regulatory protein mutants show a high level of concurrent expression in tumor cells, suggesting that hitting multiple nodes releases key Rac1-regulated pathways from normal control. Even while the identified mutations often lie in known GEF and GAP regulatory domains, as well as in lipid or protein interaction domains, no systematic analyses have been completed to identify hotspot mutations or determine their pathogenicity in ovarian cancer. Nevertheless, some insights can be drawn from a handful of analyses of regulatory protein overexpression [109,148,149], truncation [150] or altered splice variants [40]; see also review [30].

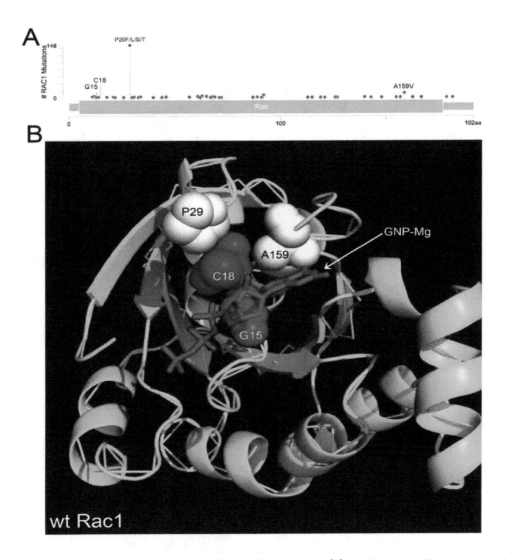

Figure 2. Pathogenic Cancer Mutations in Rac1. Rac1 gain of function mutations occur with low frequency (0.2–1%) in multiple cancer types, though as yet none have been found in serous ovarian cancer. (**A**) There are 239 pathogenic mutations in Rac1, resulting in missense substitutions at 46 amino acid residues. Melanoma has the highest frequency of Rac1 mutations, leading to substitutions at proline 29 and constitutive activation through GEF-independent fast nucleotide exchange. (**B**) Thirteen of the missense mutants are likely oncogenic (G12R/V/E, G15S, C18S/Y, P29F/L/S/T, Q61R/K, A159V) evidenced by recurrence at hotspots, paralogous with oncogenic mutations in Ras, or affecting residues that are clustered in the 3D structure close to the nucleotide binding site. Shown is the proximity of 4 point mutants in the crystal structure of wild-type Rac1 (PDB 3th5) rendered with MacPyMOL: PyMOL v1.5.0.5 (Schrödinger LLC).

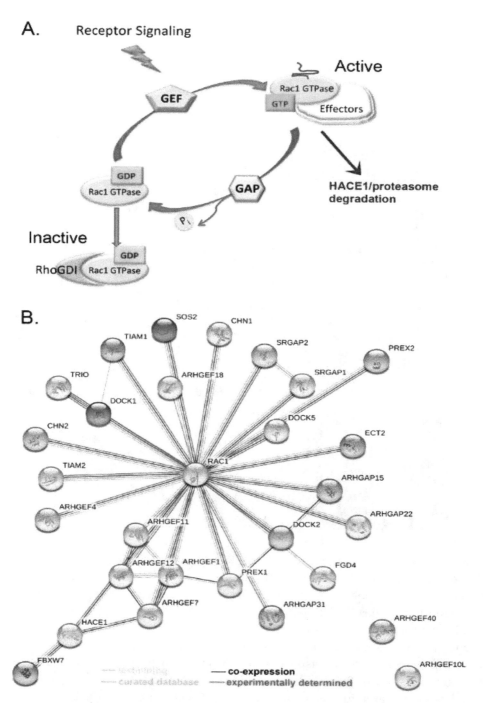

Figure 3. Rac1 Regulatory Network in Ovarian Cancer. Rac1 integrates signals downstream of tyrosine kinase receptors, adhesion molecules and G-protein coupled receptors and has nuclear functions. **(A)** There are over 40 GEF and GAP proteins involved in the regulation of Rac1 activity through the stimulation of nucleotide binding (GEFs) and hydrolysis (GAPs). Activated Rac1 binds to effectors that recognize the unique conformation of the GTP-bound GTPase and mediate downstream physiologic responses to receptor signaling. Activated Rac1 is ubiquitinated by HACE1 or FBXW7 and targeted for proteasomal degradation, further controlling protein levels and activity. **(B)** Twenty-six Rac1 GEF and GAP proteins, HACE1 and FBXW7 ubiquitin ligases have somatic mutations in serous ovarian cancer patient samples. String network analysis places Rac1 at the core with a large array of close functional associations with Rac1 regulatory proteins whose functions in ovarian cancer largely remain to be determined.

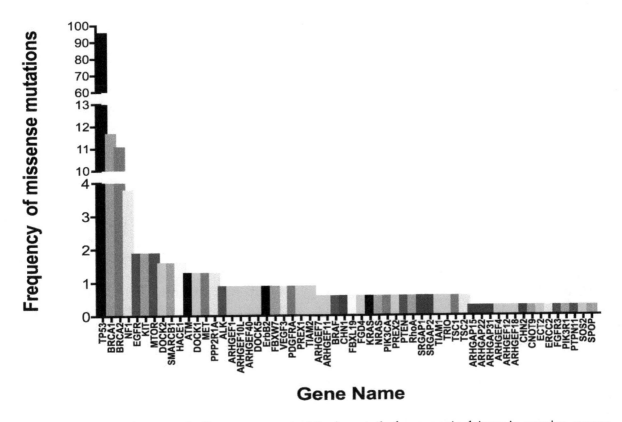

Figure 4. Rac1 regulators and effectors are part of the long tail of oncogenic drivers in ovarian cancer. A list of 54 genes with frequent missense mutations in cancers was derived from OncoKB: A precision oncology knowledge base and two recent publications on rare mutations. The cancer gene list was combined with a selected list of 28 Rac1 regulatory proteins (GEFs, GAPs, ubiquitin ligases). Plotted is the frequency of missense mutations in genes with mutation frequencies above 0 (58 of 82 analyzed) among 315 serous ovarian cancer patient samples in TCGA. The frequency for BRCA1 and BRCA2 gene mutations is the sum of somatic and germline missense mutations. For all other genes no germ line mutations are reported. Among the analyzed genes, 53 (9.2%) are Tier 1 of 574 reported in COSMIC v86; Tier 1 genes have "*documented activity relevant to cancer, plus evidence of mutations in cancer, which change the activity of the gene product in a way that promotes oncogenic transformation*". Among the Rac1 regulators only ARHGEF12 and ARHGEF10L are validated as Tier 1 and Tier 2 ("*strong indication of a role in cancer*"), respectively. Cancer genes (black and gray), Rac1 GEFs (green), Rac1 GAPs (red), ubiquitin ligases (yellow). The data show that even though missense mutations in individual Rac1 regulators occur with low frequency, there are at least 26 possible targets (10 with co-occurring alterations, $p < 0.05$) that might lead to Rac1 activation or inactivation in ovarian cancer.

Overexpression of the Rac1 GEF DOCK180 drives glioblastoma invasion through the activation of a Rac1-dependent kinase pathway [149]. A truncating mutant of PREX2 in melanoma has increased Rac1 GEF activity, and activates PI3K/AKT signaling, while abolishing binding to the PTEN tumor suppressor in melanoma [150]. An N-terminally truncated splice variant of the Vav3 GEF (Vav3.1) is a predictor of poor prognosis and platinum-response and highly expressed in ovarian cancer stem-like cell populations isolated from established cell lines [40]. These examples are supportive of a requirement for Rac1 activation in multiple cancers. Recent analyses of the metastatic TME using omental samples from patients with high grade serous ovarian cancer characterized secreted, matrix and cellular components [109]. Multivariate regression analyses of data were used to model the relationships between all TME components. Comprehensive RNA seq analysis of the TME identified 31 Rac1 GEFs, GAPS and ubiquitin ligases significantly associated with disease score by Pearson's and Spearman's tests; five GEFs and GAPs were significant based on Pearson's only (supplementary

Table 13 in [109]). Recent analyses of a large cohort of Canadian ovarian cancer patients identified variants in ARHGEF10L to be significantly associated with invasive disease [151] and three somatic missense mutations have been identified in ovarian cancer patient samples (COSMIC v86). The limited information on ARHGEF10L suggests in vitro GEF activity for RhoA, but not Rac1 or Cdc42 [152]. Since RhoA and Rac1 are often reciprocally active, connections between the two GTPases may need further analysis in ovarian cancer. Alterations in GAP expression in vivo have both activating and inhibitory effects on tumorigenesis and metastasis, likely due to dual roles as scaffolding proteins and GTP hydrolysis regulators [30]. When considering how to tackle prioritization of GEF and GAP proteins for study, categorizing potential tumor suppressive vs. promoting activity might be gained by using a ratiometric analysis of truncating/frameshift vs. missense mutations [139]. Additionally, functional analyses of select point mutants in key regulatory domains is an essential complementary effort that is necessary to understand effects on regulatory protein activity and pathway interconnections. The composite data are suggestive that Rac1 hyperactivation is an important driver in ovarian cancer and may result largely from the misregulation of GEF and GAP regulatory cascades rather than through activating mutations in Rac1 itself.

Emerging evidence suggests that Rac1 regulatory proteins function in spatially localized molecular assemblies. Such assemblies restrict Rac1 activity temporally and spatially to specific subcellular domains, which in turn restricts what downstream pathways are triggered by Rac1. In ovarian cancer, a recently described tripartite complex that includes the SOS1 GEF is essential for LPA-mediated Rac1 activation and metastasis [86]. Activation of Rac1 by the Tiam1 or PREX1 GEF proteins is spatially distinct in the cell and dictates anti- or pro-migratory responses in ovarian cancer cells [99]. The translocation of Rac1 in response to signaling and transient assembly of Rac1 GEFs at the plasma membrane can also occur through specific actin and protein based recruitment [82]. On the other hand, Rac1 forms a stable plasma membrane complex with CXCR4 independent of GTP-bound status, which is important for maintaining CXCR4 in a signaling competent conformation [153]. The PREX1 GEF is speculated to enable rapid response of Rac1 activation downstream of CXCR4 signaling. Therefore, functional studies of Rac1 and associated regulatory factors in the ovarian metastatic cascade will need to carefully consider spatiotemporal organization.

4.3. Rac1b Splice Variant

The constitutively active Rac1b splice variant mRNA level [113] and protein levels are moderate to high in the majority of serous papillary ovarian adenocarcinoma cells (Figure 5). Interestingly, Rac1b is also differentially expressed in underlying stromal cells in malignant serous papillary ovarian adenocarcinoma tissue as compared to normal ovary. The prognostic or diagnostic significance of overexpression of canonical Rac1 in ovarian cancer and/or the potential role(s) of the hyperactivated, fast cycling Rac1b isoform remain open questions. We analyzed RAC1 mRNA expression data for 298 Stage III primary serous ovarian cancer patient samples in TCGA using isoform analysis tools [154,155]. The results demonstrate that high total RAC1 mRNA expression is associated with worse outcomes (Figure 6A,B) and concur with a report that analyzed Rac1 as a risk factor in a cohort of 150 Chinese ovarian cancer patients [47]. High expression of the canonical RAC1 isoform also trended to worse outcomes but was not statistically significant (Figure 6C). The impact of RAC1b isoform expression on ovarian patient survival has not been reported and was of particular interest. Rac1b protein drives tumor cell proliferation and EMT and is upregulated by MMP3, a known survival risk factor in breast, lung, and pancreatic cancers [124,156–158]. High mRNA expression of the fast cycling and constitutively active RAC1b isoform does not predict ovarian cancer patient survival and trended toward higher survival probability (Figure 6D [113,120–122,129,130,155]); the finding was consistent irrespective of various groupings, treatment as a continuous variable or when expressed as a fraction of total RAC1 mRNA expression. The only other study assessing the significance of RAC1b isoform expression measured the prognostic value of RAC1b in progression free and overall survival [159]. Findings were based on quantitative RT-PCR analyses of 157 metastatic colorectal cancer patient samples following relapse after first line chemotherapy. In contrast to our findings in primary ovarian tumors, fractional RAC1b overexpression was significantly associated with poor progression free (HR 0.54, $p = 0.49$) and overall survival (HR 0.53, $p = 0.039$) in metastatic colorectal cancer patients. Similar to the ovarian cancer patients, RAC1b expression was not mutually exclusive and 152/157 (97%) of the metastatic colorectal patients had higher canonical RAC1 than RAC1b expression. To date there are no studies that have distinguished the functions of Rac1 and Rac1b overexpression or activity in the absence of endogenous protein, in part due to the essentiality of Rac1 function [128,160]. Together, these data indicate that overexpression and aberrant Rac1 and/or Rac1b activity are closely tied to malignant ovarian cancer and further dissection of their respective roles in tumor microenvironment responsiveness, metastasis and relapse is warranted.

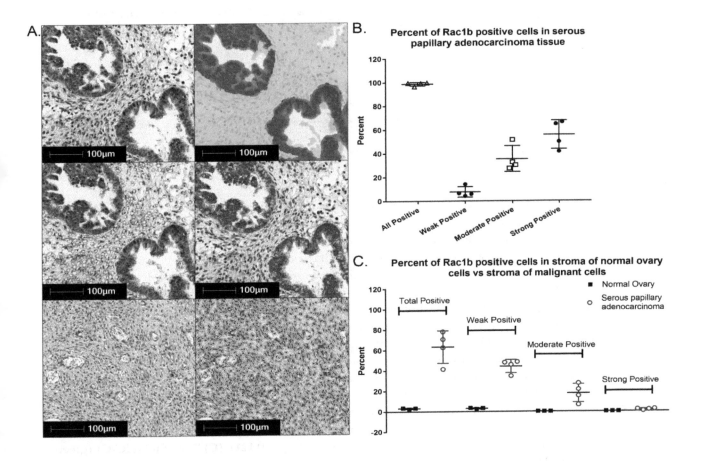

Figure 5. The constitutively active Rac1b splice variant is overexpressed in ovarian cancer. Ovarian cancer tissue microarrays were stained for Rac1b, a constitutively active Rac1 splice variant. Slides were imaged using an Aperio slide scanner and analysis was performed using HALO software. (**A**) Top panel: Malignant tissue stained with DAB for Rac1b. Analysis to identify tumor cells (red) and stromal cells (green). Middle panel: Quantification of the amount of Rac1b expression in tumor cells (right) vs. stromal cells (left) in malignant tissue. Blue-no staining, yellow-weak staining, orange-moderate staining, red-strong staining. Bottom panel: Quantification of Rac1b expression in stromal cells in normal ovary tissue, colors as for middle panel. (**B**) The majority of serous papillary ovarian adenocarcinoma cells were moderately to strongly positive for Rac1b, while stromal cells were weakly positive. (**C**) Quantitative comparisons of normal ovary tissue and serous papillary ovarian adenocarcinoma tissue evidences an elevated expression of Rac1b in the stromal cells adjacent to the malignant tumor cells relative to normal tissue.

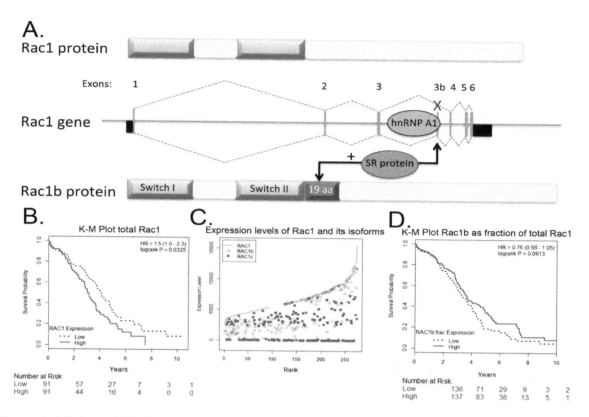

Figure 6. High total RAC1 expression predicts reduced ovarian cancer patient survival. (**A**) Rac1 undergoes regulated splicing in response to growth factor signaling, which is subject to positive and negative regulation by hnRNP A1 and SR protein. The resulting splice variant is called Rac1b and contains a 19 amino acid insert adjacent to the Switch II region. Rac1b is a fast cycling, constitutively active and frequently overexpressed in cancer, including ovarian cancer. (**B**) Kaplan-Meier plot of high vs. low total RAC1 mRNA expression. TCGA datasets for total and RAC1 isoform mRNA expression in ovarian cancer patients from ISOexpresso; uc003spx.3 (canonical RAC1) and uc003spw.3 (RAC1b containing exon 3b/4). Analyses were restricted to 298 patients with Stage III and Stage IV disease. Patients were divided into 3 groups based on total Rac1 expression. Upper tertile values represent high total Rac1 expression and lower tertile values represent low expression, middle values were excluded. Patients with high RAC1 expression have worse survival outcomes than those with low RAC1 expression (HR = 1.5, p = 0.0325); analogous results obtained using data direct from TCGA and CASViewer. No evidence for an association between isoform RAC1b and survival outcomes (HR = 0.96, p = 0.82, not shown). Higher expression of the canonical RAC1 isoform trended to lower survival probability, though was not statistically significant (HR = 1.37, p = 0.121). (**C**) Plot of total RAC1 (green line), canonical RAC1c (blue diamond), and RAC1b (red square) expression in each patient ranked according to expression levels. (**D**) Kaplan-Meier plot of RAC1b as a fraction of total RAC1, with two groups defined based on median expression. High RAC1b expression (HR = 0.76, p = 0.0913).

5. Potential Benefits of Targeting Aberrant Rac1 Activity in Ovarian Cancer

The broad impact of Rac1 on tumor cell behavior has led to consideration of Rac1 as a potential therapeutic target [25,28,95,161–163]. In ovarian cancer cell lines, knock down of Rac1 expression decreased fibronectin production [13], reversed EMT as measured by increased E-cadherin and decreased vimentin expression [46,47], inhibited tumor cell migration and invasion [47] and reduced tumor growth in a xenograft model [47]. An inhibitor of Rac1 (NSC23766) decreased ovarian tumor cell migration, invasion and matrix-metalloproteinase production [48,49,95].

Although a number of small molecule inhibitors have been developed to inhibit Rac1 activity (e.g., NSC23766, EHT 1864, EHop-016 and its derivative MBQ-167), these agents have not been translated to human use [66,164–166]. A high-throughput screen of the Prestwick library of off patent, FDA-approved drugs identified activators and inhibitors of Rho GTPases [95]. The resultant findings coupled with cheminformatics approaches identified the R-enantiomers of a limited number of non-steroidal anti-inflammatory drugs (NSAIDs), R-naproxen and R-ketorolac, as inhibitors of Rac1 [95]. The S-enantiomers are pharmacologic NSAIDs based on cyclooxygenase (COX) inhibition. GTPase inhibition by the R-enantiomers represents a previously unidentified pharmacologic activity. R-naproxen and R-ketorolac inhibit serum and EGF-stimulated Rac1 and Cdc42 activation and downstream signaling through a proposed allosteric mechanism [48,95]. R-ketorolac was tested using ovarian tumor cell lines and primary ovarian tumor cells isolated from patient ascites fluids [48]. R-ketorolac was an effective Rac1 inhibitor and decreased downstream signaling as demonstrated by reduction of PAK1 and PAK2 phosphorylation. R-ketorolac inhibited Rac1-dependent cellular functions in ovarian cancer cell lines and primary cells including inhibition of growth factor-stimulated formation of filopodia, cell adhesion to fibronectin and type I collagen, development of invadopodia and tumor cell migration [48]. The inhibitory effects of R-ketorolac in cells are comparable to those of established Rac1 and Cdc42 selective inhibitors [48,167].

In Phase 0 human studies, ovarian cancer patients received racemic ketorolac for its FDA-approved indication in postoperative analgesia [113] then blood and peritoneal fluids were collected at intervals for 24h. After administration of the racemic drug, R-ketorolac was detected in patient peritoneal fluids. The concentration of R-ketorolac was sufficient to inhibit Rac1 activity in cells retrieved from the peritoneal compartment of these post-surgical ovarian cancer patients. Potential benefit of R-ketorolac is suggested by the results of a medical record review to compare the ovarian cancer–specific survival of ovarian cancer patients who did or did not receive ketorolac [113]. The medical record review revealed increased survival of patients receiving ketorolac and this observation is consistent with other reports of improved clinical outcomes associated with ketorolac usage in breast cancer patients [168–170]. The overall findings suggest that ovarian cancer patients may benefit from inhibition of Rac1 in the clinical setting.

6. Other Ovarian Tumor Microenvironments: Extraperitoneal Dissemination and Bone Niche as a Sanctuary Site and Potential Reservoir for Relapse

While ovarian cancer metastasis is largely confined to the peritoneal cavity and localized to the omentum, there is strong evidence for extra-peritoneal dissemination [171,172]. As illustrated in preceding sections, Rac1 plays a critical role in the key processes that impact tumor dissemination and as such, Rac1 may contribute to ovarian tumor cell escape from the peritonium. Particularly in advanced disease, ovarian carcinoma can spread to distant organs by both hematogenous dissemination and lymphatic invasion [173]. In a well-designed parabiosis study, ovarian tumor cells were found to spread in anastomosed mice within two weeks of ovary injection [18], clearly illustrating hematogenous spread of the disease. Additionally, circulating tumor cells (CTCs) are frequently detected in patients [53,174]. In fact, CTCs were detected in 90% (98/109) of newly diagnosed ovarian cancer patients, where the number of CTCs correlated with disease stage and was altered with treatment [175]. Lymph node involvement of the disease is also common and has been proposed as a potential prognostic factor with site-specific prognostic differences identified between the ovary and lymph node [176]. However, this study was unable to rule out the "safe haven" hypothesis for metastatic ovarian tumor cells in retroperitoneal lymph nodes and suggested that lymph node dissection after complete cytoreduction is warranted pending further prospective data collection [176]. Interestingly, recent work comparing the survival of patients with distant lymph node metastases to patients with pleural metastases or other distant ovarian cancer metastases found increased survival in women having lymph nodes as their only distant metastatic site [177]. A follow up study investigating the relationship between site-specific patterns of distant metastases and overall survival also found that patients with lymph node metastasis had the longest survival when compared to women with other metastatic disease [173]. Collectively, these data suggest that disease dissemination through the lymphatics may have a less aggressive phenotype than disease that spreads hematogenously. Future studies will be necessary to quantitatively compare the aggressive nature of ovarian cancer cells with respect to their route of disease dissemination.

Once outside the peritoneum, other common sites of distant metastatic ovarian cancer include the liver, lung, and bone [6]. While frank bone metastases are rare in ovarian cancer [173,178], prognosis of cases with bone metastasis is poor. A recent publication [179] followed up on previous observations of bone marrow disseminated tumor cells (DTCs) in ovarian cancer patients [51,52,180,181] and affirmed that bone DTCs correlated with reduced progression free and overall survival [182,183]. Bone marrow was isolated from 79 ovarian cancer patients pre- and post-platinum-based chemotherapy. Bone DTCs were detected in 42% and 41% of patients before and after chemotherapy, respectively, illustrating the chemoresistance of cells in the bone niche [179]. Alterations in the bone microenvironment caused by irradiation and cisplatin therapy can further promote and increase metastatic spread that may be ameliorated by non-steroidal anti-inflammatory agents [184]. Additionally, tumor secreted factors such as CCL2 can activate cells in the bone marrow promoting a premetastatic niche and paving the way for successful tumor dissemination at a secondary site [98]. The predominant signaling axis that promotes bone marrow homing is the CXCR4/SDF-1α signaling cascade [185]. The expression and secretion of SDF-1α is abundant in the bone marrow microenvironment (expressed by osteoblasts and endothelial cells) and promotes the homing and maintenance of CXCR4+ cells within the bone marrow. In addition to driving hematopoietic cells as well as breast and prostate cancer cells to the bone [186–189], CXCR4/SDF-1α signaling has also been shown to promote ovarian cancer metastasis and is a predictor of poor prognosis in ovarian cancer [190,191]. Overexpression of CXCR4 is associated with cisplatin resistant ovarian cancer [192] as well as the peritoneal [193], hematogenous [194] and lymph node [195] dissemination of the disease. Moreover, CXCR4 can modulate cancer cell migration through interactions with the downstream effector Rac1 [196]. In fact, blocking or silencing of CXCR4 was found to significantly reduce RhoA and Rac-1/Cdc42 expression levels and decrease ovarian cancer cell migration [197]. Additionally, CXCR4 blockade reduced ovarian tumor growth in animal models [198,199]. Therefore, CXCR4 appears to be a shared signaling mechanism that facilitates homing and engraftment within the peritoneal cavity and the bone marrow microenvironment. How Rac1 specifically influences ovarian tumor cells within these two separate environments remains to be explored.

Ovarian cancer metastasis has long been studied in the context of the peritoneal compartment where the bulk of the tumor grows. However, as we improve our systemic and palliative therapy for ovarian cancer patients, an increasing occurrence of unusual distant metastases is being reported. Despite compelling human findings, the overall significance of the bone niche with respect to ovarian cancer prognosis remains ill-defined and suggests that a shift in research focus to understudied metastatic sites such as the bone will be critical to improving patient outcomes. Moreover, the bone marrow dissemination of ovarian cancer cells has been largely overlooked as a potential mechanism for relapse, where the persistence of tumor cells in the protected bone niche could contribute to disease recurrence. Therefore, future studies should be directed at identifying factors that enable tumor cells to be harbored in specialized niche sites that include the bone. By targeting bone marrow-resident tumor cells, we may uncover mechanistic strategies to eradicate distant tumor cell reservoirs that contribute to ovarian cancer relapse and poor overall patient survival.

7. Conclusions

Ovarian cancer remains a leading cause of death in women resulting from gynecologic malignancy principally due to recurrent, drug resistant disease, and limited options for targeted therapies. Greater understanding of signaling proteins that mediate tumor microenvironmental drivers of disease and resistance may provide new avenues for therapeutic development. Rac1 is at the nexus of numerous signaling pathways stimulated by the ovarian cancer TME and has broad roles in cancer beyond the well-recognized regulation of actin remodeling, tumor cell adhesion and migration. Rac1-dependent functions in EMT, stem cell phenotypes, angiogenesis and chemoresistance all have high relevance to ovarian cancer. Although more research is needed regarding specific contributions of aberrant Rac1 activity in ovarian cancer and disease dissemination with respect to specialized microenvironments, current knowledge suggests benefits of targeting Rac1, alone or in combination, for disease treatment.

Author Contributions: Conceptualization, L.G.H., J.M.G. and A.W.-N.; Methodology, A.W.-N.; Formal Analysis, H.K.; Investigation, M.R.R.; Data Curation, A.W.-N.; Writing—Original Draft Preparation, L.G.H., J.M.G. and A.W.-N.; Writing—Review & Editing, L.G.H., J.M.G., H.K., M.R.R., A.W.-N.; Visualization, H.K., A.W.-N., M.R.R.; Supervision, L.G.H., J.M.G. and A.W.-N.; Project Administration, L.G.H., J.M.G. and A.W.-N.; Funding Acquisition, L.G.H., J.M.G. and A.W.-N.

Acknowledgments: Rac1b imaging and analyses were conducted using the University of New Mexico Pathology Dept. & Comprehensive Cancer Center Human Tissue Repository & Tissue Analysis Shared Resource. We thank Fred Schultz, M.A. for Aperio scanning of IHC slides and training in the use of Halo quantitative imaging software (Indica Labs).

References

1. Christie, E.L.; Bowtell, D.D.L. Acquired chemotherapy resistance in ovarian cancer. *Ann. Oncol.* **2017**, *28*, viii13–viii15. [CrossRef] [PubMed]

2. DiSilvestro, P.; Alvarez Secord, A. Maintenance treatment of recurrent ovarian cancer: Is it ready for prime time? *Cancer Treat. Rev.* **2018**, *69*, 53–65. [CrossRef] [PubMed]

3. Kroeger, P.T., Jr.; Drapkin, R. Pathogenesis and heterogeneity of ovarian cancer. *Curr. Opin. Obstet. Gynecol.* **2017**, *29*, 26–34. [CrossRef] [PubMed]

4. Previs, R.A.; Sood, A.K.; Mills, G.B.; Westin, S.N. The rise of genomic profiling in ovarian cancer. *Expert Rev. Mol. Diagn.* **2016**, *16*, 1337–1351. [CrossRef] [PubMed]

5. Kim, S.; Kim, B.; Song, Y.S. Ascites modulates cancer cell behavior, contributing to tumor heterogeneity in ovarian cancer. *Cancer Sci.* **2016**, *107*, 1173–1178. [CrossRef] [PubMed]

6. Thibault, B.; Castells, M.; Delord, J.P.; Couderc, B. Ovarian cancer microenvironment: Implications for cancer dissemination and chemoresistance acquisition. *Cancer Metastasis Rev.* **2014**, *33*, 17–39. [CrossRef] [PubMed]

7. Ghoneum, A.; Afify, H.; Salih, Z.; Kelly, M.; Said, N. Role of tumor microenvironment in ovarian cancer pathobiology. *Oncotarget* **2018**, *9*, 22832–22849. [CrossRef] [PubMed]

8. Ghoneum, A.; Afify, H.; Salih, Z.; Kelly, M.; Said, N. Role of tumor microenvironment in the pathobiology of ovarian cancer: Insights and therapeutic opportunities. *Cancer Med.* **2018**. [CrossRef] [PubMed]

9. Weidle, U.H.; Birzele, F.; Kollmorgen, G.; Rueger, R. Mechanisms and Targets Involved in Dissemination of Ovarian Cancer. *Cancer Genom. Proteom.* **2016**, *13*, 407–423. [CrossRef]

10. Worzfeld, T.; Pogge von Strandmann, E.; Huber, M.; Adhikary, T.; Wagner, U.; Reinartz, S.; Muller, R. The Unique Molecular and Cellular Microenvironment of Ovarian Cancer. *Front. Oncol.* **2017**, *7*, 24. [CrossRef] [PubMed]

11. Steinkamp, M.P.; Winner, K.K.; Davies, S.; Muller, C.; Zhang, Y.; Hoffman, R.M.; Shirinifard, A.; Moses, M.; Jiang, Y.; Wilson, B.S. Ovarian tumor attachment, invasion, and vascularization reflect unique microenvironments in the peritoneum: Insights from xenograft and mathematical models. *Front. Oncol* **2013**, *3*, 97. [CrossRef] [PubMed]

12. Giridhar, P.V.; Funk, H.M.; Gallo, C.A.; Porollo, A.; Mercer, C.A.; Plas, D.R.; Drew, A.F. Interleukin-6 receptor enhances early colonization of the murine omentum by upregulation of a mannose family receptor, LY75, in ovarian tumor cells. *Clin. Exp. Metastasis* **2011**, *28*, 887–897. [CrossRef] [PubMed]

13. Kenny, H.A.; Chiang, C.Y.; White, E.A.; Schryver, E.M.; Habis, M.; Romero, I.L.; Ladanyi, A.; Penicka, C.V.; George, J.; Matlin, K.; et al. Mesothelial cells promote early ovarian cancer metastasis through fibronectin secretion. *J. Clin. Investig.* **2014**, *124*, 4614–4628. [CrossRef] [PubMed]

14. Nieman, K.M.; Kenny, H.A.; Penicka, C.V.; Ladanyi, A.; Buell-Gutbrod, R.; Zillhardt, M.R.; Romero, I.L.; Carey, M.S.; Mills, G.B.; Hotamisligil, G.S.; et al. Adipocytes promote ovarian cancer metastasis and provide energy for rapid tumor growth. *Nat. Med.* **2011**, *17*, 1498–1503. [CrossRef] [PubMed]

15. McGrail, D.J.; Kieu, Q.M.; Dawson, M.R. The malignancy of metastatic ovarian cancer cells is increased on soft matrices through a mechanosensitive Rho-ROCK pathway. *J. Cell Sci.* **2014**, *127*, 2621–2626. [CrossRef] [PubMed]

16. Lungchukiet, P.; Sun, Y.; Kasiappan, R.; Quarni, W.; Nicosia, S.V.; Zhang, X.; Bai, W. Suppression of epithelial ovarian cancer invasion into the omentum by 1alpha,25-dihydroxyvitamin D3 and its receptor. *J. Steroid Biochem. Mol. Biol.* **2015**, *148*, 138–147. [CrossRef] [PubMed]

17. Khan, S.M.; Funk, H.M.; Thiolloy, S.; Lotan, T.L.; Hickson, J.; Prins, G.S.; Drew, A.F.; Rinker-Schaeffer, C.W. In vitro metastatic colonization of human ovarian cancer cells to the omentum. *Clin. Exp. Metastasis* **2010**, *27*, 185–196. [CrossRef] [PubMed]

18. Pradeep, S.; Kim, S.W.; Wu, S.Y.; Nishimura, M.; Chaluvally-Raghavan, P.; Miyake, T.; Pecot, C.V.; Kim, S.J.; Choi, H.J.; Bischoff, F.Z.; et al. Hematogenous metastasis of ovarian cancer: Rethinking mode of spread. *Cancer Cell* **2014**, *26*, 77–91. [CrossRef] [PubMed]

19. Cerami, E.; Gao, J.; Dogrusoz, U.; Gross, B.E.; Sumer, S.O.; Aksoy, B.A.; Jacobsen, A.; Byrne, C.J.; Heuer, M.L.; Larsson, E.; et al. The cBio cancer genomics portal: An open platform for exploring multidimensional cancer genomics data. *Cancer Discov.* **2012**, *2*, 401–404. [CrossRef] [PubMed]

20. Cook, D.R.; Rossman, K.L.; Der, C.J. Rho guanine nucleotide exchange factors: Regulators of Rho GTPase activity in development and disease. *Oncogene* **2014**, *33*, 4021–4035. [CrossRef] [PubMed]

21. Haga, R.B.; Ridley, A.J. Rho GTPases: Regulation and roles in cancer cell biology. *Small GTPases* **2016**, *7*, 207–221. [CrossRef] [PubMed]

22. Bid, H.K.; Roberts, R.D.; Manchanda, P.K.; Houghton, P.J. RAC1: An emerging therapeutic option for targeting cancer angiogenesis and metastasis. *Mol. Cancer Ther.* **2013**, *12*, 1925–1934. [CrossRef] [PubMed]

23. Cardama, G.A.; Gonzalez, N.; Maggio, J.; Menna, P.L.; Gomez, D.E. Rho GTPases as therapeutic targets in cancer (Review). *Int. J. Oncol.* **2017**, *51*, 1025–1034. [CrossRef] [PubMed]

24. Hodge, R.G.; Ridley, A.J. Regulating Rho GTPases and their regulators. *Nat. Rev. Mol. Cell Biol.* **2016**, *17*, 496–510. [CrossRef] [PubMed]

25. Jansen, S.; Gosens, R.; Wieland, T.; Schmidt, M. Paving the Rho in cancer metastasis: Rho GTPases and beyond. *Pharmacol. Ther.* **2018**, *183*, 1–21. [CrossRef] [PubMed]

26. Lawson, C.D.; Ridley, A.J. Rho GTPase signaling complexes in cell migration and invasion. *J. Cell Biol.* **2018**, *217*, 447–457. [CrossRef] [PubMed]

27. Porter, A.P.; Papaioannou, A.; Malliri, A. Deregulation of Rho GTPases in cancer. *Small GTPases* **2016**, *7*, 123–138. [CrossRef] [PubMed]

28. Zandvakili, I.; Lin, Y.; Morris, J.C.; Zheng, Y. Rho GTPases: Anti- or pro-neoplastic targets? *Oncogene* **2017**, *36*, 3213–3222. [CrossRef] [PubMed]

29. Troeger, A.; Williams, D.A. Hematopoietic-specific Rho GTPases Rac2 and RhoH and human blood disorders. *Exp. Cell Res.* **2013**, *319*, 2375–2383. [CrossRef] [PubMed]

30. Kazanietz, M.G.; Caloca, M.J. The Rac GTPase in Cancer: From Old Concepts to New Paradigms. *Cancer Res.* **2017**, *77*, 5445–5451. [CrossRef] [PubMed]

31. Maldonado, M.D.M.; Dharmawardhane, S. Targeting Rac and Cdc42 GTPases in Cancer. *Cancer Res.* **2018**, *78*, 3101–3111. [CrossRef] [PubMed]

32. Sadok, A.; Marshall, C.J. Rho GTPases: Masters of cell migration. *Small GTPases* **2014**, *5*, e29710. [CrossRef] [PubMed]

33. Orgaz, J.L.; Herraiz, C.; Sanz-Moreno, V. Rho GTPases modulate malignant transformation of tumor cells. *Small GTPases* **2014**, *5*, e29019. [CrossRef] [PubMed]

34. Akunuru, S.; Palumbo, J.; Zhai, Q.J.; Zheng, Y. Rac1 targeting suppresses human non-small cell lung adenocarcinoma cancer stem cell activity. *PLoS ONE* **2011**, *6*, e16951. [CrossRef] [PubMed]

35. Wang, J.Y.; Yu, P.; Chen, S.; Xing, H.; Chen, Y.; Wang, M.; Tang, K.; Tian, Z.; Rao, Q.; Wang, J. Activation of Rac1 GTPase promotes leukemia cell chemotherapy resistance, quiescence and niche interaction. *Mol. Oncol.* **2013**, *7*, 907–916. [CrossRef] [PubMed]

36. Yoon, C.H.; Hyun, K.H.; Kim, R.K.; Lee, H.; Lim, E.J.; Chung, H.Y.; An, S.; Park, M.J.; Suh, Y.; Kim, M.J.; et al. The small GTPase Rac1 is involved in the maintenance of stemness and malignancies in glioma stem-like cells. *FEBS Lett.* **2011**, *585*, 2331–2338. [CrossRef] [PubMed]

37. Cardama, G.A.; Alonso, D.F.; Gonzalez, N.; Maggio, J.; Gomez, D.E.; Rolfo, C.; Menna, P.L. Relevance of small GTPase Rac1 pathway in drug and radio-resistance mechanisms: Opportunities in cancer therapeutics. *Crit. Rev. Oncol. Hematol.* **2018**, *124*, 29–36. [CrossRef] [PubMed]

38. Lou, S.; Wang, P.; Yang, J.; Ma, J.; Liu, C.; Zhou, M. Prognostic and Clinicopathological Value of Rac1 in Cancer Survival: Evidence from a Meta-Analysis. *J. Cancer* **2018**, *9*, 2571–2579. [CrossRef] [PubMed]

39. Nayak, R.C.; Chang, K.H.; Vaitinadin, N.S.; Cancelas, J.A. Rho GTPases control specific cytoskeleton-dependent functions of hematopoietic stem cells. *Immunol. Rev.* **2013**, *256*, 255–268. [CrossRef] [PubMed]

40. Reimer, D.; Boesch, M.; Wolf, D.; Marth, C.; Sopper, S.; Hatina, J.; Altevogt, P.; Parson, W.; Hackl, H.; Zeimet, A.G. Truncated isoform Vav3.1 is highly expressed in ovarian cancer stem cells and clinically relevant in predicting prognosis and platinum-response. *Int. J. Cancer* **2018**, *142*, 1640–1651. [CrossRef] [PubMed]

41. Klymenko, Y.; Kim, O.; Stack, M.S. Complex Determinants of Epithelial: Mesenchymal Phenotypic Plasticity in Ovarian Cancer. *Cancers* **2017**, *9*, 104. [CrossRef] [PubMed]

42. Deng, J.; Wang, L.; Chen, H.; Hao, J.; Ni, J.; Chang, L.; Duan, W.; Graham, P.; Li, Y. Targeting epithelial-mesenchymal transition and cancer stem cells for chemoresistant ovarian cancer. *Oncotarget* **2016**, *7*, 55771–55788. [CrossRef] [PubMed]

43. Barbolina, M.V.; Moss, N.M.; Westfall, S.D.; Liu, Y.; Burkhalter, R.J.; Marga, F.; Forgacs, G.; Hudson, L.G.; Stack, M.S. Microenvironmental regulation of ovarian cancer metastasis. *Cancer Treat. Res.* **2009**, *149*, 319–334. [PubMed]

44. da Silva-Diz, V.; Lorenzo-Sanz, L.; Bernat-Peguera, A.; Lopez-Cerda, M.; Munoz, P. Cancer cell plasticity: Impact on tumor progression and therapy response. *Semin. Cancer Biol.* **2018**. [CrossRef] [PubMed]

45. Zhang, Y.; Weinberg, R.A. Epithelial-to-mesenchymal transition in cancer: Complexity and opportunities. *Front. Med.* **2018**. [CrossRef] [PubMed]

46. Fang, D.; Chen, H.; Zhu, J.Y.; Wang, W.; Teng, Y.; Ding, H.F.; Jing, Q.; Su, S.B.; Huang, S. Epithelial-mesenchymal transition of ovarian cancer cells is sustained by Rac1 through simultaneous activation of MEK1/2 and Src signaling pathways. *Oncogene* **2017**, *36*, 1546–1558. [CrossRef] [PubMed]

47. Leng, R.; Liao, G.; Wang, H.; Kuang, J.; Tang, L. Rac1 expression in epithelial ovarian cancer: Effect on cell EMT and clinical outcome. *Med. Oncol.* **2015**, *32*, 329. [CrossRef] [PubMed]

48. Guo, Y.; Kenney, S.R.; Muller, C.Y.; Adams, S.; Rutledge, T.; Romero, E.; Murray-Krezan, C.; Prekeris, R.; Sklar, L.A.; Hudson, L.G.; et al. R-Ketorolac Targets Cdc42 and Rac1 and Alters Ovarian Cancer Cell Behaviors Critical for Invasion and Metastasis. *Mol. Cancer Ther.* **2015**, *14*, 2215–2227. [CrossRef] [PubMed]

49. Zhou, G.; Peng, F.; Zhong, Y.; Chen, Y.; Tang, M.; Li, D. Rhein suppresses matrix metalloproteinase production by regulating the Rac1/ROS/MAPK/AP-1 pathway in human ovarian carcinoma cells. *Int. J. Oncol.* **2017**, *50*, 933–941. [CrossRef] [PubMed]

50. Romero-Laorden, N.; Olmos, D.; Fehm, T.; Garcia-Donas, J.; Diaz-Padilla, I. Circulating and disseminated tumor cells in ovarian cancer: A systematic review. *Gynecol. Oncol.* **2014**, *133*, 632–639. [CrossRef] [PubMed]

51. Fehm, T.; Banys, M.; Rack, B.; Janni, W.; Marth, C.; Blassl, C.; Hartkopf, A.; Trope, C.; Kimmig, R.; Krawczyk, N.; et al. Pooled analysis of the prognostic relevance of disseminated tumor cells in the bone marrow of patients with ovarian cancer. *Int. J. Gynecol. Cancer* **2013**, *23*, 839–845. [CrossRef] [PubMed]

52. Fehm, T.; Becker, S.; Bachmann, C.; Beck, V.; Gebauer, G.; Banys, M.; Wallwiener, D.; Solomayer, E.F. Detection of disseminated tumor cells in patients with gynecological cancers. *Gynecol. Oncol.* **2006**, *103*, 942–947. [CrossRef] [PubMed]

53. Gasparri, M.L.; Savone, D.; Besharat, R.A.; Farooqi, A.A.; Bellati, F.; Ruscito, I.; Panici, P.B.; Papadia, A. Circulating tumor cells as trigger to hematogenous spreads and potential biomarkers to predict the prognosis in ovarian cancer. *Tumour Biol. J. Int. Soc. Oncodev. Biol. Med.* **2016**, *37*, 71–75. [CrossRef] [PubMed]

54. Yeung, T.L.; Leung, C.S.; Yip, K.P.; Au Yeung, C.L.; Wong, S.T.; Mok, S.C. Cellular and molecular processes in ovarian cancer metastasis. A Review in the Theme: Cell and Molecular Processes in Cancer Metastasis. *Am. J. Physiol. Cell Physiol.* **2015**, *309*, C444–C456. [CrossRef] [PubMed]

55. Zhou, Y.; Bian, B.; Yuan, X.; Xie, G.; Ma, Y.; Shen, L. Prognostic Value of Circulating Tumor Cells in Ovarian Cancer: A Meta-Analysis. *PLoS ONE* **2015**, *10*, e0130873. [CrossRef] [PubMed]

56. Blassl, C.; Kuhlmann, J.D.; Webers, A.; Wimberger, P.; Fehm, T.; Neubauer, H. Gene expression profiling of single circulating tumor cells in ovarian cancer—Establishment of a multi-marker gene panel. *Mol. Oncol.* **2016**, *10*, 1030–1042. [CrossRef] [PubMed]

57. Nwani, N.G.; Sima, L.E.; Nieves-Neira, W.; Matei, D. Targeting the Microenvironment in High Grade Serous Ovarian Cancer. *Cancers* **2018**, *10*, 266. [CrossRef] [PubMed]

58. Monk, B.J.; Minion, L.E.; Coleman, R.L. Anti-angiogenic agents in ovarian cancer: Past, present, and future. *Ann. Oncol.* **2016** *27*, i33–i39. [CrossRef] [PubMed]

59. Hansen, J.M.; Coleman, R.L.; Sood, A.K. Targeting the tumour microenvironment in ovarian cancer. *Eur. J. Cancer* **2016**, *56*, 131–143. [CrossRef] [PubMed]

60. Nohata, N.; Uchida, Y.; Stratman, A.N.; Adams, R.H.; Zheng, Y.; Weinstein, B.M.; Mukouyama, Y.S.; Gutkind, J.S. Temporal-specific roles of Rac1 during vascular development and retinal angiogenesis. *Dev. Biol.* **2016**, *411*, 183–194. [CrossRef] [PubMed]

61. Galan Moya, E.M.; Le Guelte, A.; Gavard, J. PAKing up to the endothelium. *Cell. Signal.* **2009**, *21*, 1727–1737. [CrossRef] [PubMed]

62. Abraham, S.; Scarcia, M.; Bagshaw, R.D.; McMahon, K.; Grant, G.; Harvey, T.; Yeo, M.; Esteves, F.O.; Thygesen, H.H.; Jones, P.F.; et al. A Rac/Cdc42 exchange factor complex promotes formation of lateral filopodia and blood vessel lumen morphogenesis. *Nat. Commun.* **2015**, *6*, 7286. [CrossRef] [PubMed]

63. Fryer, B.H.; Field, J. Rho, Rac, Pak and angiogenesis: Old roles and newly identified responsibilities in endothelial cells. *Cancer Lett.* **2005**, *229*, 13–23. [CrossRef] [PubMed]

64. Soga, N.; Connolly, J.O.; Chellaiah, M.; Kawamura, J.; Hruska, K.A. Rac regulates vascular endothelial growth factor stimulated motility. *Cell Commun. Adhes.* **2001**, *8*, 1–13. [CrossRef] [PubMed]

65. Xue, Y.; Bi, F.; Zhang, X.; Pan, Y.; Liu, N.; Zheng, Y.; Fan, D. Inhibition of endothelial cell proliferation by targeting Rac1 GTPase with small interference RNA in tumor cells. *Biochem. Biophys. Res. Commun.* **2004**, *320*, 1309–1315. [CrossRef] [PubMed]

66. Humphries-Bickley, T.; Castillo-Pichardo, L.; Hernandez-O'Farrill, E.; Borrero-Garcia, L.D.; Forestier-Roman, I.; Gerena, Y.; Blanco, M.; Rivera-Robles, M.J.; Rodriguez-Medina, J.R.; Cubano, L.A.; et al. Characterization of a Dual Rac/Cdc42 Inhibitor MBQ-167 in Metastatic Cancer. *Mol. Cancer Ther.* **2017**, *16*, 805–818. [CrossRef] [PubMed]

67. Castillo-Pichardo, L.; Humphries-Bickley, T.; De La Parra, C.; Forestier-Roman, I.; Martinez-Ferrer, M.; Hernandez, E.; Vlaar, C.; Ferrer-Acosta, Y.; Washington, A.V.; Cubano, L.A.; et al. The Rac Inhibitor EHop-016 Inhibits Mammary Tumor Growth and Metastasis in a Nude Mouse Model. *Transl. Oncol.* **2014**, *7*, 546–555. [CrossRef] [PubMed]

68. Nagahashi, M.; Ramachandran, S.; Rashid, O.M.; Takabe, K. Lymphangiogenesis: A new player in cancer progression. *World J. Gastroenterol.* **2010**, *16*, 4003–4012. [CrossRef] [PubMed]

69. Schulz, M.M.; Reisen, F.; Zgraggen, S.; Fischer, S.; Yuen, D.; Kang, G.J.; Chen, L.; Schneider, G.; Detmar, M. Phenotype-based high-content chemical library screening identifies statins as inhibitors of in vivo lymphangiogenesis. *Proc. Natl. Acad. Sci. USA* **2012**, *109*, E2665–E2674. [CrossRef] [PubMed]

70. Sorensen, E.W.; Gerber, S.A.; Sedlacek, A.L.; Rybalko, V.Y.; Chan, W.M.; Lord, E.M. Omental immune aggregates and tumor metastasis within the peritoneal cavity. *Immunol. Res.* **2009**, *45*, 185–194. [CrossRef] [PubMed]

71. Kuerti, S.; Oliveira-Ferrer, L.; Milde-Langosch, K.; Schmalfeldt, B.; Legler, K.; Woelber, L.; Prieske, K.; Mahner, S.; Trillsch, F. VEGF-C expression attributes the risk for lymphatic metastases to ovarian cancer patients. *Oncotarget* **2017**, *8*, 43218–43227. [CrossRef] [PubMed]

72. Hisamatsu, T.; Mabuchi, S.; Sasano, T.; Kuroda, H.; Takahashi, R.; Matsumoto, Y.; Kawano, M.; Kozasa, K.; Takahashi, K.; Sawada, K.; et al. The significance of lymphatic space invasion and its association with vascular endothelial growth factor-C expression in ovarian cancer. *Clin. Exp. Metastasis* **2015**, *32*, 789–798. [CrossRef] [PubMed]

73. Wang, Y.; Nakayama, M.; Pitulescu, M.E.; Schmidt, T.S.; Bochenek, M.L.; Sakakibara, A.; Adams, S.; Davy, A.; Deutsch, U.; Luthi, U.; et al. Ephrin-B2 controls VEGF-induced angiogenesis and lymphangiogenesis. *Nature* **2010**, *465*, 483–486. [CrossRef] [PubMed]

74. Liu, S.; Li, Y.; Qi, W.; Zhao, Y.; Huang, A.; Sheng, W.; Lei, B.; Lin, P.; Zhu, H.; Li, W.; et al. Expression of Tiam1 predicts lymph node metastasis and poor survival of lung adenocarcinoma patients. *Diagn. Pathol.* **2014**, *9*, 69. [CrossRef] [PubMed]

75. Zhong, D.; Li, Y.; Peng, Q.; Zhou, J.; Zhou, Q.; Zhang, R.; Liang, H. Expression of Tiam1 and VEGF-C correlates with lymphangiogenesis in human colorectal carcinoma. *Cancer Biol. Ther.* **2009**, *8*, 689–695. [CrossRef] [PubMed]

76. Lim, J.J.; Yang, K.; Taylor-Harding, B.; Wiedemeyer, W.R.; Buckanovich, R.J. VEGFR3 inhibition chemosensitizes ovarian cancer stemlike cells through down-regulation of BRCA1 and BRCA2. *Neoplasia* **2014**, *16*, 343–353. [CrossRef] [PubMed]

77. Hofbauer, S.W.; Krenn, P.W.; Ganghammer, S.; Asslaber, D.; Pichler, U.; Oberascher, K.; Henschler, R.; Wallner, M.; Kerschbaum, H.; Greil, R.; et al. Tiam1/Rac1 signals contribute to the proliferation and chemoresistance, but not motility, of chronic lymphocytic leukemia cells. *Blood* **2014**, *123*, 2181–2188. [CrossRef] [PubMed]

78. Ikram, M.; Lim, Y.; Baek, S.Y.; Jin, S.; Jeong, Y.H.; Kwak, J.Y.; Yoon, S. Co-targeting of Tiam1/Rac1 and Notch ameliorates chemoresistance against doxorubicin in a biomimetic 3D lymphoma model. *Oncotarget* **2018**, *9*, 2058–2075. [CrossRef] [PubMed]

79. Steg, A.D.; Bevis, K.S.; Katre, A.A.; Ziebarth, A.; Dobbin, Z.C.; Alvarez, R.D.; Zhang, K.; Conner, M.; Landen, C.N. Stem cell pathways contribute to clinical chemoresistance in ovarian cancer. *Clin. Cancer Res.* **2012**, *18*, 869–881. [CrossRef] [PubMed]

80. Huang, R.Y.; Chung, V.Y.; Thiery, J.P. Targeting pathways contributing to epithelial-mesenchymal transition (EMT) in epithelial ovarian cancer. *Curr. Drug Targets* **2012**, *13*, 1649–1653. [CrossRef] [PubMed]

81. Ahmed, N.; Abubaker, K.; Findlay, J.; Quinn, M. Epithelial mesenchymal transition and cancer stem cell-like phenotypes facilitate chemoresistance in recurrent ovarian cancer. *Curr. Cancer Drug Targets* **2010**, *10*, 268–278. [CrossRef] [PubMed]

82. Bustelo, X.R.; Ojeda, V.; Barreira, M.; Sauzeau, V.; Castro-Castro, A. Rac-ing to the plasma membrane: The long and complex work commute of Rac1 during cell signaling. *Small GTPases* **2012**, *3*, 60–66. [CrossRef] [PubMed]

83. Vazquez-Prado, J.; Bracho-Valdes, I.; Cervantes-Villagrana, R.D.; Reyes-Cruz, G. Gbetagamma Pathways in Cell Polarity and Migration Linked to Oncogenic GPCR Signaling: Potential Relevance in Tumor Microenvironment. *Mol. Pharmacol.* **2016**, *90*, 573–586. [CrossRef] [PubMed]

84. Xu, Y. Lysophospholipid Signaling in the Epithelial Ovarian Cancer Tumor Microenvironment. *Cancers* **2018**, *10*, 227. [CrossRef] [PubMed]

85. Devine, K.M.; Smicun, Y.; Hope, J.M.; Fishman, D.A. S1P induced changes in epithelial ovarian cancer proteolysis, invasion, and attachment are mediated by Gi and Rac. *Gynecol. Oncol.* **2008**, *110*, 237–245. [CrossRef] [PubMed]

86. Chen, H.; Wu, X.; Pan, Z.K.; Huang, S. Integrity of SOS1/EPS8/ABI1 tri-complex determines ovarian cancer metastasis. *Cancer Res.* **2010**, *70*, 9979–9990. [CrossRef] [PubMed]

87. Ward, J.D.; Dhanasekaran, D.N. LPA Stimulates the Phosphorylation of p130Cas via Galphai2 in Ovarian Cancer Cells. *Genes Cancer* **2012**, *3*, 578–591. [CrossRef] [PubMed]

88. Ward, J.D.; Ha, J.H.; Jayaraman, M.; Dhanasekaran, D.N. LPA-mediated migration of ovarian cancer cells involves translocalization of Galphai2 to invadopodia and association with Src and beta-pix. *Cancer Lett.* **2015**, *356*, 382–391. [CrossRef] [PubMed]

89. Fritz, R.D.; Pertz, O. The dynamics of spatio-temporal Rho GTPase signaling: Formation of signaling patterns. *F1000Research* **2016**, *5*. [CrossRef] [PubMed]

90. Yang, C.; Liu, Y.; Lemmon, M.A.; Kazanietz, M.G. Essential role for Rac in heregulin beta1 mitogenic signaling: A mechanism that involves epidermal growth factor receptor and is independent of ErbB4. *Mol. Cell. Biol.* **2006**, *26*, 831–842. [CrossRef] [PubMed]

91. Zhu, G.; Fan, Z.; Ding, M.; Zhang, H.; Mu, L.; Ding, Y.; Zhang, Y.; Jia, B.; Chen, L.; Chang, Z.; et al. An EGFR/PI3K/AKT axis promotes accumulation of the Rac1-GEF Tiam1 that is critical in EGFR-driven tumorigenesis. *Oncogene* **2015**, *34*, 5971–5982. [CrossRef] [PubMed]

92. Davies, S.; Holmes, A.; Lomo, L.; Steinkamp, M.P.; Kang, H.; Muller, C.Y.; Wilson, B.S. High incidence of ErbB3, ErbB4, and MET expression in ovarian cancer. *Int. J. Gynecol. Pathol.* **2014**, *33*, 402–410. [CrossRef] [PubMed]

93. Lopez-Haber, C.; Barrio-Real, L.; Casado-Medrano, V.; Kazanietz, M.G. Heregulin/ErbB3 Signaling Enhances CXCR4-Driven Rac1 Activation and Breast Cancer Cell Motility via Hypoxia-Inducible Factor 1alpha. *Mol. Cell. Biol.* **2016**, *36*, 2011–2026. [CrossRef] [PubMed]

94. Li, W.; Xiong, X.; Abdalla, A.; Alejo, S.; Zhu, L.; Lu, F.; Sun, H. HGF-induced formation of the MET-AXL-ELMO2-DOCK180 complex promotes RAC1 activation, receptor clustering, and cancer cell migration and invasion. *J. Biol. Chem.* **2018**. [CrossRef] [PubMed]

95. Oprea, T.I.; Sklar, L.A.; Agola, J.O.; Guo, Y.; Silberberg, M.; Roxby, J.; Vestling, A.; Romero, E.; Surviladze, Z.; Waller, A.; et al. Novel Activities of Select NSAID R-Enantiomers against Rac1 and Cdc42 GTPases. *PLoS ONE* **2015** *10*, e0142812. [CrossRef] [PubMed]

96.   Tan, W.; Palmby, T.R.; Gavard, J.; Amornphimoltham, P.; Zheng, Y.; Gutkind, J.S. An essential role for Rac1 in endothelial cell function and vascular development. *FASEB J.* **2008**, *22*, 1829–1838. [CrossRef] [PubMed]

97.   Hoang, M.V.; Nagy, J.A.; Senger, D.R. Active Rac1 improves pathologic VEGF neovessel architecture and reduces vascular leak: Mechanistic similarities with angiopoietin-1. *Blood* **2011**, *117*, 1751–1760. [CrossRef] [PubMed]

98.   Peinado, H.; Zhang, H.; Matei, I.R.; Costa-Silva, B.; Hoshino, A.; Rodrigues, G.; Psaila, B.; Kaplan, R.N.; Bromberg, J.F.; Kang, Y.; et al. Pre-metastatic niches: Organ-specific homes for metastases. *Nat. Rev. Cancer* **2017**, *17*, 302–317. [CrossRef] [PubMed]

99.   Marei, H.; Carpy, A.; Woroniuk, A.; Vennin, C.; White, G.; Timpson, P.; Macek, B.; Malliri, A. Differential Rac1 signalling by guanine nucleotide exchange factors implicates FLII in regulating Rac1-driven cell migration. *Nat. Commun.* **2016**, *7*, 10664. [CrossRef] [PubMed]

100. Xu, S.; Yang, Y.; Dong, L.; Qiu, W.; Yang, L.; Wang, X.; Liu, L. Construction and characteristics of an E-cadherin-related three-dimensional suspension growth model of ovarian cancer. *Sci. Rep.* **2014**, *4*, 5646. [CrossRef] [PubMed]

101. Shishido, A.; Mori, S.; Yokoyama, Y.; Hamada, Y.; Minami, K.; Qian, Y.; Wang, J.; Hirose, H.; Wu, X.; Kawaguchi, N.; et al. Mesothelial cells facilitate cancer stemlike properties in spheroids of ovarian cancer cells. *Oncol. Rep.* **2018**, *40*, 2105–2114. [PubMed]

102. Ween, M.P.; Oehler, M.K.; Ricciardelli, C. Role of versican, hyaluronan and CD44 in ovarian cancer metastasis. *Int. J. Mol. Sci.* **2011**, *12*, 1009–1029. [CrossRef] [PubMed]

103. Chen, C.; Zhao, S.; Karnad, A.; Freeman, J.W. The biology and role of CD44 in cancer progression: Therapeutic implications. *J. Hematol. Oncol.* **2018**, *11*, 64. [CrossRef] [PubMed]

104. Cai, J.; Tang, H.; Xu, L.; Wang, X.; Yang, C.; Ruan, S.; Guo, J.; Hu, S.; Wang, Z. Fibroblasts in omentum activated by tumor cells promote ovarian cancer growth, adhesion and invasiveness. *Carcinogenesis* **2012**, *33*, 20–29. [CrossRef] [PubMed]

105. Curtis, M.; Kenny, H.A.; Ashcroft, B.; Mukherjee, A.; Johnson, A.; Zhang, Y.; Helou, Y.; Batlle, R.; Liu, X.; Gutierrez, N.; et al. Fibroblasts Mobilize Tumor Cell Glycogen to Promote Proliferation and Metastasis. *Cell MeTable* **2018**. [CrossRef] [PubMed]

106. Raptis, L.; Arulanandam, R.; Geletu, M.; Turkson, J. The R(h)oads to Stat3: Stat3 activation by the Rho GTPases. *Exp. Cell Res.* **2011**, *317*, 1787–1795. [CrossRef] [PubMed]

107. Savant, S.S.; Sriramkumar, S.; O'Hagan, H.M. The Role of Inflammation and Inflammatory Mediators in the Development, Progression, Metastasis, and Chemoresistance of Epithelial Ovarian Cancer. *Cancers* **2018**, *10*, 251. [CrossRef] [PubMed]

108. Lawson, C.D.; Burridge, K. The on-off relationship of Rho and Rac during integrin-mediated adhesion and cell migration. *Small GTPases* **2014**, *5*, e27958. [CrossRef] [PubMed]

109. Pearce, O.M.T.; Delaine-Smith, R.M.; Maniati, E.; Nichols, S.; Wang, J.; Bohm, S.; Rajeeve, V.; Ullah, D.; Chakravarty, P.; Jones, R.R.; et al. Deconstruction of a Metastatic Tumor Microenvironment Reveals a Common Matrix Response in Human Cancers. *Cancer Discov.* **2018**, *8*, 304–319. [CrossRef] [PubMed]

110. Montfort, A.; Pearce, O.; Maniati, E.; Vincent, B.G.; Bixby, L.; Bohm, S.; Dowe, T.; Wilkes, E.H.; Chakravarty, P.; Thompson, R.; et al. A Strong B-cell Response Is Part of the Immune Landscape in Human High-Grade Serous Ovarian Metastases. *Clin. Cancer Res.* **2017**, *23*, 250–262. [CrossRef] [PubMed]

111. Flies, D.B.; Higuchi, T.; Harris, J.C.; Jha, V.; Gimotty, P.A.; Adams, S.F. Immune checkpoint blockade reveals the stimulatory capacity of tumor-associated CD103(+) dendritic cells in late-stage ovarian cancer. *Oncoimmunology* **2016**, *5*, e1185583. [CrossRef] [PubMed]

112. Higuchi, T.; Flies, D.B.; Marjon, N.A.; Mantia-Smaldone, G.; Ronner, L.; Gimotty, P.A.; Adams, S.F. CTLA-4 Blockade Synergizes Therapeutically with PARP Inhibition in BRCA1-Deficient Ovarian Cancer. *Cancer Immunol. Res.* **2015**, *3*, 1257–1268. [CrossRef] [PubMed]

113. Guo, Y.; Kenney, S.R.; Cook, L.; Adams, S.F.; Rutledge, T.; Romero, E.; Oprea, T.I.; Sklar, L.A.; Bedrick, E.; Wiggins, C.L.; et al. A Novel Pharmacologic Activity of Ketorolac for Therapeutic Benefit in Ovarian Cancer Patients. *Clin. Cancer Res.* **2015**, *21*, 5064–5072. [CrossRef] [PubMed]

114. Hodis, E.; Watson, I.R.; Kryukov, G.V.; Arold, S.T.; Imielinski, M.; Theurillat, J.P.; Nickerson, E.; Auclair, D.; Li, L.; Place, C.; et al. A landscape of driver mutations in melanoma. *Cell* **2012**, *150*, 251–263. [CrossRef] [PubMed]

115. Davis, M.J.; Ha, B.H.; Holman, E.C.; Halaban, R.; Schlessinger, J.; Boggon, T.J. RAC1P29S is a spontaneously activating cancer-associated GTPase. *Proc. Natl. Acad. Sci. USA* **2013**, *110*, 912–917. [CrossRef] [PubMed]

116. Kumar, A.; Rajendran, V.; Sethumadhavan, R.; Purohit, R. Molecular dynamic simulation reveals damaging impact of RAC1 F28L mutation in the switch I region. *PLoS ONE* **2013**, *8*, e77453. [CrossRef] [PubMed]

117. Chang, M.T.; Asthana, S.; Gao, S.P.; Lee, B.H.; Chapman, J.S.; Kandoth, C.; Gao, J.; Socci, N.D.; Solit, D.B.; Olshen, A.B.; et al. Identifying recurrent mutations in cancer reveals widespread lineage diversity and mutational specificity. *Nat. Biotechnol.* **2016**, *34*, 155–163. [CrossRef] [PubMed]

118. Gao, J.; Chang, M.T.; Johnsen, H.C.; Gao, S.P.; Sylvester, B.E.; Sumer, S.O.; Zhang, H.; Solit, D.B.; Taylor, B.S.; Schultz, N.; et al. 3D clusters of somatic mutations in cancer reveal numerous rare mutations as functional targets. *Genome Med.* **2017**, *9*, 4. [CrossRef] [PubMed]

119. Marei, H.; Malliri, A. GEFs: Dual regulation of Rac1 signaling. *Small GTPases* **2017**, *8*, 90–99. [CrossRef] [PubMed]

120. Jordan, P.; Brazao, R.; Boavida, M.G.; Gespach, C.; Chastre, E. Cloning of a novel human Rac1b splice variant with increased expression in colorectal tumors. *Oncogene* **1999**, *18*, 6835–6839. [CrossRef] [PubMed]

121. Schnelzer, A.; Prechtel, D.; Knaus, U.; Dehne, K.; Gerhard, M.; Graeff, H.; Harbeck, N.; Schmitt, M.; Lengyel, E. Rac1 in human breast cancer: Overexpression, mutation analysis, and characterization of a new isoform, Rac1b. *Oncogene* **2000**, *19*, 3013–3020. [CrossRef] [PubMed]

122. Singh, A.; Karnoub, A.E.; Palmby, T.R.; Lengyel, E.; Sondek, J.; Der, C.J. Rac1b, a tumor associated, constitutively active Rac1 splice variant, promotes cellular transformation. *Oncogene* **2004**, *23*, 9369–9380. [CrossRef] [PubMed]

123. Matos, P.; Jordan, P. Expression of Rac1b stimulates NF-kappaB-mediated cell survival and G1/S progression. *Exp. Cell Res.* **2005**, *305*, 292–299. [CrossRef] [PubMed]

124. Radisky, D.C.; Levy, D.D.; Littlepage, L.E.; Liu, H.; Nelson, C.M.; Fata, J.E.; Leake, D.; Godden, E.L.; Albertson, D.G.; Nieto, M.A.; et al. Rac1b and reactive oxygen species mediate MMP-3-induced EMT and genomic instability. *Nature* **2005**, *436*, 123–127. [CrossRef] [PubMed]

125. Orlichenko, L.; Geyer, R.; Yanagisawa, M.; Khauv, D.; Radisky, E.S.; Anastasiadis, P.Z.; Radisky, D.C. The 19-amino acid insertion in the tumor-associated splice isoform Rac1b confers specific binding to p120 catenin. *J. Biol. Chem.* **2010**, *285*, 19153–19161. [CrossRef] [PubMed]

126. Silva, A.L.; Carmo, F.; Bugalho, M.J. RAC1b overexpression in papillary thyroid carcinoma: A role to unravel. *Eur. J. Endocrinol. Eur. Fed. Endocr. Soc.* **2013**, *168*, 795–804. [CrossRef] [PubMed]

127. Zhou, C.; Licciulli, S.; Avila, J.L.; Cho, M.; Troutman, S.; Jiang, P.; Kossenkov, A.V.; Showe, L.C.; Liu, Q.; Vachani, A.; et al. The Rac1 splice form Rac1b promotes K-ras-induced lung tumorigenesis. *Oncogene* **2013**, *32*, 903–909. [CrossRef] [PubMed]

128. Li, G.; Ying, L.; Wang, H.; Wei, S.S.; Chen, J.; Chen, Y.H.; Xu, W.P.; Jie, Q.Q.; Zhou, Q.; Li, Y.G.; et al. Rac1b enhances cell survival through activation of the JNK2/c-JUN/Cyclin-D1 and AKT2/MCL1 pathways. *Oncotarget* **2016**, *7*, 17970–17985. [CrossRef] [PubMed]

129. Fu, X.D. Both sides of the same coin: Rac1 splicing regulating by EGF signaling. *Cell Res.* **2017**, *27*, 455–456. [CrossRef] [PubMed]

130. Wang, F.; Fu, X.; Chen, P.; Wu, P.; Fan, X.; Li, N.; Zhu, H.; Jia, T.T.; Ji, H.; Wang, Z.; et al. SPSB1-mediated HnRNP A1 ubiquitylation regulates alternative splicing and cell migration in EGF signaling. *Cell Res.* **2017**, *27*, 540–558. [CrossRef] [PubMed]

131. Gao, J.; Aksoy, B.A.; Dogrusoz, U.; Dresdner, G.; Gross, B.; Sumer, S.O.; Sun, Y.; Jacobsen, A.; Sinha, R.; Larsson, E.; et al. Integrative analysis of complex cancer genomics and clinical profiles using the cBioPortal. *Sci. Signal.* **2013**, *6*, pl1. [CrossRef] [PubMed]

132. Krauthammer, M.; Kong, Y.; Ha, B.H.; Evans, P.; Bacchiocchi, A.; McCusker, J.P.; Cheng, E.; Davis, M.J.; Goh, G.; Choi, M.; et al. Exome sequencing identifies recurrent somatic RAC1 mutations in melanoma. *Nat. Genet.* **2012**, *44*, 1006–1014. [CrossRef] [PubMed]

133. DeLano, W.L. *PyMOL: An Open-Source Molecular Graphics Tool*; Delano Scientific: San Carlos, CA, USA, 2002.

134. Kawazu, M.; Ueno, T.; Kontani, K.; Ogita, Y.; Ando, M.; Fukumura, K.; Yamato, A.; Soda, M.; Takeuchi, K.; Miki, Y.; et al. Transforming mutations of RAC guanosine triphosphatases in human cancers. *Proc. Natl. Acad. Sci. USA* **2013**, *110*, 3029–3034. [CrossRef] [PubMed]

135. Watson, I.R.; Li, L.; Cabeceiras, P.K.; Mahdavi, M.; Gutschner, T.; Genovese, G.; Wang, G.; Fang, Z.; Tepper, J.M.; Stemke-Hale, K.; et al. The RAC1 P29S hotspot mutation in melanoma confers resistance to pharmacological inhibition of RAF. *Cancer Res.* **2014**, *74*, 4845–4852. [CrossRef] [PubMed]

136. Cheung, H.W.; Cowley, G.S.; Weir, B.A.; Boehm, J.S.; Rusin, S.; Scott, J.A.; East, A.; Ali, L.D.; Lizotte, P.H.; Wong, T.C.; et al. Systematic investigation of genetic vulnerabilities across cancer cell lines reveals lineage-specific dependencies in ovarian cancer. *Proc. Natl. Acad. Sci. USA* **2011**, *108*, 12372–12377. [CrossRef] [PubMed]

137. Cowley, G.S.; Weir, B.A.; Vazquez, F.; Tamayo, P.; Scott, J.A.; Rusin, S.; East-Seletsky, A.; Ali, L.D.; Gerath, W.F.; Pantel, S.E.; et al. Parallel genome-scale loss of function screens in 216 cancer cell lines for the identification of context-specific genetic dependencies. *Sci. Data* **2014**, *1*, 140035. [CrossRef] [PubMed]

138. Cancer Genome Atlas Research Network. Integrated genomic analyses of ovarian carcinoma. *Nature* **2011**, *474*, 609–615. [CrossRef] [PubMed]

139. Vogelstein, B.; Papadopoulos, N.; Velculescu, V.E.; Zhou, S.; Diaz, L.A., Jr.; Kinzler, K.W. Cancer genome landscapes. *Science* **2013**, *339*, 1546–1558. [CrossRef] [PubMed]

140. Zoughlami, Y.; van Stalborgh, A.M.; van Hennik, P.B.; Hordijk, P.L. Nucleophosmin1 is a negative regulator of the small GTPase Rac1. *PLoS ONE* **2013**, *8*, e68477. [CrossRef] [PubMed]

141. Payapilly, A.; Malliri, A. Compartmentalisation of RAC1 signalling. *Curr. Opin. Cell Biol.* **2018**, *54*, 50–56. [CrossRef] [PubMed]

142. Mettouchi, A.; Lemichez, E. Ubiquitylation of active Rac1 by the E3 ubiquitin-ligase HACE1. *Small GTPases* **2012**, *3*, 102–106. [CrossRef] [PubMed]

143. Szklarczyk, D.; Franceschini, A.; Wyder, S.; Forslund, K.; Heller, D.; Huerta-Cepas, J.; Simonovic, M.; Roth, A.; Santos, A.; Tsafou, K.P.; et al. STRING v10: Protein-protein interaction networks, integrated over the tree of life. *Nucleic Acids Res.* **2015**, *43*, D447–D452. [CrossRef] [PubMed]

144. Bamford, S.; Dawson, E.; Forbes, S.; Clements, J.; Pettett, R.; Dogan, A.; Flanagan, A.; Teague, J.; Futreal, P.A.; Stratton, M.R.; et al. The COSMIC (Catalogue of Somatic Mutations in Cancer) database and website. *Br. J. Cancer* **2004**, *91*, 355–358. [CrossRef] [PubMed]

145. Chakravarty, D.; Gao, J.; Phillips, S.M.; Kundra, R.; Zhang, H.; Wang, J.; Rudolph, J.E.; Yaeger, R.; Soumerai, T.; Nissan, M.H.; et al. OncoKB: A Precision Oncology Knowledge Base. *JCO Precis. Oncol.* **2017**, *2017*. [CrossRef] [PubMed]

146. Armenia, J.; Wankowicz, S.A.M.; Liu, D.; Gao, J.; Kundra, R.; Reznik, E.; Chatila, W.K.; Chakravarty, D.; Han, G.C.; Coleman, I.; et al. The long tail of oncogenic drivers in prostate cancer. *Nat. Genet.* **2018**, *50*, 645–651. [CrossRef] [PubMed]

147. Futreal, P.A.; Coin, L.; Marshall, M.; Down, T.; Hubbard, T.; Wooster, R.; Rahman, N.; Stratton, M.R. A census of human cancer genes. *Nat. Rev. Cancer* **2004**, *4*, 177–183. [CrossRef] [PubMed]

148. Ryan, M.B.; Finn, A.J.; Pedone, K.H.; Thomas, N.E.; Der, C.J.; Cox, A.D. ERK/MAPK Signaling Drives Overexpression of the Rac-GEF, PREX1, in BRAF- and NRAS-Mutant Melanoma. *Mol. Cancer Res. MCR* **2016**, *14*, 1009–1018. [CrossRef] [PubMed]

149. Misek, S.A.; Chen, J.; Schroeder, L.; Rattanasinchai, C.; Sample, A.; Sarkaria, J.N.; Gallo, K.A. EGFR Signals through a DOCK180-MLK3 Axis to Drive Glioblastoma Cell Invasion. *Mol. Cancer Res. MCR* **2017**, *15*, 1085–1095. [CrossRef] [PubMed]

150. Lissanu Deribe, Y.; Shi, Y.; Rai, K.; Nezi, L.; Amin, S.B.; Wu, C.C.; Akdemir, K.C.; Mahdavi, M.; Peng, Q.; Chang, Q.E.; et al. Truncating PREX2 mutations activate its GEF activity and alter gene expression regulation in NRAS-mutant melanoma. *Proc. Natl. Acad. Sci. USA* **2016**, *113*, E1296–E1305. [CrossRef] [PubMed]

151. Earp, M.; Tyrer, J.P.; Winham, S.J.; Lin, H.Y.; Chornokur, G.; Dennis, J.; Aben, K.K.H.; Anton-Culver, H.; Antonenkova, N.; Bandera, E.V.; et al. Variants in genes encoding small GTPases and association with epithelial ovarian cancer susceptibility. *PLoS ONE* **2018**, *13*, e0197561. [CrossRef] [PubMed]

152. Winkler, S.; Mohl, M.; Wieland, T.; Lutz, S. GrinchGEF—A novel Rho-specific guanine nucleotide exchange factor. *Biochem. Biophys. Res. Commun.* **2005**, *335*, 1280–1286. [CrossRef] [PubMed]

153. Zoughlami, Y.; Voermans, C.; Brussen, K.; van Dort, K.A.; Kootstra, N.A.; Maussang, D.; Smit, M.J.; Hordijk, P.L.; van Hennik, P.B. Regulation of CXCR4 conformation by the small GTPase Rac1: Implications for HIV infection. *Blood* **2012**, *119*, 2024–2032. [CrossRef] [PubMed]

154. Han, S.; Kim, D.; Kim, Y.; Choi, K.; Miller, J.E.; Kim, D.; Lee, Y. CAS-viewer: Web-based tool for

splicing-guided integrative analysis of multi-omics cancer data. *BMC Med Genom.* **2018**, *11*, 25. [CrossRef] [PubMed]

155. Yang, I.S.; Son, H.; Kim, S.; Kim, S. ISOexpresso: A web-based platform for isoform-level expression analysis in human cancer. *BMC Genom.* **2016**, *17*, 631. [CrossRef] [PubMed]

156. Mehner, C.; Miller, E.; Khauv, D.; Nassar, A.; Oberg, A.L.; Bamlet, W.R.; Zhang, L.; Waldmann, J.; Radisky, E.S.; Crawford, H.C.; et al. Tumor cell-derived MMP3 orchestrates Rac1b and tissue alterations that promote pancreatic adenocarcinoma. *Mol. Cancer Res. MCR* **2014**, *12*, 1430–1439. [CrossRef] [PubMed]

157. Mehner, C.; Miller, E.; Nassar, A.; Bamlet, W.R.; Radisky, E.S.; Radisky, D.C. Tumor cell expression of MMP3 as a prognostic factor for poor survival in pancreatic, pulmonary, and mammary carcinoma. *Genes Cancer* **2015**, *6*, 480–489. [PubMed]

158. Stallings-Mann, M.L.; Waldmann, J.; Zhang, Y.; Miller, E.; Gauthier, M.L.; Visscher, D.W.; Downey, G.P.; Radisky, E.S.; Fields, A.P.; Radisky, D.C. Matrix metalloproteinase induction of Rac1b, a key effector of lung cancer progression. *Sci. Transl. Med.* **2012**, *4*, 142ra195. [CrossRef] [PubMed]

159. Alonso-Espinaco, V.; Cuatrecasas, M.; Alonso, V.; Escudero, P.; Marmol, M.; Horndler, C.; Ortego, J.; Gallego, R.; Codony-Servat, J.; Garcia-Albeniz, X.; et al. RAC1b overexpression correlates with poor prognosis in KRAS/BRAF WT metastatic colorectal cancer patients treated with first-line FOLFOX/XELOX chemotherapy. *Eur. J. Cancer* **2014**, *50*, 1973–1981. [CrossRef] [PubMed]

160. Huff, L.P.; Decristo, M.J.; Trembath, D.; Kuan, P.F.; Yim, M.; Liu, J.; Cook, D.R.; Miller, C.R.; Der, C.J.; Cox, A.D. The Role of Ect2 Nuclear RhoGEF Activity in Ovarian Cancer Cell Transformation. *Genes Cancer* **2013**, *4*, 460–475. [CrossRef] [PubMed]

161. Lin, Y.; Zheng, Y. Approaches of targeting Rho GTPases in cancer drug discovery. *Expert Opin. Drug Discov.* **2015**, *10*, 991–1010. [CrossRef] [PubMed]

162. Pajic, M.; Herrmann, D.; Vennin, C.; Conway, J.R.; Chin, V.T.; Johnsson, A.K.; Welch, H.C.; Timpson, P. The dynamics of Rho GTPase signaling and implications for targeting cancer and the tumor microenvironment. *Small GTPases* **2015**, *6*, 123–133. [CrossRef] [PubMed]

163. Smithers, C.C.; Overduin, M. Structural Mechanisms and Drug Discovery Prospects of Rho GTPases. *Cells* **2016**, *5*, 26. [CrossRef] [PubMed]

164. Nassar, N.; Cancelas, J.; Zheng, J.; Williams, D.A.; Zheng, Y. Structure-function based design of small molecule inhibitors targeting Rho family GTPases. *Curr. Top. Med. Chem.* **2006**, *6*, 1109–1116. [CrossRef] [PubMed]

165. Dharmawardhane, S.; Hernandez, E.; Vlaar, C. Development of EHop-016: A small molecule inhibitor of Rac. *Enzymes* **2013**, *33 Pt A*, 117–146.

166. Shutes, A.; Onesto, C.; Picard, V.; Leblond, B.; Schweighoffer, F.; Der, C.J. Specificity and mechanism of action of EHT 1864, a novel small molecule inhibitor of Rac family small GTPases. *J. Biol. Chem.* **2007**, *282*, 35666–35678. [CrossRef] [PubMed]

167. Hong, L.; Kenney, S.R.; Phillips, G.K.; Simpson, D.; Schroeder, C.E.; Noth, J.; Romero, E.; Swanson, S.; Waller, A.; Strouse, J.J.; et al. Characterization of a Cdc42 protein inhibitor and its use as a molecular probe. *J. Biol. Chem.* **2013**, *288*, 8531–8543. [CrossRef] [PubMed]

168. Forget, P.; Bentin, C.; Machiels, J.P.; Berliere, M.; Coulie, P.G.; De Kock, M. Intraoperative use of ketorolac or diclofenac is associated with improved disease-free survival and overall survival in conservative breast cancer surgery. *Br. J. Anaesth.* **2014**. [CrossRef] [PubMed]

169. Retsky, M.; Demicheli, R.; Hrushesky, W.J.; Forget, P.; De Kock, M.; Gukas, I.; Rogers, R.A.; Baum, M.; Sukhatme, V.; Vaidya, J.S. Reduction of breast cancer relapses with perioperative non-steroidal anti-inflammatory drugs: New findings and a review. *Curr. Med. Chem.* **2013**, *20*, 4163–4176. [CrossRef] [PubMed]

170. Forget, P.; Vandenhende, J.; Berliere, M.; Machiels, J.P.; Nussbaum, B.; Legrand, C.; De Kock, M. Do intraoperative analgesics influence breast cancer recurrence after mastectomy? A retrospective analysis. *Anesth. Analg.* **2010**, *110*, 1630–1635. [CrossRef] [PubMed]

171. Bowtell, D.D.; Bohm, S.; Ahmed, A.A.; Aspuria, P.J.; Bast, R.C., Jr.; Beral, V.; Berek, J.S.; Birrer, M.J.; Blagden, S.; Bookman, M.A.; et al. Rethinking ovarian cancer II: Reducing mortality from high-grade serous ovarian cancer. *Nat. Rev. Cancer* **2015**, *15*, 668–679. [CrossRef] [PubMed]

172. Lengyel, E. Ovarian cancer development and metastasis. *Am. J. Pathol.* **2010**, *177*, 1053–1064. [CrossRef] [PubMed]

173. Deng, K.; Yang, C.; Tan, Q.; Song, W.; Lu, M.; Zhao, W.; Lou, G.; Li, Z.; Li, K.; Hou, Y. Sites of distant metastases and overall survival in ovarian cancer: A study of 1481 patients. *Gynecol. Oncol.* **2018**, *150*, 460–465. [CrossRef] [PubMed]

174. Obermayr, E.; Bednarz-Knoll, N.; Orsetti, B.; Weier, H.U.; Lambrechts, S.; Castillo-Tong, D.C.; Reinthaller, A.; Braicu, E.I.; Mahner, S.; Sehouli, J.; et al. Circulating tumor cells: Potential markers of minimal residual disease in ovarian cancer? a study of the OVCAD consortium. *Oncotarget* **2017**, *8*, 106415–106428. [CrossRef] [PubMed]

175. Zhang, X.; Li, H.; Yu, X.; Li, S.; Lei, Z.; Li, C.; Zhang, Q.; Han, Q.; Li, Y.; Zhang, K.; et al. Analysis of Circulating Tumor Cells in Ovarian Cancer and Their Clinical Value as a Biomarker. *Cell. Physiol. Biochem. Int. J. Exp. Cell. Physiol. Biochem. Pharmacol.* **2018**, *48*, 1983–1994. [CrossRef] [PubMed]

176. Keyver-Paik, M.D.; Arden, J.M.; Luders, C.; Thiesler, T.; Abramian, A.; Hoeller, T.; Hecking, T.; Ayub, T.H.; Doeser, A.; Kaiser, C.; et al. Impact of Chemotherapy on Retroperitoneal Lymph Nodes in Ovarian Cancer. *Anticancer Res.* **2016**, *36*, 1815–1824. [PubMed]

177. Hjerpe, E.; Staf, C.; Dahm-Kahler, P.; Stalberg, K.; Bjurberg, M.; Holmberg, E.; Borgfeldt, C.; Tholander, B.; Hellman, K.; Kjolhede, P.; et al. Lymph node metastases as only qualifier for stage IV serous ovarian cancer confers longer survival than other sites of distant disease—A Swedish Gynecologic Cancer Group (SweGCG) study. *Acta Oncol.* **2018**, *57*, 331–337. [CrossRef] [PubMed]

178. Sehouli, J.; Olschewski, J.; Schotters, V.; Fotopoulou, C.; Pietzner, K. Prognostic role of early versus late onset of bone metastasis in patients with carcinoma of the ovary, peritoneum and fallopian tube. *Ann. Oncol.* **2013**, *24*, 3024–3028. [CrossRef] [PubMed]

179. Chebouti, I.; Blassl, C.; Wimberger, P.; Neubauer, H.; Fehm, T.; Kimmig, R.; Kasimir-Bauer, S. Analysis of disseminated tumor cells before and after platinum based chemotherapy in primary ovarian cancer. Do stem cell like cells predict prognosis? *Oncotarget* **2016**. [CrossRef] [PubMed]

180. Pantel, K.; Alix-Panabieres, C. Bone marrow as a reservoir for disseminated tumor cells: A special source for liquid biopsy in cancer patients. *BoneKEy Rep.* **2014**, *3*, 584. [CrossRef] [PubMed]

181. Banys, M.; Solomayer, E.F.; Becker, S.; Krawczyk, N.; Gardanis, K.; Staebler, A.; Neubauer, H.; Wallwiener, D.; Fehm, T. Disseminated tumor cells in bone marrow may affect prognosis of patients with gynecologic malignancies. *Int. J. Gynecol. Cancer* **2009**, *19*, 948–952. [CrossRef] [PubMed]

182. Wimberger, P.; Heubner, M.; Otterbach, F.; Fehm, T.; Kimmig, R.; Kasimir-Bauer, S. Influence of platinum-based chemotherapy on disseminated tumor cells in blood and bone marrow of patients with ovarian cancer. *Gynecol. Oncol.* **2007**, *107*, 331–338. [CrossRef] [PubMed]

183. Wimberger, P.; Roth, C.; Pantel, K.; Kasimir-Bauer, S.; Kimmig, R.; Schwarzenbach, H. Impact of platinum-based chemotherapy on circulating nucleic acid levels, protease activities in blood and disseminated tumor cells in bone marrow of ovarian cancer patients. *Int. J. Cancer* **2011**, *128*, 2572–2580. [CrossRef] [PubMed]

184. Gunjal, P.M.; Schneider, G.; Ismail, A.A.; Kakar, S.S.; Kucia, M.; Ratajczak, M.Z. Evidence for induction of a tumor metastasis-receptive microenvironment for ovarian cancer cells in bone marrow and other organs as an unwanted and underestimated side effect of chemotherapy/radiotherapy. *J. Ovarian Res.* **2015**, *8*, 20. [CrossRef] [PubMed]

185. Sharma, M.; Afrin, F.; Satija, N.; Tripathi, R.P.; Gangenahalli, G.U. Stromal-derived factor-1/CXCR4 signaling: Indispensable role in homing and engraftment of hematopoietic stem cells in bone marrow. *Stem Cells Dev.* **2011**, *20*, 933–946. [CrossRef] [PubMed]

186. Gupta, N.; Duda, D.G. Role of stromal cell-derived factor 1alpha pathway in bone metastatic prostate cancer. *J. Biomed. Res.* **2016**, *30*, 181–185. [PubMed]

187. Lapidot, T.; Kollet, O. The essential roles of the chemokine SDF-1 and its receptor CXCR4 in human stem cell homing and repopulation of transplanted immune-deficient NOD/SCID and NOD/SCID/B2m(null) mice. *Leukemia* **2002**, *16*, 1992–2003. [CrossRef] [PubMed]

188. Peled, A.; Petit, I.; Kollet, O.; Magid, M.; Ponomaryov, T.; Byk, T.; Nagler, A.; Ben-Hur, H.; Many, A.; Shultz, L.; et al. Dependence of human stem cell engraftment and repopulation of NOD/SCID mice on CXCR4. *Science* **1999**, *283*, 845–848. [CrossRef] [PubMed]

189. Price, T.T.; Burness, M.L.; Sivan, A.; Warner, M.J.; Cheng, R.; Lee, C.H.; Olivere, L.; Comatas, K.; Magnani, J.; Kim Lyerly, H.; et al. Dormant breast cancer micrometastases reside in specific bone marrow niches that regulate their transit to and from bone. *Sci. Transl. Med.* **2016**, *8*, 340ra373. [CrossRef] [PubMed]

190. Liu, C.F.; Liu, S.Y.; Min, X.Y.; Ji, Y.Y.; Wang, N.; Liu, D.; Ma, N.; Li, Z.F.; Li, K. The prognostic value of CXCR4 in ovarian cancer: A meta-analysis. *PLoS ONE* **2014**, *9*, e92629. [CrossRef] [PubMed]

191. Guo, Q.; Gao, B.L.; Zhang, X.J.; Liu, G.C.; Xu, F.; Fan, Q.Y.; Zhang, S.J.; Yang, B.; Wu, X.H. CXCL12-CXCR4 Axis Promotes Proliferation, Migration, Invasion, and Metastasis of Ovarian Cancer. *Oncol. Res.* **2015**, *22*, 247–258. [CrossRef] [PubMed]

192. Li, J.; Jiang, K.; Qiu, X.; Li, M.; Hao, Q.; Wei, L.; Zhang, W.; Chen, B.; Xin, X. Overexpression of CXCR4 is significantly associated with cisplatin-based chemotherapy resistance and can be a prognostic factor in epithelial ovarian cancer. *BMB Rep.* **2014**, *47*, 33–38. [CrossRef] [PubMed]

193. Kajiyama, H.; Shibata, K.; Terauchi, M.; Ino, K.; Nawa, A.; Kikkawa, F. Involvement of SDF-1alpha/CXCR4 axis in the enhanced peritoneal metastasis of epithelial ovarian carcinoma. *Int. J. Cancer* **2008**, *122*, 91–99. [CrossRef] [PubMed]

194. Figueras, A.; Alsina-Sanchis, E.; Lahiguera, A.; Abreu, M.; Muinelo-Romay, L.; Moreno-Bueno, G.; Casanovas, O.; Graupera, M.; Matias-Guiu, X.; Vidal, A.; et al. A Role for CXCR4 in Peritoneal and Hematogenous Ovarian Cancer Dissemination. *Mol. Cancer Ther.* **2018**, *17*, 532–543. [CrossRef] [PubMed]

195. Guo, L.; Cui, Z.M.; Zhang, J.; Huang, Y. Chemokine axes CXCL12/CXCR4 and CXCL16/CXCR6 correlate with lymph node metastasis in epithelial ovarian carcinoma. *Chin. J. Cancer* **2011**, *30*, 336–343. [CrossRef] [PubMed]

196. Arnaud, M.P.; Vallee, A.; Robert, G.; Bonneau, J.; Leroy, C.; Varin-Blank, N.; Rio, A.G.; Troadec, M.B.; Galibert, M.D.; Gandemer, V. CD9, a key actor in the dissemination of lymphoblastic leukemia, modulating CXCR4-mediated migration via RAC1 signaling. *Blood* **2015**, *126*, 1802–1812. [CrossRef] [PubMed]

197. Mao, T.L.; Fan, K.F.; Liu, C.L. Targeting the CXCR4/CXCL12 axis in treating epithelial ovarian cancer. *Gene Ther.* **2017**, *24*, 621–629. [CrossRef] [PubMed]

198. Ray, P.; Lewin, S.A.; Mihalko, L.A.; Schmidt, B.T.; Luker, K.E.; Luker, G.D. Noninvasive imaging reveals inhibition of ovarian cancer by targeting CXCL12-CXCR4. *Neoplasia* **2011**, *13*, 1152–1161. [CrossRef] [PubMed]

199. Righi, E.; Kashiwagi, S.; Yuan, J.; Santosuosso, M.; Leblanc, P.; Ingraham, R.; Forbes, B.; Edelblute, B.; Collette, B.; Xing, D.; et al. CXCL12/CXCR4 blockade induces multimodal antitumor effects that prolong survival in an immunocompetent mouse model of ovarian cancer. *Cancer Res.* **2011**, *71*, 5522–5534. [CrossRef] [PubMed]

6

The Endometriotic Tumor Microenvironment in Ovarian Cancer

Jillian R. Hufgard Wendel, Xiyin Wang and Shannon M. Hawkins *

Department of Obstetrics and Gynecology, Indiana University School of Medicine, Indianapolis, IN 46202, USA;
jhufgard@iu.edu (J.R.H.W.); xw49@iu.edu (X.W.)
* Correspondence: shhawkin@iu.edu

Abstract: Women with endometriosis are at increased risk of developing ovarian cancer, specifically ovarian endometrioid, low-grade serous, and clear-cell adenocarcinoma. An important clinical caveat to the association of endometriosis with ovarian cancer is the improved prognosis for women with endometriosis at time of ovarian cancer staging. Whether endometriosis-associated ovarian cancers develop from the molecular transformation of endometriosis or develop because of the endometriotic tumor microenvironment remain unknown. Additionally, how the presence of endometriosis improves prognosis is also undefined, but likely relies on the endometriotic microenvironment. The unique tumor microenvironment of endometriosis is composed of epithelial, stromal, and immune cells, which adapt to survive in hypoxic conditions with high levels of iron, estrogen, and inflammatory cytokines and chemokines. Understanding the unique molecular features of the endometriotic tumor microenvironment may lead to impactful precision therapies and/or modalities for prevention. A challenge to this important study is the rarity of well-characterized clinical samples and the limited model systems. In this review, we will describe the unique molecular features of endometriosis-associated ovarian cancers, the endometriotic tumor microenvironment, and available model systems for endometriosis-associated ovarian cancers. Continued research on these unique ovarian cancers may lead to improved prevention and treatment options.

Keywords: ovarian cancer; endometriosis; tumor microenvironment; miRNA molecules; genes; hypoxia; inflammation; model systems

1. Introduction

Endometriosis is a debilitating disease that is estimated to affect up to 5 million U.S. women and girls. Endometriosis results in considerable morbidity, including pelvic pain, multiple operations, infertility, and negative effects on psychosocial quality of life [1–5]. Unfortunately, endometriosis is also a significant risk factor for development of ovarian cancer [6]. The presence of endometriosis increases the risk of ovarian endometrioid, low-grade serous, and clear-cell adenocarcinoma by up to 8.9-fold but not high-grade serous adenocarcinoma [7–12]. Thus, ovarian endometrioid, low-grade serous, and clear-cell adenocarcinomas are considered endometriosis-associated ovarian cancers. Ovarian cancer is considered a top-five cancer killer in U.S. women, claiming more than 14,000 lives in 2015 [13]. Therefore, 5 million U.S. women and girls with endometriosis are at risk for developing deadly ovarian cancer. Fortunately, ovarian endometrioid and clear-cell adenocarcinoma represent roughly 20% of all ovarian cancers and account for less than 10% of deaths [14–16]. Clinically, studies suggest that co-occurrence of endometriosis with ovarian cancer is associated with an improved prognosis [17–20]. Important factors in this improved prognosis include discovery at early age and early stage disease in women with endometriosis at time of ovarian cancer staging [21–24], but may also represent the unique biology from the endometriotic tumor microenvironment. This review will focus on the contributions of the endometriotic tumor microenvironment to ovarian cancer biology.

2. Unique Molecular Features of Endometriosis-Associated Ovarian Cancer

Each histotype of epithelial ovarian cancer is thought to arise from a distinct precursor lesion. For example, endometriosis is thought to give rise to both ovarian endometrioid and clear-cell adenocarcinomas [25]. Recently, sophisticated proteomic tracing studies suggest that ovarian endometrioid adenocarcinomas arise from secretory cells of endometriosis or the endometrium, while ovarian clear-cell adenocarcinomas arise from ciliated cells. Importantly, it is hypothesized that the unique cellular environment dictates the development of ciliated or secretory cells, which then gain mutations to become malignant [26]. Recently, next-generation sequencing studies showed mutations in cancer-driver genes (i.e., AT-rich interaction domain 1A (ARID1A), Phosphatidylinositol-4, 5-bisphosphate 3-kinase catalytic subunit alpha (PIK3CA), and Kirsten rat sarcoma viral oncogene homolog (KRAS)) in deep infiltrating endometriotic lesions, supporting the idea that the endometriotic microenvironment facilitates mutations [27]. Because deep infiltrating endometriotic lesions do not pose a risk of malignant transformation, the unique contributions of driver mutations in these particular endometriotic lesions are still relatively unknown [27]. Interestingly, these mutations in cancer-driver genes were only present in glandular epithelium and not underlying stroma [27]. These data support the idea that both epithelium and stromal populations of deep infiltrating endometriosis do not represent similar clonal populations. Further, this data may represent the idea that unique stromal populations are recruited to the area [28,29]. Detailed studies of unique genetic contributions of both epithelial and/or stromal compartments in malignant transformation are needed.

Studies examining endometriotic lesions and ovarian cancer from the same patient have shown concordant mutations in ARID1A, phosphatase and tensin homolog (PTEN), PIK3CA, and KRAS, suggesting that mutations in endometriosis cause a predisposition to ovarian cancer [30–33]. Mutations in KRAS and ARID1A have been discovered in endometriosis, including ovarian endometriosis and deep infiltrating endometriosis [27,34]. Loss of ARID1A is higher in atypical endometriosis and non-atypical endometriosis adjacent to ovarian cancer than non-atypical endometriotic distal lesions [30,32,35–39]. In general, both endometrioid and clear cell ovarian cancer with or without endometriosis have common high frequency mutations in ARID1A, PIK3CA, catenin betat 1 (CTNNB1), PTEN, and KRAS [33,40–45]. In terms of unique molecular features, 29% of low-grade ovarian endometrioid adenocarcinomas with concurrent endometriosis contained mutations in KRAS compared to 3% of low-grade endometrioid adenocarcinomas lacking endometriosis [33]. Importantly, Ishikawa et al. showed high frequency of ARID1A mutations and one patient with both ARID1A and KRAS mutations in endometriosis-associated ovarian cancers [43]. The contributions of both ARID1A and KRAS warrant further study in terms of endometriosis, the endometriotic tumor microenvironment, and endometriosis-associated ovarian cancer.

In terms of low-grade serous tumors, an A to T substitution in BRAF has been identified in 36–68% of low-grade serous ovarian cancers and is associated with improved prognosis [46–48]. Additionally, increased expression of B-raf proto-oncogene, serine/threonine kinase (BRAF) was also noted in eutopic and ectopic endometrium of women with endometriosis when compared to control endometrium [49]. The contributions of BRAF to endometriosis and endometriosis-associated ovarian cancers, specifically, low-grade serous ovarian cancers are understudied.

In addition to mutational changes, epigenetic changes play a role in both endometriosis and endometriosis-associated ovarian cancers. Methylation changes in both endometriosis and endometriosis-associated ovarian cancer have recently been reviewed [50,51]. Along those lines, endometriosis tissues have decrease expression of ten-eleven translocation genes (TET1, TET2, and TET3), which convert 5-methylcytosine to 5-hydroxymethlcytosine and play a role in changes in levels of 5-hydroxymethylcytosine marks in endometriosis tissues and blood [52]. Unfortunately, the authors did not assess 5-hydroxymethlcytosine marks in specific genes. Further studies are needed in endometriosis-associated ovarian cancer to examine changes in these and other alternative DNA marks. MicroRNA (miRNA) molecules, which are also considered epigenetic changes, are dysregulated in endometriosis (reviewed in [53]). While dysregulated miRNAs in epithelial ovarian cancers have been recently reviewed [54,55], dysregulated miRNA molecules in endometriosis-associated ovarian cancers have not been individually reviewed. Given that miRNA molecules can be secreted from cells, we have included miRNA molecules under endometriotic tumor microenvironment (below).

A challenge to studies on the endometriotic tumor microenvironment is the rarity of clinical samples of ovarian cancer with concurrent endometriosis and the rigor of details provided for patient characterization. Given over 22,000 women will be diagnosed with ovarian cancer in 2016 [13], only 10% will be endometrioid and roughly 10% will be clear-cell [14–16]. Additionally, a majority of women with endometriosis-associated ovarian cancers do not have endometriosis at time of staging. Roughly 30% of ovarian endometrioid or clear-cell adenocarcinomas will have concurrent endometriosis, further narrowing the number of tumors to study with concurrent endometriosis [56–59]. Many studies do not describe the patient population in terms of absence or presence of endometriosis, leaving readers to believe that the women may not have endometriosis, which may not be accurate. Efforts for data harmonization for rare tumors may improve reproducibility. Using well-characterized samples, Banz et al. used transcriptome microarray analysis to evaluate normal ovary, endometriomas, and endometrioid ovarian cancer with and without endometriosis [60]. The results showed a small group of cytokines dysregulated in ovarian cancers with endometriosis, consistent with the inflammatory milieu of endometriosis [60]. Additionally, Zhang et al. showed a unique gene signature in ovarian endometrioid adenocarcinoma with concurrent endometriosis compared to ovarian endometrioid adenocarcinoma without concurrent endometriosis [61]. Highly dysregulated signaling pathways included nuclear factor kappa B (NFkB), transforming growth factor beta (TGFβ), and KRAS signaling [61]. Most likely there are contributions from genetics and epigenetics that may be mediated from the endometriotic tumor microenvironment [62]. However, further studies are needed to examine how endometriosis affects ovarian cancer.

3. The Unique Endometriotic Tumor Microenvironment

While the pathogenesis of endometriosis is still largely poorly understood, the most accepted theory is the implantation theory following retrograde menstruation (reviewed in [63]). Most menstruating women have retrograde menstruation [64], but only 10% have endometriosis [1–3], suggesting that unique conditions occur in women with endometriosis. The endometriotic microenvironment contains multiple cell types—endometrial epithelial cells, stromal fibroblasts, endothelial cells, and immune cells—as well as inflammatory mediators, metabolic waste products such as iron from the breakdown of red blood cells, steroid hormones, and small RNA molecules. Thus, it is not surprising that the conditions found in endometriosis are also advantageous to the growth and development of ovarian cancer. However, very little is known about how these stressful conditions directly affect ovarian cancer. In this section, we will describe these important factors within the scope of endometriosis and how these important factors pertain to ovarian cancer. Figure 1 summarizes graphically key players in the endometriotic tumor microenvironment as it pertains to ovarian cancer.

3.1. Hypoxia and Endothelial Cells

Hypoxia is thought to be critical to the survival and invasion of endometriotic cells through multiple mechanisms including autophagy [65–68], TGFβ signaling [69], and signal transducer and activator of transcription 3 (STAT3) signaling [70–72]. In endometriosis, hypoxia stabilizes hypoxia inducible factor-1α (HIF1A) which downregulates dual-specificity phosphatase-2 (DUSP2) directly and indirectly through miR-20a [73]. Ultimately, this downregulation leads to increased angiogenesis and proliferation through activation of extracellular signal-regulated kinase (ERK) signaling cascades [73,74]. As such, molecular immunohistochemistry shows a high correlation between precursor endometriosis lesions and matched clear-cell adenocarcinomas for expression of HIF1A and phosphorylated mechanistic target of rapamycin kinase (P-mTOR) [75]. Importantly, vascular endothelial growth factor (VEGF), leptin (LEP), cysteine rich angiongenic inducer 61

(CYR61), and osteopontin (SPP1) work together in response to hypoxia to establish a local vascular network within the endometriotic lesion [74]. In addition to neoangiogenesis mediated through HIF1A, as endometriotic lesions undergo hypoxia and inflammation from repeated menstrual cycles, the expression of tissue factor increases. Tissue factor is a critical protein for extrinsic coagulation cascade, leading to hypercoagulation. Clinically, women with clear-cell ovarian cancer have more frequent venous thromboembolism [76]. Hypoxia may also lead to cellular proliferation through estrogen receptor, leptin, and prostaglandin modulation [77]. These studies suggest that the hypoxic microenvironment of endometriosis plays a role in not only the potentiation of endometriosis by promoting cell proliferation and nutrient availability through vascularization but may also play roles in outcomes for women with clear-cell ovarian cancer. The increased expression of HIF1A in endometriosis may represent a novel therapeutic target for endometriosis or ovarian cancer [78].

3.2. Fibroblasts and Extracellular Matrix Components

Endometriosis is pathologically complex, containing endometrial epithelial and stromal fibroblasts outside the uterine cavity, alongside invading hemosiderin-laden macrophages [79]. The endometriotic extracellular matrix (ECM) plays a significant role in paracrine/autocrine signaling between epithelial and stromal cells [80–83]. Studies have shown unique functional properties of primary cultures of human endometrial stromal fibroblasts from women with endometriosis compared to cultures from women without endometriosis. Specifically, fibroblast cultures from women with endometriosis have a deficiency in decidualization, the differentiation process by which the uterus prepares for pregnancy [84]. Additionally, these fibroblasts from women with endometriosis have increased ERK signaling, high proliferative potential from progesterone resistance, and acquire an inflammatory phenotype [85–89]. While the importance of stromal-epithelial crosstalk is noted in embryo implantation in the uterus [80], the role of similar crosstalk in endometriosis or epithelial ovarian cancers is still understudied but may represent a key component of the endometriotic tumor microenvironment.

To examine the tumor microenvironment in ovarian cancer, Zhang et al. used computer-aided image analysis and showed that the number of cancer-associated fibroblasts, as indicated by cells positive for smooth muscle antigen, was higher in epithelial ovarian cancers compared to benign adnexal masses. Unfortunately, the specific histology of ovarian cancers and the pathology of the benign adnexal masses were not described in these studies. Large numbers of similarly staining cancer-associated fibroblasts were also found in omental metastatic lesions [90]. Co-culture of cancer-associated fibroblast with ovarian cancer cell lines (SKOV3, CAOV3) led to increased invasion and migration when compared to ovarian cancer cell lines grown in co-culture with normal fibroblasts [90]. One of the main questions regarding cancer-associated fibroblasts is how and why they are becoming activated to benefit tumor cells. Mitra et al. proposed that ovarian cancer cells reprogram fibroblasts into cancer-associated fibroblasts through miRNA expression changes [91]. Specifically, cancer-associated fibroblasts have a significant downregulation of miR-31 and miR-214 and upregulation of miR-155. C-C motif ligand 5 (CCL5), a chemokine known to be highly upregulated in ovarian cancers, is a direct target of miR-214. Similarly, endometriomas have high expression of chemokines and dysregulated miRNA expression [92]. Advancements in the understanding of the role of non-epithelial ovarian cancer cells in ovarian cancer may lead to better treatments which block tumor promotion brought on by tumor adjacent cells.

3.3. Immune Cells and Inflammatory Mediators

Dysregulated inflammation plays a key role in endometriosis-associated pathology [93]. For example, Capobianco and Rovere-Querini provide an in-depth review of the role of macrophages in endometriosis, showing a relationship between components of the endometriotic microenvironment such as high iron, hypoxia, and angiogenesis with macrophage recruitment and activation [94]. Additionally, a syngeneic mouse model of endometriosis showed that endometriotic lesions failed to grow without macrophages, and if macrophages were removed after implantation, angiogenesis was halted, blocking the progression of the endometriotic lesion [95]. Further, Canet et al. suggest that retainment of a specific macrophage population in endometriomas, the cell division cycle 42 (CDC42)-positive population, protects endometriomas from malignant transformation [96]. Similarly, platelet factor 4 (PF4) also known as chemokine (C-X-C Motif) ligand 4 (CXCL4) is highly expressed on macrophages in endometriomas, but not on tumor-associated macrophages of clear cell ovarian cancers [97]. Thus, specific details of the macrophage population in endometriosis and ovarian cancer are important and require further study.

Transcriptomic work on endometriomas showed that the inflammatory cytokine transforming growth factor beta 1 (TGFβ1), regulates other inflammatory mediators relevant to endometriosis, including tumor necrosis factor alpha (TNFα) and interleukin-6 (IL6) [92]. These inflammatory mediators are highly elevated in peritoneal fluid from women with endometriosis [98–101]. The acute and chronic inflammation of endometriosis is a response to the invading tissue, leading to the release of regulated on activation normal T cell expressed and secreted (RANTES), monocyte chemotactic protein-1 (MCP1), and interleukin-8 (IL8), which act as chemoattractants recruiting more macrophages to the area [102]. In terms of the endometriotic tumor microenvironment, the promotion of tumor invasion via macrophages may be dependent on TNFα [103], which is elevated in women with endometriosis [98,99]. Along the same lines, work using an estrogen receptor beta (ERβ)-overexpressing syngeneic mouse model of endometriosis suggests that non-genomic effects of ERβ play a role in the TNFα-mediated dysregulation of endometriosis progression [104]. Encouragingly, treatment of a syngeneic mouse model of endometriosis with a long-acting TNFα-blocking agent decreased endometriotic implant size [105]. However, treatment of women with rectovaginal nodules with infliximab, a TNFα monoclonal antibody, had no improved clinical effect over placebo [106]. Understanding the immune response to misplaced endometrial tissue will be a large factor in understanding the onset and progression of endometriosis and lead to a better understanding of how endometriosis creates a unique and potentially tumor-promoting microenvironment.

3.4. Altered Metabolism

Endometriotic cysts contain blood. When blood is metabolized, heme and iron are released into the microenvironment [107]. Because of this, endometriotic cysts contain higher iron levels than other benign ovarian cysts [108]. Consequently, an iron-rich microenvironment can lead to increased proliferation, DNA synthesis, and adhesion, and promote chronic inflammation, allowing for the spread of endometriosis [107]. High iron also leads to excessive oxidative stress, which creates a microenvironment conducive to the induction of mutations and has been linked to cancer development in the liver and lung [107,109]. Shigetomi et al. outlines how endometriotic cells under oxidative stress from excess iron are able to bypass cell cycle checkpoints after DNA damage by overexpressing hepatocyte nuclear factor-1 beta (HNF1B), which activates forkhead box transcription factors and alters miRNA expression promoting cell survival [110]. Due to the excess iron exposure, endometriotic cysts have higher expression of lactose dehydogenase, lipid peroxidase, and 8-hydroxy-2′-deoxyguanosine. High expression of these markers of oxidative stress link endometriosis, high iron, and higher frequencies of gene mutations [108]. These data corroborate the hypothesis that endometriosis produces a high iron microenvironment that may lead to increased DNA damage through oxidative stress, but also promotes cell survival, leading to a highly mutated subpopulation of cells that continue to grow [111].

Alongside high iron levels, endometriotic peritoneal fluid has elevated lactate. Further, endometriotic lesions express high levels of glycolysis genes compared to eutopic endometrium [112]. Increased expression of HNF1α in the endometriotic peritoneum leads to the conversion of glucose to lactate in a process known as the "Warburg Effect," known for its promotion of cell survival in stressful microenvironments [113]. Lipidomics has also been pursued for understanding the metabolomic profile of the endometriotic microenvironment. Lipid profiling studies on endometrial aspirates have shown a reduction of saturated diacylglycerols and triacylglycerols in endometriosis patients compared to healthy controls [114]. In fact, this study generated a panel of 123 metabolites which were differentially expressed in endometriosis women and correctly identified 86% of samples to either the endometriosis or control group [114]. A similar study on endometrial biopsies used five lipid metabolites as biomarkers and were able to predict endometriosis with 75% specificity and 90.5% sensitivity [115]. A true model of the endometriotic tumor microenvironment should include increased iron levels, higher levels of glycolysis-associated proteins, and endometriosis-associated lipidomic profiles.

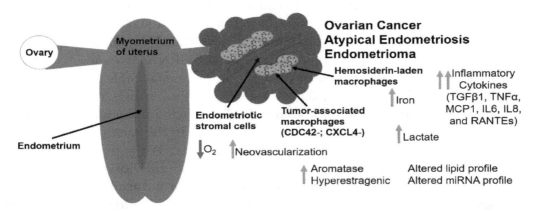

Figure 1. Composition of the endometriotic tumor microenvironment. Endometriosis represents a pathologically benign disease. Endometriosis may be classified into endometriomas, superficial peritoneal disease, or deep infiltrating endometriosis (invasion > 5 mm). Although deep infiltrating endometriosis is invading, typically into the muscularis layer of the bowel, it is clinically not associated with ovarian cancer. Endometriomas are epithelial lined cysts of the ovary, which can be filled with a brown cyst fluid, and thus the name "chocolate cysts." Endometriomas can be associated with ovarian cancer, with atypical endometriomas having a higher risk of malignant transformation. Atypical endometriomas are characterized by epithelial cells with enlarged hyperchromatic and pleomorphic nuclei, with cellular crowding and high nuclear-to-cytoplasmic ratio. The altered endometriotic tumor microenvironment may lead to malignant transformation or propagation of proliferative potential [107]. RANTES: regulated on activation normal T cell expressed and secreted; MCP1: monocyte chemotactic protein-1; IL: interleukin; TGFβ1: transforming growth factor beta 1; TNFα: tumor necrosis factor alpha; CDC42: cell division cycle 42; CXCL4: chemokine (C-X-C motif) ligand 4.

3.5. Steroid Hormones

Endometriosis is an estrogen-responsive disorder with lesion-level hyperestrogenism. Specifically, endometriotic tissue differs from eutopic endometrial tissue by the high expression of aromatase (CYP19A1) and 17β-hydroxysteroid-dehydrogenase (17β-HSD) type 1 and the absence of 17β-HSD type 2 [107,116]. Aromatase converts androstenedione or testosterone to estrone and estradiol at the level of the endometriotic microenvironment. High levels of estradiol have been linked to IL8 and RANTES production, which facilitate proliferation, inflammation, and feedback to increased expression of aromatase [107,117]. Aromatase activity is also stimulated through prostaglandin E$_2$, an inflammatory product of cyclooxygenase 1 and 2 (COX1/2), found in endometriotic lesions in high levels [118]. Inhibitors of prostaglandin E2 receptor show promising effects in a xenograft model of endometriosis [119]. At the endometriotic lesion level, there is significant feed forward production and maintenance of estrogen, associated with pro-tumorigenic qualities. Medical management of endometriosis with oral contraceptives lowers overall steroid hormone levels. This may explain why the protection from combined oral contraceptive therapy on ovarian cancer risk is more robust for women with endometriosis (odds ratio 0.21 (0.08–0.58), $p = 0.003$) compared to non-endometriosis population (odds ratio 0.47 (0.37–0.61, $p < 0.001$)) [120]. Thus, the role of steroid hormones on endometriosis-associated ovarian cancers needs further study.

3.6. Small RNA Molecules

Small RNA molecules are non-coding RNA molecules that can play an important role in the post-transcriptional regulation of gene expression. Multiple groups of small RNAs have been identified, such as microRNAs (miRNAs), small nucleolar RNA (snoRNAs), small interfering RNAs (siRNAs), and Piwi-interacting RNA (piRNAs) [121]. The most studied type of small RNA molecules in endometriosis-associated ovarian cancers are miRNAs. In general, miRNAs regulate gene expression by mRNA cleavage and translational repression [122,123]. Studies have shown that miRNAs are frequently dysregulated in endometriosis and endometriosis-associated ovarian cancers (reviewed in [53–55]). Compilation of dysregulated miRNAs in ovarian endometrioid and clear-cell adenocarcinomas, as well as endometriosis (Supplemental Table S1) shows dysregulated miRNA molecules for each tissue type [53,55,124–133]. Figure 2 shows the number of miRNAs dysregulated in ovarian clear-cell and endometrioid adenocarcinomas, and endometriosis tissues. Supplemental Table S1 details the specific miRNA molecules in the each unique and overlapping group. MiR-126 was found downregulated in all three groups. While the function of miR-126 is still unknown, miR-126 was significantly downregulated in endometriosis compared with eutopic endometrium [134]. Additionally, downregulation of miR-126 induced non-ovarian cancer cell proliferation, migration, and invasion, mediated through numerous validated targets, such as PI3K, KRAS, and VEGF. Reduced levels of miR-126 were a significant predictor of poor survival of cancer patients, although women with ovarian cancer were not included in the study [135]. Thus, miR-126 may play a role in endometriosis and ovarian cancer, even though these functional studies did not have ovarian cancer samples with concurrent endometriosis.

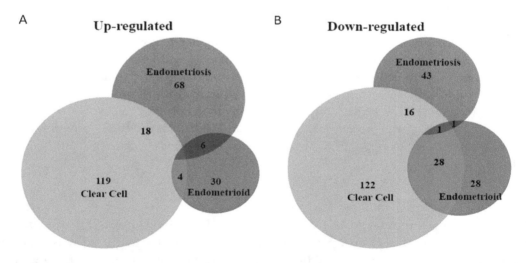

Figure 2. Venn diagram of overlap of number of miRNAs differentially expressed in endometriosis and ovarian clear-cell and endometrioid adenocarcinoma. The miRNAs differentially expressed are depicted in three overlapping circles. The numbers indicate the miRNA counts that are unique or in common between the groups. (**A**) Upregulated miRNAs; (**B**) downregulated miRNAs. Supplemental Table S1 details the miRNAs in each group above.

MiR-30a, miR-30c, miR-31, miR-532-5p, and miR-885-5p were upregulated in clear cell ovarian cancer by multiple studies [124–127,131,132]. MiR-30 was found to be 5-fold overexpressed in ovarian clear-cell adenocarcinoma [132]. Sestito et al. showed that overexpression of miR-30a delayed tumor formation in xenograft tumors, and overexpression of miR-30a sensitized ovarian cancer cells to chemotherapy [136]. Downregulation of miR-532 was associated with poor survival in women with ovarian cancer, and overexpression of miR-532 suppressed the proliferative and invasive capacity of the ovarian cancer cell lines, ES2 and SKOV-3, and inhibited tumor growth in vivo [137]. Endometrioid ovarian cancer had the shortest list of dysregulated miRNAs (Figure 2 and Supplemental Table S1). MiR-200 family miRNAs (miR-200a, -200b, -200c, -141, and -429) were upregulated in ovarian cancer and may play crucial roles in ovarian cancer metastasis, diagnosis, and treatment [126,129,130,138].

4. Model Systems for Studying Rare Ovarian Cancers

Multiple model systems have been employed to study endometriosis and endometriosis-associated ovarian cancers (reviewed in [139,140]). This review will highlight the tumor microenvironment of the genetically engineered mouse models of endometriosis-associated ovarian cancers. We have chosen to focus on spontaneous models instead of transplant models (reviewed in [140]). Because there has yet to be a comprehensive mouse model that replicates ovarian cancer with endometriosis, this review will also focus on the role of immortalized cell lines, xenograft models, co-culture systems, and three-dimensional (3D) models.

4.1. Genetically Engineered Mouse Models

4.1.1. Candidate Genes in Genetically Engineered Mouse Models

High-grade serous ovarian cancer is a genomically complex disease [141] and although neither endometrioid nor clear-cell ovarian cancer have been as extensively profiled, they are likely complex as well. For the study of genetically engineered mouse models, fortunately, both endometrioid and clear cell ovarian cancer have high frequency mutations in only a handful of genes: *ARID1A*, *PIK3CA*, *CTNNB1*, *PTEN*, and *KRAS* [33,40–42,44,45]. Use of traditional *Cre* recombinase technology with candidate-gene floxed alleles has had mixed results in terms of single gene knockout developing endometriosis-associated ovarian cancers. Table 1 lists the promoters driving *Cre* recombinase, and Table 2 details the brief rationale behind the use of specific genes in these mouse models. Table 3 lists these genes with combinations of tissue-specific promoters driving *Cre* recombinase. Despite the promising allele targets and the tissue-specific promoters driving *Cre* recombinase, there are no genetic mouse models of endometriosis and concurrent ovarian cancer. Investigators have created genetically engineered mouse models, which developed ovarian low-grade serous, clear-cell, or endometrioid adenocarcinoma (Table 3). However, none of these models have concurrent endometriosis. This suggests that different genetic combinations are required to model concurrent endometriosis and ovarian cancer. The discussion below highlights the role of the microenvironment of each model, and how this microenvironment may be playing a role in ovarian cancer development. Even though the presented models do not completely represent the endometriotic tumor microenvironment, they are still useful for understanding development of endometrioid or clear-cell ovarian cancer.

Table 1. *Cre* recombinase promoters and site of effects.

Cre	Gene Promoter	Location of Expression	Ref.
Adenovirus (Ad)	Cytomegalovirus	Injection site	[142]
Amhr2	Anti-Müllerian hormone receptor type 2	Oviduct: stroma Uterus: stroma and smooth muscle cells Ovary: granulosa cells and ovarian surface epithelium	[143,144]
Cyp19	Cytochrome P450 family 19	Granulosa cells of antral follicles and luteal cells	[145]
Ovgp1	Oviductal glycoprotein 1	Non-ciliated oviductal epithelial cells	[146]
Pax8	Paired box gene 8	Fallopian tube, cervix, uterus, and endometrium	[147]
Pgr	Progesterone receptor	Oviduct: epithelium Uterus: epithelium, stroma, myometrium Ovary: time-limited granulosa cells	[148]

Table 2. Genes important in mouse models of endometriosis-associated ovarian cancer.

Mouse Allele	Gene Name and Mouse Ref	Effect of *Cre* Recombination	Endometriosis-Associated Ovarian Cancer Implications and Ref.
Arid1a^f/f	AT-rich interactive domain 1A	ARID1A loss	46–95% of clear-cell and 30% of endometrioid tumors have loss of ARID1A [30,43–45]
Apc^f/f	Adenomatous polyposis coli	Overexpression of β-catenin	Mutations in APC lead to activation of β-catenin which is frequently activated in endometriosis-associated ovarian cancers [149]
Ctnnb1^f/f	Catenin beta-1	Overexpression of β-catenin	16–54% of endometroid ovarian cancers have mutations in β-catenin, leading to nuclear localization, and activation of wingless integration site (WNT) signaling [150–153]
Kras^lsl-G12D	Kirsten rat sarcoma	Expression of oncogenic Kras	29% of low-grade endometrioid ovarian tumors with concurrent endometriosis [33]
MUC1^+/-	Mucin 1	Expression human MUC1 in mouse	Expressed in endometrium and endometriosis; potential biomarker for endometriosis or ovarian cancer [154]
Pik3ca^H1047R	Phosphatidylinositol-4,5-bisphosphate 3-kinase catalytic subunit alpha	Mutation in Pik3ca kinase domain	20% of clear-cell and 20% of endometrioid ovarian cancers with mutations [155]
Pten^f/f	Phosphatase and tensin homolog	PTEN loss and activation of AKT	20% of clear-cell and 20% of endometrioid cancers [156]

Table 3. Mouse models with implications in endometriosis and endometriosis-associated ovarian cancers.

Genotype	Phenotype	Penetrance	Details	Ref.
Arid1a^f/f;Ad^Cre (Ovarian bursa)	No cancer	0/29 with adnexal masses / 0/42 with adnexal masses	No endometriosis	[157,158]
Arid1a^f/f;Amhr2^Cre	No cancer	0/20 with adnexal masses	No endometriosis	[159]
Arid1a^f/f;Pgr^Cre	No cancer	0/20 with adnexal masses	No endometriosis	[160]
Pten^f/f;Ad^Cre (Ovarian bursa)	No cancer	0/5 with adnexal masses / 0/63 with adnexal masses	No endometriosis	[158,161]
Pten^f/f;Ad^Cre (Infundibulum to ovarian bursa)	Low penetrance endometrioid ovarian cancer at 26 weeks	8/13 with ovarian endometriosis like lesions / 1/13 with ovarian cancer by 26 weeks	Endometriosis-like lesions of ovary (lacked stromal component)	[162]
Pten^f/f;Cyp19^Cre	No cancer	0/4 with adnexal masses	No endometriosis	[163]
Pten^f/f;Amhr2^Cre	Granulosa cell tumor	5/70 with ovarian cancers by 7 months	No endometriosis	[164]
Pten^f/f;Apc^f/f;Ovgp1^Cre	Endometrioid ovarian carcinoma	10/15 with ovarian cancers	Metastatic lesions	[146]
Pten^f/f;Pax8^Cre	Endometrioid oviductal adenocarcinoma	3/4 with oviductal cancers by 7 months	Oviductal tumors metastasized to ovary	[147]

Table 3. *Cont.*

Genotype	Phenotype	Penetrance	Details	Ref.
$Pik3ca^{H1047R};Ad^{Cre}$ (Ovarian bursa)	No cancer	0/6 with adnexal masses	4/5 ovarian surface epithelium hyperplasia (microscopic)	[157]
$Kras^{G12D};Ad^{Cre}$ (Infundibulum to ovarian bursa)	15/15 endometriosis-like lesions of ovary	15/15 with endometriosis-like lesions of ovary	Endometriosis-like lesions of ovary (lacked stromal component)	[162]
$Kras^{G12D};Ad^{Cre}$ (Uterotubal injection to ovarian bursa)	7/15 with peritoneal endometriosis	7/15 with peritoneal endometriosis	Peritoneal endometriosis	[162]
$Kras^{G12D};Ad^{Cre}$ (IP injection)	No cancer	0/13 with adnexal masses	No endometriosis	[162]
$Kras^{G12D};Amhr2^{Cre}$	No cancer	0/4 with adnexal masses	No endometriosis Abnormal follicles	[145,163]
$Kras^{G12D};Cyp19^{Cre}$		0/4 with adnexal masses	No endometriosis Abnormal follicles	[145,163]
$Kras^{G12D};Pgr^{Cre}$	No cancer	0/3 with adnexal masses	No endometriosis	[163]
$Ctnnb1^{f/f};Amhr2^{Cre}$	Endometrioid ovarian carcinoma	5/6 with ovarian cancer by 6 months	No endometriosis	[165]
$Arid1a^{f/f};Pik3ca^{H1047R};Ad^{Cre}$ (Ovarian bursa)	Poorly differentiated clear-cell ovarian carcinoma	23/30 with ovarian cancer by 7 weeks	77% penetrance No endometriosis Aggressive metastatic tumors	[157]
$Arid1a^{f/f};Pten^{f/f};Ad^{Cre}$ (Ovarian bursa)	5/13 endometrioid ovarian carcinoma 8/13 undifferentiated adenocarcinoma	13/22 with ovarian cancer by 9 months	59% penetrance No endometriosis Aggressive undifferentiated tumors	[158]
$Apc^{f/f};Pgr^{Cre}$	Endometrioid ovarian carcinoma	12/43 with ovarian cancer	No endometriosis 16% endometrioid ovarian cysts	[166]
$Pten^{f/f};Apc^{f/f};Ad^{Cre}$ (Ovarian bursa)	Endometrioid ovarian carcinoma	29/29 with ovarian cancer	100% penetrance No endometriosis Aggressive metastatic tumors	[161]
$Pten^{f/f};Apc^{f/f};Pik3ca^{H1047R};Ad^{Cre}$ (Ovarian bursa)	Endometrioid ovarian carcinoma	11/11 with ovarian cancer	No endometriosis Aggressive metastatic tumors	[167]
$Kras^{G12D};Pten^{f/f};Ad^{Cre}$ (Infundibulum to ovarian bursa)	Endometrioid ovarian carcinoma	9/9 with ovarian cancer by 12 weeks	100% penetrance Aggressive metastatic disease No endometriosis	[162]
$MUC1^{+/-};Kras^{G12D};Ad^{Cre}$ (Ovarian bursa)	Endometriosis-like lesions of ovary	No ovarian cancer	endometriosis-like lesions of ovary	[168]
$Ctnnb1^{f/f};Pten^{f/f};Amhr2^{Cre}$	Endometrioid ovarian carcinoma	5/5 with ovarian cancer by 6 weeks	No endometriosis	[165]
$Kras^{G12D};Pten^{f/f};Amhr2^{Cre}$	Low grade ovarian serous papillary adenocarcinomas	100% with ovarian tumors by 10 weeks	No endometriosis	[143,163]
$Kras^{G12D};Pten^{f/f};Pgr^{Cre}$	No cancer	0/3 with adnexal masses	No endometriosis	[163]
$Kras^{G12D};Pten^{f/f};Cyp19^{Cre}$	No cancer	0/3 with adnexal masses	No endometriosis	[163]

4.1.2. Endometriosis

The only genetically engineered mouse model to spontaneously develop endometriosis with a single gene change is a highly innovative mouse model developed by Dinulescu et al. [162]. Using an oncogenic *KRAS* knock-in allele mouse (*Kras^G12D*), peritoneal endometriosis developed after injection of adenovirus-driven *Cre* (Ad^Cre^) through the uterotubal junction to infect the ovarian bursa. This true peritoneal endometriosis model contained glandular epithelium and stromal components validated by molecular immunohistochemistry to cytokeratin 7, 8, and 20, estrogen receptor, progesterone receptor, smooth muscle actin, and CD10 [162]. Conversely, when Ad^Cre^ was injected through the infundibulum to the ovarian bursa, the model develops ovarian endometriosis-like lesions without the stromal component [162]. A transplantation experiment hints that the peritoneal endometriosis is uterine or tubal in origin while the ovarian endometriosis-like lesions are ovarian surface epithelium derived [162]. While long-term follow up showed no development of ovarian cancer, future studies into the molecular lineage using secretory or ciliary markers may allow better definition of cell of origin [26,62]. A similar mouse model adds human mucin 1 (*MUC1*) to oncogenic *Kras^G12D* with Ad^Cre^ intrabursal injection [168]. This mouse model similarly exhibits endometriosis-like lesions of the ovary. Importantly, these mice developed an immune response to MUC1 with high numbers of CD4+ Foxp3+ regulatory T cells in para-aortic lymph nodes compared to uninjected mice without lesions [168]. Models which recapitulate the immune response are needed to study the endometriotic tumor microenvironment.

Because mice do not normally menstruate, modeling retrograde menstruation requires significant manipulation. In homologous mouse models of endometriosis, endometrium from an estrogen-primed donor mouse is injected into a syngeneic estrogen-treated recipient mouse. However, homologous mouse models such as these grow poorly without exogenous estrogen [162]. A variation is the menstrual mouse model. In this model, the donor mouse undergoes significant hormonal manipulation followed by a stimulation of the uterus leading to decidualization. Hormone withdrawal leads to degeneration of the endometrium with leukocyte invasion, similar to menstruation in women [169–171]. Donor sloughed endometrium is then placed into recipient syngeneic mouse. Using this approach, Cheng et al. placed oncogenic *Kras^G12V* endometrial tissue into the subcuticular ventral abdomen of syngeneic mice without exogenous hormonal stimulation or matrix [172]. These lesions contained glandular epithelium, stroma, immune cells, extracellular matrix, and blood vessels with both estrogen receptor alpha and beta expression [172]. Similarly, Greaves et al. used a similar approach with endometrial tissue from a menstrual model of wild type mice. Using hormonally stimulated receptor mice, injection of tissue intraperitoneal with this non-genetically modified endometrial tissue leads to peritoneal endometriosis [173]. Again, these tissues were histologically and molecularly similar to human endometriosis [173]. Hormonal levels (i.e., endogenous versus exogenous high levels), tissue placement (i.e., subcuticular versus intraperitoneal), and genetic changes important to endometriosis-associated ovarian cancers (i.e., oncogenic *KRAS*, loss of function *ARID1A*) must be considered when using these menstrual endometriosis models. Additionally, genetically engineered mouse models that are unable to undergo decidualization such as *Pgr^Cre^;Arid1a^f/f^* mice [160] do not allow such studies.

4.1.3. Clear Cell Ovarian Cancer

Poorly differentiated clear-cell ovarian carcinoma develops at 7.5 weeks post-injection in *Ad^Cre^;Arid1a^f/f^;Pik3ca*^*H1047R*^ female mice with 77% penetrance and with 57% of injected mice having peritoneal metastasis [157]. Similar deletion of *ARID1A* alone or with knock-in of *Pik3ca* mutations showed ovarian surface epithelium hyperplasia but no endometriosis [157,158]. Although clear cell features are present two weeks post-injection, endometriotic-like lesions are not described [157]. Microarray analysis, comparing primary ovarian tumors to contralateral un-injected ovary, found almost 600 genes dysregulated with significant enrichment in immune system function [157]. Consistent with an endometriotic tumor microenvironment, IL6 signaling was found to be increased in the primary tumors, peritoneal metastases, body fluids, and ascites [157]. IL6 signaling and tumor cell growth was blocked with IL6 neutralizing antibodies. While IL6 expression was also implicated in normal ovarian surface epithelium hyperplasia with *ARID1A* deletion or *Pik3ca* mutation alone, the combination further enhanced IL6 production [157]. Cross-species, global gene expression profiling showed similar dysregulated genes in this mouse model compared to ovarian clear-cell adenocarcinoma from women [174]. Together these data suggest that the deletion of *ARID1A* and mutation in $Pik3ca^{*H1057R}$ results in increased IL6 expression leading to the ovarian surface epithelial hyperplasia and eventually clear cell ovarian cancer. These tumor cells perpetuate IL6 production, creating a positive feedback loop of increased IL6 and increased cell (normal and cancerous) proliferation [157,174]. This interaction highlights how the tumor and its microenvironment can interact with one another to generate a more tumor-promoting environment.

4.1.4. Endometrioid

ARID1A, *PIK3CA*, *CTNNB1*, *PTEN*, and *KRAS* [33,40–42,44,45] are commonly mutated in both endometrioid and clear cell ovarian cancers from women. However, manipulation of these genes in mice typically results in endometrioid but not clear cell ovarian cancer. On injection of adenovirus-driven Cre (Ad^{Cre}) into the ovarian bursa through the infundibulum of $Pten^{f/f};Kras^{G12D}$ female mice generated female mice with 100% penetrance of highly aggressive and metastatic endometrioid ovarian cancer at 12 weeks. Interestingly, this mouse model has ovarian endometriosis-like lesions with either addition of oncogenic $Kras^{G12D}$ or deletion of *Pten* alone, but only results in endometrioid ovarian cancer when both *Pten* and $Kras^{G12D}$ are simultaneously mutated [162].

A mouse model targeting both *Pten* and *Apc* resulted in endometrioid ovarian cancer with high penetrance and metastatic disease [161]. Unfortunately, this conditional knockout (Ad^{Cre}) did not result in endometriosis, which may be due to the early (6-week post-injection) tumor development [161]. Another model of endometrioid carcinoma in mice utilized a double conditional knockout of *Pten* and *Arid1a* and intrabursal Ad^{Cre} injection to show a progression of ovarian surface epithelium hyperplasia, endometrioid carcinoma, and finally poorly differentiated carcinoma [158]. The well-differentiated endometrioid carcinoma was confined to the ovaries, suggesting the place of origin, while the undifferentiated tumors had metastasized into the peritoneal cavity [158]. Guan et al. hypothesizes that *ARID1A* plays a role in both tumor initiation and progression but requires the collaborative second hit of *Pten* to produce tumors [158]. Although the hyperplasia was not linked to endometriosis in these mice, it does speak to an environment of uncontrolled cellular proliferation giving rise to endometrioid ovarian cancer when left untreated.

High nuclear β-catenin levels have uniquely been found in endometrioid ovarian cancer from women, where this nuclear accumulation leads to activation of the WNT pathway [149]. Gain-of-function deletion of exon 3 of *Ctnnb1* leads to stable β-catenin expression in mice [175]. $Amhr2^{Cre}Ctnnb1^{f/f}$ female mice have aggressive endometrioid ovarian cancers with 100% penetrance by 6 months. Addition of *Pten* deletion to this model allows for tumors that are even more aggressive by 6 weeks [165]. Similar to deletion of exon 3 of *Ctnnb1*, deletion of *Apc* leads to stable β-catenin and WNT signaling activation [149]. Only with deletion of *Pten* did mice develop ovarian tumors [161]. To model the progression of type I tumors to the more aggressive type II tumors, Wu et al. (2013) added $Pik3ca^{E545K/+}$ to $Apc^{f/f}\ Pten^{f/f}$ mice with Ad^{Cre} and showed peritoneal and lung metastasis [167].

While these models used $Amhr2^{Cre}$ or Ad^{Cre} to focus genetic changes in the ovarian surface epithelium, other studies have created conditional genetic changes in the oviduct. When *Apc* and *Pten* were concurrently deleted in the fallopian tube using $Ovgp1^{Cre}$, endometrioid tumors of the ovaries developed in 10 of 15 mice, with 50% of those resulting in metastasis to the lungs or omentum [146]. Deletion of *Pten* in the fallopian tube by *Pax8^{Cre}* also resulted in endometrioid tumors. Specifically, 75% of female mice developed primary tumors in the fallopian tube by 7 months, and 75% of tumor-burdened mice had metastasis to the ovaries [147]. Deletion of *Apc* with *Pgr^{Cre}* female mice revealed tumors in both the oviduct and ovaries. Specifically, 25 of 40 female mice developed endometrioid oviductal tumors, one of 43 developed granulosa cell tumors, and 12 of 43 developed endometrioid ovarian tumors. While these female mice had simple ovarian cysts, the authors did not specifically denominate them as endometriosis [166]. Taken together, these mouse models suggest that the oviduct and/or the ovary may be involved in endometrioid cancer development in the mouse.

4.1.5. Low-Grade Serous Ovarian Cancer

Addition of oncogenic *Kras* (*Kras^{G12D}*) with either *Amhr2^{Cre}* or *Cyp19^{Cre}* resulted in ovaries with abnormal follicles, which were non-tumorigenic but also non-mitotic and non-apoptotic [145]. Deletion of *Pten* using *Amhr2^{Cre}* did result in increased proliferation and increased cell survival of ovarian surface epithelium [163]. However, the loss of the tumor suppressor *Pten* alone is not tumorigenic in somatic cells of the ovary. When *Pten* is deleted in the context of oncogenic *Kras* with *Amhr2^{Cre}*, there is development of low-grade serous papillary cystadenocarcinoma [163]. Although no endometriosis was noted, these mice were shown to have ovarian surface epithelium hyperplasia and abnormal follicle-derived ovarian lesions. Mullany et al. continued work on the *Kras^{G12D}*;*Pten^{f/f}*;*Amhr2^{Cre}* mice and showed that ovarian surface epithelium cells, removed from mutant mice prior to tumor formation, developed into tumors when grown in soft agar [143]. This key result suggests that *Kras* and *Ptell* play a significant role in the development of tumors in the ovarian surface epithelium, and the genetic mutations are the primary driver, since tumor formation occurred even outside of the ovarian microenvironment [143].

4.2. Other Models

4.2.1. Immortalized Cell Lines

Immortalized human ovarian cancer cell lines have been widely used for studying molecular mechanisms of ovarian cancer. Ovarian cancer cell lines are used to study cancer biology, connecting genetic and epigenetic alterations to cancer development, progression, and drug response. Importantly, ovarian cancer cell lines have been developed from different histological and molecular subtypes of ovarian cancer. Unfortunately, molecular characterization has revealed that common ovarian cancer cell lines (i.e., SKOV3, HEYA8) do not molecularly represent the histology of tumor of origin. The number of cell lines derived from either endometrioid or clear cell ovarian cancers is more limited than high-grade serous cell lines. However, molecular profiling, including attention to gene mutations common in these endometriosis-associated ovarian cancers (i.e., *ARID1A*, *PIK3CA*, *CTNNB1*, *PTEN*, and *KRAS*) and mutations common in high-grade serous (i.e., TP53), have allowed better molecular and biological distinction [176–182]. Table 4 shows the common endometrioid and clear-cell ovarian cancer cell lines, including lines that were not derived from endometriosis-associated ovarian cancers, but which may molecularly represent non-high grade serous cell lines. Even fewer cell endometriotic cell lines exist, with 12Z cells being the only widely shared epithelial-like endometriosis immortalized cell line [183]. For rigor and reproducibility, additional well-characterized endometriotic cell lines and possibly ovarian cancer cell lines derived from women with endometriosis need to be created.

Table 4. Endometriosis and endometriosis-associated ovarian cancer cell lines.

Cell Line	Original Derivation	Putative Histotype by Molecular Studies	Genetic Mutations	Genetic Gains	Ref.
11Z	Red peritoneal endometriotic lesion	Benign	Unknown	Unknown	[183]
12Z	Red peritoneal endometriotic lesion	Benign (epithelial-like)	Unknown	Unknown	[183]
EEC16	Benign endometriotic lesion (epithelial-like)	Benign	Unknown	Unknown	[184]
EMosis-CC/TERT	Benign endometriotic lesion (epithelial-like)	Benign	Unknown	Unknown	[185]
22B	Red peritoneal endometriotic lesion (Stromal/fibroblast-like)	Benign	Unknown	Unknown	[183]
Hs 832(C).T (CRL-7566)	Benign endometriotic ovarian cyst	Benign	Unknown	Unknown	ATCC
OVTOKO	Clear-cell (spleen metastasis)	Clear-cell	None	ERRB2, HNF1B, MET, PPM1D, STAT3, TP53, YAP1, ZNF217, CDKN2A, CDKN2B	[177–179,182]
OVMANA	Clear-cell (primary tumor)	Clear-cell	BRCA2, PIK3CA, ARID1A	ARID1A, MET, PPM1D, TP53, ZNF217	[178,179,182,186]
TOV21G	Clear-cell (primary tumor)	Clear-cell	KRAS, PTEN, PIK3CA, CTNNB1, ARID1A, TPX2		[178–182,187]
RMG-1	Clear-cell (ascites)	Clear-cell	TP53*	ERBB2	[178,179,182,188]
RMG-2	Clear-cell	Clear-cell	PPP2R1A, ARID1A	ERBB2, HNF1B, MET, PIK3CA, PPM1D, STAT3, ZNF217, CDKN2A, CDKN2B	[179]
OCC1	Clear-cell	Clear-cell			[189]
JHOC-5	Clear-cell (pelvic metastasis)	Clear-cell		ARID1A, ERBB2, HNF1B, MET, PIK3CA, PPM1D, STAT2, ZNF217, CDKN2A, CDKN2B	[178,179,182,190]
JHOC-7	Clear-cell	Clear-cell	PIK3CA	ARID1A, HNF1B, PIK3CA, PPM1D, STAT3, ZNF217	[179]

Table 4. *Cont.*

Cell Line	Original Derivation	Putative Histotype by Molecular Studies	Genetic Mutations	Genetic Gains	Ref.
JHOC-9	Clear-cell	Clear-cell	PTEN, ARID1A	HNF1B, ZNF217	[179]
ES2	Poorly differentiated clear-cell (primary tumor)	Endometrioid/Clear-cell	BRAF, TP53, APC, MYC		[178–182,191]
OVISE	Clear-cell (pelvic metastasis)	Endometrioid/Clear-cell	ARID1A		[177–179,182]
OVSAYO	Clear-cell	Serous	TP53		[179]
TOV112D	Endometrioid (primary tumor)	Endometrioid	CTNNB1, TP53		[179–182,187]
OVK18	Endometrioid (ascites)	Endometrioid	TP53, PTEN, KRAS, ARID1A		[178,182,192]
SNU-251	Endometrioid	Endometrioid	BRCA1		[193]
2008	Endometrioid	Atypical non-serous	TP53		[179]
IGROV1	Endometrioid with serous/clear cell (primary tumor)	Endometrioid/Clear-cell	PTEN, TP53, ARID1A, BRCA1, BRCA2, PIK3CA, TPX2		[178–180,182,194]
59M	Endometrioid with clear cell (ascites)	Endometrioid/Clear-cell	TP53	MYC	[178,180,182,193,195]
COV362	Endometrioid (pleural effusion)	Serous	TP53, BRCA1, RB1*, EGFR, APC	MYC	[178,180,182,196]
A2780	Unknown adenocarcinoma	Endometrioid	PTEN, ARID1A, PIK3CA, BRAF		[178–182,197]
HEYA8	Moderately differentiated papillary serous (peritoneal metastasis)	Unlikely serous	KRAS, BRAF		[178,179,182,198]
SKOV3	Well differentiated, adenocarcinoma (ascites)	Endometrioid/Clear-cell	PIK3CA, ARID1A	ERBB2	[178–182,199]

* Homozygous deletion.

4.2.2. Xenograft Models

Implantation of immortalized human cell lines typically requires immunocompromised mice. A Japanese group created telomerase transformed endometriosis epithelial cell lines and confirmed cellular growth, steroid hormone response, and lack of malignant transformation in nude mice [185]. Further, these cells have been used in xenograft models to study treatment effects of small molecular inhibitors in endometriosis [104,200]. However, limited distribution outside Japan has restricted the use of these cells for studies of endometriosis-associated ovarian cancers. A similarly developed endometriotic epithelial cell line (EEC16) does not grow in SCID mice [184].

In terms of the endometriotic tumor microenvironment, Komiyama et al. placed normal endometrium of women without endometriosis into SCID mice. RMG-1 cells, a clear-cell ovarian cancer cell line, were grown in mice then transplanted into mice with or without endometrial implants. Although the tumors weighed less when grown with endometrium, proliferation was significantly higher in mice with transplanted endometrium. Additionally, these tumors expressed high levels of TGFβ and IL6. Addition of normal human endometrium changed the xenograft model to a more endometriotic microenvironment [201].

4.2.3. Three Dimensional (3D) and Co-Culture Models

Immortalized cell lines in monolayer two-dimensional (2D) culture fail to recapitulate the complexity of tumor tissue. Tumors are three-dimensional (3D) structures, surrounded by other cell types and a unique extracellular matrix (ECM) that is biologically optimized for growth of each cell type [202]. To recapitulate this for in vitro model systems, immortalized cell lines can be grown in Matrigel, ultra-low-adhesive plates, or a hanging drop. Using these methods, many immortalized cell lines will form 3D spheroids. Three-dimensional spheroid models can be highly instructive towards the understanding of current drug resistance and new therapeutics because they better mimic the way 3D tumors or de novo spheroids interact with the surrounding microenvironment. Specifically, the architecture of spheroids results in non-heterogeneity of nutrient and drug penetration, which can cause differential responses to varying layers of the spheroid. For example, Lee et al. compared 31 ovarian cancer cell lines in both 2D monolayer and 3D spheroids to primary tumors. Three-dimensional spheroids showed slower rates of proliferation and decreased drug sensitivity than the same cells grown in 2D [202]. Additionally, these 3D spheroids mimicked histological characteristics of primary tumors. Although the authors did not perform genome-wide transcriptomic analysis, candidate biomarkers such as mucin 16, cell surface associated (CA125), Wilms Tumor 1 (WT1), estrogen receptor, Paired box gene 8 (PAX8), and β-catenin were examined by IHC on a tissue microarray composed of 2D and 3D samples. The expression of these biomarkers correlated well with expression in primary tumors [202]. These data suggest that 3D spheroid models alter the microenvironment in a potentially more biological way compared to other in vitro systems. Additionally, Lal-Nag et al. used high-throughput screening to test multiple oncological drugs against the HEYA8 cell line. The cells responded differently to various drugs if they were grown in monolayer, in the process of forming spheroids, or already in pre-formed spheroids. This work establishes that the dimensionality of ovarian cancer cells plays a role in how they respond to their environment [203]. Similarly, Chowwanadisai et al. created cisplatin-resistant ovarian cancer spheroids by treating cells with sub-threshold doses of cisplatin, which resulted in a mesenchymal-enriched gene expression signature [204]. While molecular changes within spheroids may play a role in chemotherapy resistance, size of spheroids, similar to remaining disease after debulking surgery, plays a role in response. Tanenbaum et al. [205] showed that small spheroids treated with either short-term high-dose or prolonged low-dose cisplatin underwent significant shrinkage. Importantly, large spheroids preferentially responded to short-term high doses of cisplatin [205]. The investigators did not explore if the remaining cells became chemotherapy-resistant [205]. Although immortalized cell lines from endometrioid or clear cell ovarian cancers have not been extensively tested in 3D culture, we anticipate that they would behave similarly.

In addition to single cell types within 3D spheroids, co-culture systems can be useful. For example, endometrial epithelial cells are inhibited at a rate of 65–80% when grown in co-culture with endometrial stromal cells, highlighting the need for complex co-culture models [206]. Additionally, co-culture models of epithelial and stromal endometriosis cells show that stromal cells are responsible for metabolism of iron. The authors hypothesize that storage of iron by stromal cells is protective against malignant transformation of epithelial cells. Specifically, a lack of stromal cells and an abundance of epithelial cells, which cannot metabolize iron, leads to oxidative damage and oncogenic change [207]. This hypothesis fits with data from Anglesio et al. showing tumorigenic mutations in *KRAS* in epithelial cells of endometriosis but not stromal cells [27]. Similarly, co-culture of macrophages with endometriotic epithelial or endometriotic stromal cells leads to an increase in invasion that is more robust in epithelial than stromal cells [208]. Three-dimensional organoids made from endometrium and decidua have been developed simultaneously by two independent laboratories and represent promising models for in vitro study [209,210]. Development of additional endometriotic tumor microenvironment models are needed to study ovarian cancer cells within spheroids, 3D organoids, or co-culture systems.

5. Future of Precision Therapy for/or Prevention of Ovarian Cancer

Endometriosis is a known risk factor for ovarian cancer [41]. However, early treatment of endometriosis represents a known prevention strategy for ovarian cancer. For example, a woman on oral contraceptive therapy has a more robust protection against ovarian cancer if she has endometriosis than if she does not [120]. While treatment of endometriosis with contraceptives is effective, women desiring fertility do not enjoy the side of effects of contraception, and when medical management is stopped, 73% of women have return of symptoms. Additionally, surgical treatment of endometriosis with removal of one or both ovaries results in significant decrease in ovarian cancer risk. However, 55% of women undergoing local resection of endometriosis will have at least one more surgery over the course of seven years [211,212]. Morbidity associated with multiple operations makes selection of timing for endometriosis surgery important in pre-menopausal women. New treatments for endometriosis are needed. Importantly, discovery of new treatments for endometriosis should be a priority for ovarian cancer funding agencies as these therapies may lead to prevention of ovarian cancer.

In terms of therapy highlighting the importance of the molecular signaling between cells within tumors, Mok et al. used a systems biology approach to study individual cell types. Machine learning with large databases of drugs and molecular effects highlighted an FDA-approved drug for potential targeted treatment. While this study used high-grade serous ovarian tumors, it brings forward the importance of non-epithelial ovarian cancer cells in cancer treatment [213]. Importantly, the study focused on TGFβ signaling pathways [213]. Endometriosis also has dysregulated TGFβ signaling pathways [92]. Similar treatment of endometriosis may prevent ovarian cancer.

6. Conclusions

The Gynecologic Cancers Steering Committee of the National Institutes of Health (NIH) proposed strategic priorities for ovarian cancer. These research priorities focus on discovery of biomarkers, identification of cancer subsets to drive treatment recommendations, immunotherapy, combination therapies, and manipulation of the host-tumor microenvironment. While these priorities are not specific for a particular histotype, they are highly applicable to both the more common high-grade serous and less common endometriosis-associated ovarian cancers and warrant further study in endometriosis-associated ovarian cancer models.

Author Contributions: J.R.H.W., X.W. and S.M.H. constructed the outline of the review, synthesized and referenced the works included, and wrote the manuscript.

References

1. Bulun, S.E. Endometriosis. *N. Engl. J. Med.* **2009**, *360*, 268–279. [CrossRef] [PubMed]
2. Giudice, L.C.; Kao, L.C. Endometriosis. *Lancet* **2004**, *364*, 1789–1799. [CrossRef]
3. Buck Louis, G.M.; Hediger, M.L.; Peterson, C.M.; Croughan, M.; Sundaram, R.; Stanford, J.; Chen, Z.; Fujimoto, V.Y.; Varner, M.W.; Trumble, A.; et al. Incidence of endometriosis by study population and diagnostic method: The endo study. *Fertil. Steril.* **2011**, *96*, 360–365. [CrossRef] [PubMed]
4. DiVasta, A.D.; Vitonis, A.F.; Laufer, M.R.; Missmer, S.A. Spectrum of symptoms in women diagnosed with endometriosis during adolescence vs. adulthood. *Am. J. Obstet. Gynecol.* **2018**, *218*, 324.e1–324.e11. [CrossRef] [PubMed]
5. Aerts, L.; Grangier, L.; Streuli, I.; Dallenbach, P.; Marci, R.; Wenger, J.M.; Pluchino, N. Psychosocial impact of endometriosis: From co-morbidity to intervention. *Best Pract. Res. Clin. Obstet. Gynaecol.* **2018**. [CrossRef] [PubMed]
6. Pearce, C.L.; Stram, D.O.; Ness, R.B.; Stram, D.A.; Roman, L.D.; Templeman, C.; Lee, A.W.; Menon, U.; Fasching, P.A.; McAlpine, J.N.; et al. Population distribution of lifetime risk of ovarian cancer in the united states. *Cancer Epidemiol. Biomark. Prev.* **2015**, *24*, 671–676. [CrossRef] [PubMed]
7. Pearce, C.L.; Templeman, C.; Rossing, M.A.; Lee, A.; Near, A.M.; Webb, P.M.; Nagle, C.M.; Doherty, J.A.; Cushing-Haugen, K.L.; Wicklund, K.G.; et al. Association between endometriosis and risk of histological subtypes of ovarian cancer: A pooled analysis of case-control studies. *Lancet Oncol.* **2012**, *13*, 385–394. [CrossRef]
8. Nagle, C.M.; Olsen, C.M.; Webb, P.M.; Jordan, S.J.; Whiteman, D.C.; Green, A.C.; Australian Cancer Study Group; Australian Ovarian Cancer Study Group. Endometrioid and clear cell ovarian cancers: A comparative analysis of risk factors. *Eur. J. Cancer* **2008**, *44*, 2477–2484. [CrossRef] [PubMed]
9. Rossing, M.A.; Cushing-Haugen, K.L.; Wicklund, K.G.; Doherty, J.A.; Weiss, N.S. Risk of epithelial ovarian cancer in relation to benign ovarian conditions and ovarian surgery. *Cancer Causes Control* **2008**, *19*, 1357–1364. [CrossRef] [PubMed]
10. Brinton, L.A.; Gridley, G.; Persson, I.; Baron, J.; Bergqvist, A. Cancer risk after a hospital discharge diagnosis of endometriosis. *Am. J. Obstet. Gynecol.* **1997**, *176*, 572–579. [CrossRef]
11. Kobayashi, H.; Sumimoto, K.; Moniwa, N.; Imai, M.; Takakura, K.; Kuromaki, T.; Morioka, E.; Arisawa, K.; Terao, T. Risk of devloping ovarian cancer among women with ovarian endometrioma: A cohort study in shizuoka, Japan. *Int. J. Cancer* **2007**, *17*, 37–43. [CrossRef] [PubMed]
12. Somigliana, E.; Vigano, P.; Parazzini, F.; Stoppelli, S.; Giambattista, E.; Vercellini, P. Association between endometriosis and cancer: A comprehensive review and a critical analysis of clinical and epidemiological evidence. *Gynecol. Oncol.* **2006**, *101*, 331–341. [CrossRef] [PubMed]
13. Siegel, R.L.; Miller, K.D.; Jemal, A. Cancer statistics, 2018. *CA Cancer J. Clin.* **2018**, *68*, 7–30. [CrossRef] [PubMed]
14. Kurman, R.J.; Shih Ie, M. The dualistic model of ovarian carcinogenesis: Revisited, revised, and expanded. *Am. J. Pathol.* **2016**, *186*, 733–747. [CrossRef] [PubMed]
15. Reid, B.M.; Permuth, J.B.; Sellers, T.A. Epidemiology of ovarian cancer: A review. *Cancer Biol. Med.* **2017**, *14*, 9–32. [PubMed]
16. Prat, J. Pathology of borderline and invasive cancers. *Best Pract. Res. Clin. Obstet. Gynaecol.* **2017**, *41*, 15–30. [CrossRef] [PubMed]
17. Lu, J.; Tao, X.; Zhou, J.; Lu, Y.; Wang, Z.; Liu, H.; Xu, C. Improved clinical outcomes of patients with ovarian carcinoma arising in endometriosis. *Oncotarget* **2017**, *8*, 5843–5852. [CrossRef] [PubMed]
18. Dinkelspiel, H.E.; Matrai, C.; Pauk, S.; Pierre-Louis, A.; Chiu, Y.L.; Gupta, D.; Caputo, T.; Ellenson, L.H.; Holcomb, K. Does the presence of endometriosis affect prognosis of ovarian cancer? *Cancer Investig.* **2016**, *34*, 148–154. [CrossRef] [PubMed]
19. McMeekin, D.S.; Burger, R.A.; Manetta, A.; DiSaia, P.; Berman, M.L. Endometrioid adenocarcinoma of the ovary and its relationship to endometriosis. *Gynecol. Oncol.* **1995**, *59*, 81–86. [CrossRef] [PubMed]
20. Melin, A.; Lundholm, C.; Malki, N.; Swahn, M.L.; Sparen, P.; Bergqvist, A. Endometriosis as a prognostic factor for cancer survival. *Int. J. Cancer* **2011**, *129*, 948–955. [CrossRef] [PubMed]
21. Quirk, J.T.; Natarajan, N.; Mettlin, C.J. Age-specific ovarian cancer incidence rate patterns in the united states. *Gynecol. Oncol.* **2005**, *99*, 248–250. [CrossRef] [PubMed]

22. Gershenson, D.M. Treatment of ovarian cancer in young women. *Clin. Obstet. Gynecol.* **2012**, *55*, 65–74. [CrossRef] [PubMed]

23. Storey, D.J.; Rush, R.; Stewart, M.; Rye, T.; Al-Nafussi, A.; Williams, A.R.; Smyth, J.F.; Gabra, H. Endometrioid epithelial ovarian cancer: 20 years of prospectively collected data from a single center. *Cancer* **2008**, *112*, 2211–2220. [CrossRef] [PubMed]

24. Noli, S.; Cipriani, S.; Scarfone, G.; Villa, A.; Grossi, E.; Monti, E.; Vercellini, P.; Parazzini, F. Long term survival of ovarian endometriosis associated clear cell and endometrioid ovarian cancers. *Int. J. Gynecol. Cancer* **2013**, *23*, 244–248. [CrossRef] [PubMed]

25. Ahmed, A.A.; Becker, C.M.; Bast, R.C., Jr. The origin of ovarian cancer. *BJOG* **2012**, *119*, 134–136. [CrossRef] [PubMed]

26. Cochrane, D.R.; Tessier-Cloutier, B.; Lawrence, K.M.; Nazeran, T.; Karnezis, A.N.; Salamanca, C.; Cheng, A.S.; McAlpine, J.N.; Hoang, L.N.; Gilks, C.B.; et al. Clear cell and endometrioid carcinomas: Are their differences attributable to distinct cells of origin? *J. Pathol.* **2017**, *243*, 26–36. [CrossRef] [PubMed]

27. Anglesio, M.S.; Papadopoulos, N.; Ayhan, A.; Nazeran, T.M.; Noe, M.; Horlings, H.M.; Lum, A.; Jones, S.; Senz, J.; Seckin, T.; et al. Cancer-associated mutations in endometriosis without cancer. *N. Engl. J. Med.* **2017**, *376*, 1835–1848. [CrossRef] [PubMed]

28. Chui, M.H.; Wang, T.L.; Shih, I.M. Endometriosis: Benign, malignant, or something in between? *Oncotarget* **2017**, *8*, 78263–78264. [CrossRef] [PubMed]

29. Lac, V.; Huntsman, D.G. Distinct developmental trajectories of endometriotic epithelium and stroma: Implications for the origins of endometriosis. *J. Pathol.* **2018**. [CrossRef] [PubMed]

30. Wiegand, K.C.; Shah, S.P.; Al-Agha, O.M.; Zhao, Y.; Tse, K.; Zeng, T.; Senz, J.; McConechy, M.K.; Anglesio, M.S.; Kalloger, S.E.; et al. Arid1a mutations in endometriosis-associated ovarian carcinomas. *N. Engl. J. Med.* **2010**, *363*, 1532–1543. [CrossRef] [PubMed]

31. Sato, N.; Tsunoda, H.; Nishida, M.; Morishita, Y.; Takimoto, Y.; Kubo, T.; Noguchi, M. Loss of heterozygosity on 10q23.3 and mutation of the tumor suppressor gene Pten in benign endometrial cyst of the ovary: Possible sequence progression from benign endometrial cyst to endometrioid carcinoma and clear cell carcinoma of the ovary. *Cancer Res.* **2000**, *60*, 7052–7056. [PubMed]

32. Yamamoto, S.; Tsuda, H.; Takano, M.; Tamai, S.; Matsubara, O. Loss of arid1a protein expression occurs as an early event in ovarian clear-cell carcinoma development and frequently coexists with PIK3CA mutations. *Mod. Pathol.* **2012**, *25*, 615–624. [CrossRef] [PubMed]

33. Stewart, C.J.; Leung, Y.; Walsh, M.D.; Walters, R.J.; Young, J.P.; Buchanan, D.D. Kras mutations in ovarian low-grade endometrioid adenocarcinoma: Association with concurrent endometriosis. *Hum. Pathol.* **2012**, *43*, 1177–1183. [CrossRef] [PubMed]

34. Zou, Y.; Zhou, J.Y.; Guo, J.B.; Wang, L.Q.; Luo, Y.; Zhang, Z.Y.; Liu, F.Y.; Tan, J.; Wang, F.; Huang, O.P. The presence of kras, ppp2r1a and arid1a mutations in 101 Chinese samples with ovarian endometriosis. *Mutat. Res.* **2018**, *809*, 1–5. [CrossRef] [PubMed]

35. Wiegand, K.C.; Lee, A.F.; Al-Agha, O.M.; Chow, C.; Kalloger, S.E.; Scott, D.W.; Steidl, C.; Wiseman, S.M.; Gascoyne, R.D.; Gilks, B.; et al. Loss of baf250a (arid1a) is frequent in high-grade endometrial carcinomas. *J. Pathol.* **2011**, *224*, 328–333. [CrossRef] [PubMed]

36. Yamamoto, S.; Tsuda, H.; Takano, M.; Tamai, S.; Matsubara, O. Pik3ca mutations and loss of arid1a protein expression are early events in the development of cystic ovarian clear cell adenocarcinoma. *Virchows Arch.* **2012**, *460*, 77–87. [CrossRef] [PubMed]

37. Samartzis, E.P.; Samartzis, N.; Noske, A.; Fedier, A.; Caduff, R.; Dedes, K.J.; Fink, D.; Imesch, P. Loss of arid1a/baf250a-expression in endometriosis: A biomarker for risk of carcinogenic transformation? *Mod. Pathol.* **2012**, *25*, 885–892. [CrossRef] [PubMed]

38. Ayhan, A.; Mao, T.L.; Seckin, T.; Wu, C.H.; Guan, B.; Ogawa, H.; Futagami, M.; Mizukami, H.; Yokoyama, Y.; Kurman, R.J.; et al. Loss of arid1a expression is an early molecular event in tumor progression from ovarian endometriotic cyst to clear cell and endometrioid carcinoma. *Int. J. Gynecol. Cancer* **2012**, *22*, 1310–1315. [CrossRef] [PubMed]

39. Xiao, W.; Awadallah, A.; Xin, W. Loss of arid1a/baf250a expression in ovarian endometriosis and clear cell carcinoma. *Int. J. Clin. Exp. Pathol.* **2012**, *5*, 642–650. [PubMed]

40. Anglesio, M.S.; Yong, P.J. Endometriosis-associated ovarian cancers. *Clin. Obstet. Gynecol.* **2017**, *60*, 711–727. [CrossRef] [PubMed]

41. Vercellini, P.; Vigano, P.; Buggio, L.; Makieva, S.; Scarfone, G.; Cribiu, F.M.; Parazzini, F.; Somigliana, E. Perimenopausal management of ovarian endometriosis and associated cancer risk: When is medical or surgical treatment indicated? *Best Pract. Res. Clin. Obstet. Gynaecol.* **2018**. [CrossRef] [PubMed]

42. Friedlander, M.L.; Russell, K.; Millis, S.; Gatalica, Z.; Bender, R.; Voss, A. Molecular profiling of clear cell ovarian cancers: Identifying potential treatment targets for clinical trials. *Int. J. Gynecol. Cancer* **2016**, *26*, 648–654. [CrossRef] [PubMed]

43. Ishikawa, M.; Nakayama, K.; Nakamura, K.; Ono, R.; Sanuki, K.; Yamashita, H.; Ishibashi, T.; Minamoto, T.; Iida, K.; Razia, S.; et al. Affinity-purified DNA-based mutation profiles of endometriosis-related ovarian neoplasms in Japanese patients. *Oncotarget* **2018**, *9*, 14754–14763. [CrossRef] [PubMed]

44. Jones, S.; Wang, T.L.; Shih Ie, M.; Mao, T.L.; Nakayama, K.; Roden, R.; Glas, R.; Slamon, D.; Diaz, L.A., Jr.; Vogelstein, B.; et al. Frequent mutations of chromatin remodeling gene arid1a in ovarian clear cell carcinoma. *Science* **2010**, *330*, 228–231. [CrossRef] [PubMed]

45. Shibuya, Y.; Tokunaga, H.; Saito, S.; Shimokawa, K.; Katsuoka, F.; Bin, L.; Kojima, K.; Nagasaki, M.; Yamamoto, M.; Yaegashi, N.; et al. Identification of somatic genetic alterations in ovarian clear cell carcinoma with next generation sequencing. *Genes Chromosom. Cancer* **2018**, *57*, 51–60. [CrossRef] [PubMed]

46. Grisham, R.N.; Iyer, G.; Garg, K.; DeLair, D.; Hyman, D.M.; Zhou, Q.; Iasonos, A.; Berger, M.F.; Dao, F.; Spriggs, D.R. Braf mutation is associated with early stage disease and improved outcome in patients with low-grade serous ovarian cancer. *Cancer* **2013**, *119*, 548–554. [CrossRef] [PubMed]

47. Sieben, N.L.; Macropoulos, P.; Roemen, G.M.; Kolkman-Uljee, S.M.; Jan Fleuren, G.; Houmadi, R.; Diss, T.; Warren, B.; Al Adnani, M.; De Goeij, A.P.; et al. In ovarian neoplasms, braf, but not kras, mutations are restricted to low-grade serous tumours. *J. Pathol.* **2004**, *202*, 336–340. [CrossRef] [PubMed]

48. Singer, G.; Oldt, R., 3rd; Cohen, Y.; Wang, B.G.; Sidransky, D.; Kurman, R.J.; Shih Ie, M. Mutations in BRAF and KRAS characterize the development of low-grade ovarian serous carcinoma. *J. Natl. Cancer Inst.* **2003**, *95*, 484–486. [CrossRef] [PubMed]

49. Lv, X.; Wang, D.; Ma, Y.; Long, Z. Analysis of the oncogene braf mutation and the correlation of the expression of wild-type BRAF and CREB1 in endometriosis. *Int. J. Mol. Med.* **2018**, *41*, 1349–1356. [CrossRef] [PubMed]

50. Saare, M.; Krigul, K.L.; Laisk-Podar, T.; Ponandai-Srinivasan, S.; Rahmioglu, N.; Lalit Kumar, P.G.; Zondervan, K.; Salumets, A.; Peters, M. DNA methylation alterations-potential cause of endometriosis pathogenesis or a reflection of tissue heterogeneity? *Biol. Reprod.* **2018**. [CrossRef] [PubMed]

51. He, J.; Chang, W.; Feng, C.; Cui, M.; Xu, T. Endometriosis malignant transformation: Epigenetics as a probable mechanism in ovarian tumorigenesis. *Int. J. Genom.* **2018**, *2018*, 1465348. [CrossRef] [PubMed]

52. Roca, F.J.; Loomans, H.A.; Wittman, A.T.; Creighton, C.J.; Hawkins, S.M. Ten-eleven translocation genes are downregulated in endometriosis. *Curr. Mol. Med.* **2016**, *16*, 288–298. [CrossRef] [PubMed]

53. Nothnick, W.B. MicroRNAs and endometriosis: Distinguishing drivers from passengers in disease pathogenesis. *Semin. Reprod. Med.* **2017**, *35*, 173–180. [CrossRef] [PubMed]

54. Logan, M.; Hawkins, S.M. Role of microRNAs in cancers of the female reproductive tract: Insights from recent clinical and experimental discovery studies. *Clin. Sci. (Lond. Engl. 1979)* **2015**, *128*, 153–180. [CrossRef] [PubMed]

55. Wang, X.; Ivan, M.; Hawkins, S.M. The role of microRNA molecules and microRNA-regulating machinery in the pathogenesis and progression of epithelial ovarian cancer. *Gynecol. Oncol.* **2017**, *147*, 481–487. [CrossRef] [PubMed]

56. Machado-Linde, F.; Sanchez-Ferrer, M.L.; Cascales, P.; Torroba, A.; Orozco, R.; Silva Sanchez, Y.; Nieto, A.; Fiol, G. Prevalence of endometriosis in epithelial ovarian cancer. Analysis of the associated clinical features and study on molecular mechanisms involved in the possible causality. *Eur. J. Gynaecol. Oncol.* **2015**, *36*, 21–24. [PubMed]

57. Stamp, J.P.; Gilks, C.B.; Wesseling, M.; Eshragh, S.; Ceballos, K.; Anglesio, M.S.; Kwon, J.S.; Tone, A.; Huntsman, D.G.; Carey, M.S. Baf250a expression in atypical endometriosis and endometriosis-associated ovarian cancer. *Int. J. Gynecol. Cancer* **2016**, *26*, 825–832. [CrossRef] [PubMed]

58. Van Gorp, T.; Amant, F.; Neven, P.; Vergote, I.; Moerman, P. Endometriosis and the development of malignant tumours of the pelvis. A review of literature. *Best Pract. Res. Clin. Obstet. Gynaecol.* **2004**, *18*, 349–371. [CrossRef] [PubMed]

59. Fukunaga, M.; Nomura, K.; Ishikawa, E.; Ushigome, S. Ovarian atypical endometriosis: Its close association with malignant epithelial tumours. *Histopathology* **1997**, *30*, 249–255. [CrossRef] [PubMed]

60. Banz, C.; Ungethuem, U.; Kuban, R.J.; Diedrich, K.; Lengyel, E.; Hornung, D. The molecular signature of endometriosis-associated endometrioid ovarian cancer differs significantly from endometriosis-independent endometrioid ovarian cancer. *Fertil. Steril.* **2010**, *94*, 1212–1217. [CrossRef] [PubMed]

61. Zhang, C.; Wang, X.; Anaya, Y.; Parodi, L.; Chen, L.; Anderson, M.L.; Hawkins, S.M. Distinct molecular pathways in ovarian endometrioid adenocarcinoma with concurrent endometriosis. *Int. J. Cancer* **2018**, in press.

62. Kolin, D.L.; Dinulescu, D.M.; Crum, C.P. Origin of clear cell carcinoma: Nature or nurture? *J. Pathol.* **2018**, *244*, 131–134. [CrossRef] [PubMed]

63. Klemmt, P.A.B.; Starzinski-Powitz, A. Molecular and cellular pathogenesis of endometriosis. *Curr. Womens Health Rev.* **2018**, *14*, 106–116. [CrossRef] [PubMed]

64. Liu, D.T.; Hitchcock, A. Endometriosis: Its association with retrograde menstruation, dysmenorrhoea and tubal pathology. *Br. J. Obstet. Gynaecol.* **1986**, *93*, 859–862. [CrossRef] [PubMed]

65. Liu, H.; Du, Y.; Zhang, Z.; Lv, L.; Xiong, W.; Zhang, L.; Li, N.; He, H.; Li, Q.; Liu, Y. Autophagy contributes to hypoxia-induced epithelial to mesenchymal transition of endometrial epithelial cells in endometriosis. *Biol. Reprod.* **2018**. [CrossRef] [PubMed]

66. Allavena, G.; Carrarelli, P.; Del Bello, B.; Luisi, S.; Petraglia, F.; Maellaro, E. Autophagy is upregulated in ovarian endometriosis: A possible interplay with p53 and heme oxygenase-1. *Fertil. Steril.* **2015**, *103*, 1244–1251.e1. [CrossRef] [PubMed]

67. Liu, H.; Zhang, Z.; Xiong, W.; Zhang, L.; Xiong, Y.; Li, N.; He, H.; Du, Y.; Liu, Y. Hypoxia-inducible factor-1alpha promotes endometrial stromal cells migration and invasion by upregulating autophagy in endometriosis. *Reproduction* **2017**, *153*, 809–820. [CrossRef] [PubMed]

68. Xu, T.X.; Zhao, S.Z.; Dong, M.; Yu, X.R. Hypoxia responsive miR-210 promotes cell survival and autophagy of endometriotic cells in hypoxia. *Eur. Rev. Med. Pharmacol. Sci.* **2016**, *20*, 399–406. [PubMed]

69. Lin, X.; Dai, Y.; Xu, W.; Shi, L.; Jin, X.; Li, C.; Zhou, F.; Pan, Y.; Zhang, Y.; Lin, X.; et al. Hypoxia promotes ectopic adhesion ability of endometrial stromal cells via tgf-beta1/smad signaling in endometriosis. *Endocrinology* **2018**, *159*, 1630–1641. [CrossRef] [PubMed]

70. Yoo, J.Y.; Kim, T.H.; Fazleabas, A.T.; Palomino, W.A.; Ahn, S.H.; Tayade, C.; Schammel, D.P.; Young, S.L.; Jeong, J.W.; Lessey, B.A. Kras activation and over-expression of sirt1/bcl6 contributes to the pathogenesis of endometriosis and progesterone resistance. *Sci. Rep.* **2017**, *7*, 6765. [CrossRef] [PubMed]

71. Hsiao, K.Y.; Chang, N.; Tsai, J.L.; Lin, S.C.; Tsai, S.J.; Wu, M.H. Hypoxia-inhibited DUSP2 expression promotes IL-6/STAT3 signaling in endometriosis. *Am. J. Reprod. Immunol.* **2017**, *78*. [CrossRef] [PubMed]

72. Kim, B.G.; Yoo, J.Y.; Kim, T.H.; Shin, J.H.; Langenheim, J.F.; Ferguson, S.D.; Fazleabas, A.T.; Young, S.L.; Lessey, B.A.; Jeong, J.W. Aberrant activation of signal transducer and activator of transcription-3 (stat3) signaling in endometriosis. *Hum. Reprod. (Oxf. Engl.)* **2015**, *30*, 1069–1078. [CrossRef] [PubMed]

73. Lin, S.C.; Wang, C.C.; Wu, M.H.; Yang, S.H.; Li, Y.H.; Tsai, S.J. Hypoxia-induced microRNA-20a expression increases ERK phosphorylation and angiogenic gene expression in endometriotic stromal cells. *J. Clin. Endocrinol. Metab.* **2012**, *97*, E1515–E1523. [CrossRef] [PubMed]

74. Hsiao, K.Y.; Chang, N.; Lin, S.C.; Li, Y.H.; Wu, M.H. Inhibition of dual specificity phosphatase-2 by hypoxia promotes interleukin-8-mediated angiogenesis in endometriosis. *Hum. Reprod. (Oxf. Engl.)* **2014**, *29*, 2747–2755. [CrossRef] [PubMed]

75. Kato, M.; Yamamoto, S.; Takano, M.; Matsubara, O.; Furuya, K. Aberrant expression of the mammalian target of rapamycin, hypoxia-inducible factor-1alpha, and glucose transporter 1 in the development of ovarian clear-cell adenocarcinoma. *Int. J. Gynecol. Pathol.* **2012**, *31*, 254–263. [CrossRef] [PubMed]

76. Duska, L.R.; Garrett, L.; Henretta, M.; Ferriss, J.S.; Lee, L.; Horowitz, N. When 'never-events' occur despite adherence to clinical guidelines: The case of venous thromboembolism in clear cell cancer of the ovary compared with other epithelial histologic subtypes. *Gynecol. Oncol.* **2010**, *116*, 374–377. [CrossRef] [PubMed]

77. Hsiao, K.Y.; Lin, S.C.; Wu, M.H.; Tsai, S.J. Pathological functions of hypoxia in endometriosis. *Front. Biosci. (Elite Ed.)* **2015**, *7*, 309–321. [CrossRef] [PubMed]

78. Zhan, L.; Wang, W.; Zhang, Y.; Song, E.; Fan, Y.; Wei, B. Hypoxia-inducible factor-1alpha: A promising therapeutic target in endometriosis. *Biochimie* **2016**, *123*, 130–137. [CrossRef] [PubMed]

79. Meserve, E.E.; Crum, C.P. Benign conditions of the ovary. In *Diagnostic Gynecologic and Obstetric Pathology*, 3rd ed.; Crum, C.P., Haefner, H.K., Peters, W.A., III, Eds.; Elsevier, Inc.: Philadephia, PA, USA, 2018; pp. 761–799.

80. Hantak, A.M.; Bagchi, I.C.; Bagchi, M.K. Role of uterine stromal-epithelial crosstalk in embryo implantation. *Int. J. Dev. Biol.* **2014**, *58*, 139–146. [CrossRef] [PubMed]

81. Kurita, T.; Medina, R.; Schabel, A.B.; Young, P.; Gama, P.; Parekh, T.V.; Brody, J.; Cunha, G.R.; Osteen, K.G.; Bruner-Tran, K.L.; et al. The activation function-1 domain of estrogen receptor alpha in uterine stromal cells is required for mouse but not human uterine epithelial response to estrogen. *Differentiation* **2005**, *73*, 313–322. [CrossRef] [PubMed]

82. Osteen, K.G.; Rodgers, W.H.; Gaire, M.; Hargrove, J.T.; Gorstein, F.; Matrisian, L.M. Stromal-epithelial interaction mediates steroidal regulation of metalloproteinase expression in human endometrium. *Proc. Natl. Acad. Sci. USA* **1994**, *91*, 10129–10133. [CrossRef] [PubMed]

83. Valdez, J.; Cook, C.D.; Ahrens, C.C.; Wang, A.J.; Brown, A.; Kumar, M.; Stockdale, L.; Rothenberg, D.; Renggli, K.; Gordon, E.; et al. On-demand dissolution of modular, synthetic extracellular matrix reveals local epithelial-stromal communication networks. *Biomaterials* **2017**, *130*, 90–103. [CrossRef] [PubMed]

84. Aghajanova, L.; Hamilton, A.; Kwintkiewicz, J.; Vo, K.C.; Giudice, L.C. Steroidogenic enzyme and key decidualization marker dysregulation in endometrial stromal cells from women with versus without endometriosis. *Biol. Reprod.* **2009**, *80*, 105–114. [CrossRef] [PubMed]

85. Velarde, M.C.; Aghajanova, L.; Nezhat, C.R.; Giudice, L.C. Increased mitogen-activated protein kinase kinase/extracellularly regulated kinase activity in human endometrial stromal fibroblasts of women with endometriosis reduces 3′,5′-cyclic adenosine 5′-monophosphate inhibition of cyclin D1. *Endocrinology* **2009**, *150*, 4701–4712. [CrossRef] [PubMed]

86. Aghajanova, L.; Horcajadas, J.A.; Weeks, J.L.; Esteban, F.J.; Nezhat, C.N.; Conti, M.; Giudice, L.C. The protein kinase a pathway-regulated transcriptome of endometrial stromal fibroblasts reveals compromised differentiation and persistent proliferative potential in endometriosis. *Endocrinology* **2010**, *151*, 1341–1355. [CrossRef] [PubMed]

87. Aghajanova, L.; Tatsumi, K.; Horcajadas, J.A.; Zamah, A.M.; Esteban, F.J.; Herndon, C.N.; Conti, M.; Giudice, L.C. Unique transcriptome, pathways, and networks in the human endometrial fibroblast response to progesterone in endometriosis. *Biol. Reprod.* **2011**, *84*, 801–815. [CrossRef] [PubMed]

88. Aghajanova, L.; Velarde, M.C.; Giudice, L.C. The progesterone receptor coactivator hic-5 is involved in the pathophysiology of endometriosis. *Endocrinology* **2009**, *150*, 3863–3870. [CrossRef] [PubMed]

89. Barragan, F.; Irwin, J.C.; Balayan, S.; Erikson, D.W.; Chen, J.C.; Houshdaran, S.; Piltonen, T.T.; Spitzer, T.L.; George, A.; Rabban, J.T.; et al. Human endometrial fibroblasts derived from mesenchymal progenitors inherit progesterone resistance and acquire an inflammatory phenotype in the endometrial niche in endometriosis. *Biol. Reprod.* **2016**, *94*, 118. [CrossRef] [PubMed]

90. Zhang, Y.; Tang, H.; Cai, J.; Zhang, T.; Guo, J.; Feng, D.; Wang, Z. Ovarian cancer-associated fibroblasts contribute to epithelial ovarian carcinoma metastasis by promoting angiogenesis, lymphangiogenesis and tumor cell invasion. *Cancer Lett.* **2011**, *303*, 47–55. [CrossRef] [PubMed]

91. Mitra, A.K.; Zillhardt, M.; Hua, Y.; Tiwari, P.; Murmann, A.E.; Peter, M.E.; Lengyel, E. MicroRNAs reprogram normal fibroblasts into cancer-associated fibroblasts in ovarian cancer. *Cancer Discov.* **2012**, *2*, 1100–1108. [CrossRef] [PubMed]

92. Hawkins, S.M.; Creighton, C.J.; Han, D.Y.; Zariff, A.; Anderson, M.L.; Gunaratne, P.H.; Matzuk, M.M. Functional microRNA involved in endometriosis. *Mol. Endocrinol.* **2011**, *25*, 821–832. [CrossRef] [PubMed]

93. Lessey, B.A.; Kim, J.J. Endometrial receptivity in the eutopic endometrium of women with endometriosis: It is affected, and let me show you why. *Fertil. Steril.* **2017**, *108*, 19–27. [CrossRef] [PubMed]

94. Capobianco, A.; Rovere-Querini, P. Endometriosis, a disease of the macrophage. *Front. Immunol.* **2013**, *4*, 9. [CrossRef] [PubMed]

95. Bacci, M.; Capobianco, A.; Monno, A.; Cottone, L.; Di Puppo, F.; Camisa, B.; Mariani, M.; Brignole, C.; Ponzoni, M.; Ferrari, S.; et al. Macrophages are alternatively activated in patients with endometriosis and required for growth and vascularization of lesions in a mouse model of disease. *Am. J. Pathol.* **2009**, *175*, 547–556. [CrossRef] [PubMed]

96. Canet, B.; Pons, C.; Espinosa, I.; Prat, J. Cdc42-positive macrophages may prevent malignant transformation of ovarian endometriosis. *Hum. Pathol.* **2012**, *43*, 720–725. [CrossRef] [PubMed]

97. Furuya, M.; Tanaka, R.; Miyagi, E.; Kami, D.; Nagahama, K.; Miyagi, Y.; Nagashima, Y.; Hirahara, F.; Inayama, Y.; Aoki, I. Impaired CXCL4 expression in tumor-associated macrophages (tams) of ovarian cancers arising in endometriosis. *Cancer Biol. Ther.* **2012**, *13*, 671–680. [CrossRef] [PubMed]

98.   Eisermann, J.; Gast, M.J.; Pineda, J.; Odem, R.R.; Collins, J.L. Tumor necrosis factor in peritoneal fluid of women undergoing laparoscopic surgery. *Fertil. Steril.* **1988**, *50*, 573–579. [CrossRef]

99.   Calhaz-Jorge, C.; Costa, A.P.; Barata, M.; Santos, M.C.; Melo, A.; Palma-Carlos, M.L. Tumour necrosis factor alpha concentrations in the peritoneal fluid of infertile women with minimal or mild endometriosis are lower in patients with red lesions only than in patients without red lesions. *Hum. Reprod. (Oxf. Engl.)* **2000**, *15*, 1256–1260. [CrossRef]

100. Jin, C.H.; Yi, K.W.; Ha, Y.R.; Shin, J.H.; Park, H.T.; Kim, T.; Hur, J.Y. Chemerin expression in the peritoneal fluid, serum, and ovarian endometrioma of women with endometriosis. *Am. J. Reprod. Immunol.* **2015**, *74*, 379–386. [CrossRef] [PubMed]

101. Young, V.J.; Brown, J.K.; Saunders, P.T.; Duncan, W.C.; Horne, A.W. The peritoneum is both a source and target of TGF-Beta in women with endometriosis. *PLoS ONE* **2014**, *9*, e106773. [CrossRef] [PubMed]

102. Worley, M.J.; Welch, W.R.; Berkowitz, R.S.; Ng, S.W. Endometriosis-associated ovarian cancer: A review of pathogenesis. *Int. J. Mol. Sci.* **2013**, *14*, 5367–5379. [CrossRef] [PubMed]

103. Lewis, C.E.; Pollard, J.W. Distinct role of macrophages in different tumor microenvironments. *Cancer Res.* **2006**, *66*, 605–612. [CrossRef] [PubMed]

104. Han, S.J.; Jung, S.Y.; Wu, S.P.; Hawkins, S.M.; Park, M.J.; Kyo, S.; Qin, J.; Lydon, J.P.; Tsai, S.Y.; Tsai, M.J.; et al. Estrogen receptor beta modulates apoptosis complexes and the inflammasome to drive the pathogenesis of endometriosis. *Cell* **2015**, *163*, 960–974. [CrossRef] [PubMed]

105. Altan, Z.M.; Denis, D.; Kagan, D.; Grund, E.M.; Palmer, S.S.; Nataraja, S.G. A long-acting tumor necrosis factor alpha-binding protein demonstrates activity in both in vitro and in vivo models of endometriosis. *J. Pharmacol. Exp. Ther.* **2010**, *334*, 460–466. [CrossRef] [PubMed]

106. Koninckx, P.R.; Craessaerts, M.; Timmerman, D.; Cornillie, F.; Kennedy, S. Anti-TNF-alpha treatment for deep endometriosis-associated pain: A randomized placebo-controlled trial. *Hum. Reprod. (Oxf. Engl.)* **2008**, *23*, 2017–2023. [CrossRef] [PubMed]

107. Wei, J.J.; William, J.; Bulun, S. Endometriosis and ovarian cancer: A review of clinical, pathologic, and molecular aspects. *Int. J. Gynecol. Pathol.* **2011**, *30*, 553–568. [CrossRef] [PubMed]

108. Yamaguchi, K.; Mandai, M.; Toyokuni, S.; Hamanishi, J.; Higuchi, T.; Takakura, K.; Fujii, S. Contents of endometriotic cysts, especially the high concentration of free iron, are a possible cause of carcinogenesis in the cysts through the iron-induced persistent oxidative stress. *Clin. Cancer Res.* **2008**, *14*, 32–40. [CrossRef] [PubMed]

109. Mandai, M.; Matsumura, N.; Baba, T.; Yamaguchi, K.; Hamanishi, J.; Konishi, I. Ovarian clear cell carcinoma as a stress-responsive cancer: Influence of the microenvironment on the carcinogenesis and cancer phenotype. *Cancer Lett.* **2011**, *310*, 129–133. [CrossRef] [PubMed]

110. Shigetomi, H.; Higashiura, Y.; Kajihara, H.; Kobayashi, H. A potential link of oxidative stress and cell cycle regulation for development of endometriosis. *Gynecol. Endocrinol.* **2012**, *28*, 897–902. [CrossRef] [PubMed]

111. Vercellini, P.; Crosignani, P.; Somigliana, E.; Vigano, P.; Buggio, L.; Bolis, G.; Fedele, L. The 'incessant menstruation' hypothesis: A mechanistic ovarian cancer model with implications for prevention. *Hum. Reprod. (Oxf. Engl.)* **2011**, *26*, 2262–2273. [CrossRef] [PubMed]

112. Young, V.J.; Brown, J.K.; Maybin, J.; Saunders, P.T.; Duncan, W.C.; Horne, A.W. Transforming growth factor-β induced warburg-like metabolic reprogramming may underpin the development of peritoneal endometriosis. *J. Clin. Endocrinol. Metab.* **2014**, *99*, 3450–3459. [CrossRef] [PubMed]

113. Young, V.J.; Ahmad, S.F.; Brown, J.K.; Duncan, W.C.; Horne, A.W. Id2 mediates the transforming growth factor-β1-induced warburg-like effect seen in the peritoneum of women with endometriosis. *MHR Basic Sci. Reprod. Med.* **2016**, *22*, 648–654. [CrossRef] [PubMed]

114. Dominguez, F.; Ferrando, M.; Diaz-Gimeno, P.; Quintana, F.; Fernandez, G.; Castells, I.; Simon, C. Lipidomic profiling of endometrial fluid in women with ovarian endometriosisdagger. *Biol. Reprod.* **2017**, *96*, 772–779. [CrossRef] [PubMed]

115. Li, J.; Gao, Y.; Guan, L.; Zhang, H.; Sun, J.; Gong, X.; Li, D.; Chen, P.; Ma, Z.; Liang, X.; et al. Discovery of phosphatidic acid, phosphatidylcholine, and phosphatidylserine as biomarkers for early diagnosis of endometriosis. *Front. Physiol* **2018**, *9*, 14. [CrossRef] [PubMed]

116. Cheng, Y.H.; Imir, A.; Fenkci, V.; Yilmaz, M.B.; Bulun, S.E. Stromal cells of endometriosis fail to produce paracrine factors that induce epithelial 17beta-hydroxysteroid dehydrogenase type 2 gene and its

transcriptional regulator sp1: A mechanism for defective estradiol metabolism. *Am. J. Obstet. Gynecol.* **2007**, *196*, 391.e1–391.e7; discussion 391.e7–391.e8. [CrossRef] [PubMed]

117. Khorram, O.; Taylor, R.N.; Ryan, I.P.; Schall, T.J.; Landers, D.V. Peritoneal fluid concentrations of the cytokine rantes correlate with the severity of endometriosis. *Am. J. Obstet. Gynecol.* **1993**, *169*, 1545–1549. [CrossRef]

118. Tsai, S.J.; Wu, M.H.; Lin, C.C.; Sun, H.S.; Chen, H.M. Regulation of steroidogenic acute regulatory protein expression and progesterone production in endometriotic stromal cells. *J. Clin. Endocrinol. Metab.* **2001**, *86*, 5765–5773. [CrossRef] [PubMed]

119. Arosh, J.A.; Lee, J.; Balasubbramanian, D.; Stanley, J.A.; Long, C.R.; Meagher, M.W.; Osteen, K.G.; Bruner-Tran, K.L.; Burghardt, R.C.; Starzinski-Powitz, A.; et al. Molecular and preclinical basis to inhibit PGE2 receptors EP2 and EP4 as a novel nonsteroidal therapy for endometriosis. *Proc. Natl. Acad. Sci. USA* **2015**, *112*, 9716–9721. [CrossRef] [PubMed]

120. Modugno, F.; Ness, R.B.; Allen, G.O.; Schildkraut, J.M.; Davis, F.G.; Goodman, M.T. Oral contraceptive use, reproductive history, and risk of epithelial ovarian cancer in women with and without endometriosis. *Am. J. Obstet. Gynecol.* **2004**, *191*, 733–740. [CrossRef] [PubMed]

121. Hawkins, S.M.; Buchold, G.M.; Matzuk, M.M. Minireview: The roles of small rna pathways in reproductive medicine. *Mol. Endocrinol.* **2011**, *25*, 1257–1279. [CrossRef] [PubMed]

122. Bartel, D.P. MicroRNAs: Genomics, biogenesis, mechanism, and function. *Cell* **2004**, *116*, 281–297. [CrossRef]

123. Bartel, D.P.; Chen, C.Z. Micromanagers of gene expression: The potentially widespread influence of metazoan microRNAs. *Nat. Rev.* **2004**, *5*, 396–400. [CrossRef] [PubMed]

124. Yanaihara, N.; Noguchi, Y.; Saito, M.; Takenaka, M.; Takakura, S.; Yamada, K.; Okamoto, A. microRNA gene expression signature driven by miR-9 overexpression in ovarian clear cell carcinoma. *PLoS ONE* **2016**, *11*, e0162584. [CrossRef] [PubMed]

125. Zhang, X.; Guo, G.; Wang, G.; Zhao, J.; Wang, B.; Yu, X.; Ding, Y. Profile of differentially expressed miRNAs in high-grade serous carcinoma and clear cell ovarian carcinoma, and the expression of miR-510 in ovarian carcinoma. *Mol. Med. Rep.* **2015**, *12*, 8021–8031. [CrossRef] [PubMed]

126. Vilming Elgaaen, B.; Olstad, O.K.; Haug, K.B.; Brusletto, B.; Sandvik, L.; Staff, A.C.; Gautvik, K.M.; Davidson, B. Global miRNA expression analysis of serous and clear cell ovarian carcinomas identifies differentially expressed miRNAs including miR-200c-3p as a prognostic marker. *BMC Cancer* **2014**, *14*, 80. [CrossRef] [PubMed]

127. Wyman, S.K.; Parkin, R.K.; Mitchell, P.S.; Fritz, B.R.; O'Briant, K.; Godwin, A.K.; Urban, N.; Drescher, C.W.; Knudsen, B.S.; Tewari, M. Repertoire of microRNAs in epithelial ovarian cancer as determined by next generation sequencing of small RNA cDNA libraries. *PLoS ONE* **2009**, *4*, e5311. [CrossRef] [PubMed]

128. Wu, R.L.; Ali, S.; Bandyopadhyay, S.; Alosh, B.; Hayek, K.; Daaboul, M.F.; Winer, I.; Sarkar, F.H.; Ali-Fehmi, R. Comparative analysis of differentially expressed miRNAs and their downstream mRNAs in ovarian cancer and its associated endometriosis. *J Cancer Sci. Ther.* **2015**, *7*, 258–265. [PubMed]

129. Iorio, M.V.; Visone, R.; Di Leva, G.; Donati, V.; Petrocca, F.; Casalini, P.; Taccioli, C.; Volinia, S.; Liu, C.G.; Alder, H.; et al. microRNA signatures in human ovarian cancer. *Cancer Res.* **2007**, *67*, 8699–8707. [CrossRef] [PubMed]

130. Braicu, O.L.; Budisan, L.; Buiga, R.; Jurj, A.; Achimas-Cadariu, P.; Pop, L.A.; Braicu, C.; Irimie, A.; Berindan-Neagoe, I. miRNA expression profiling in formalin-fixed paraffin-embedded endometriosis and ovarian cancer samples. *Onco Targets Ther.* **2017**, *10*, 4225–4238. [CrossRef] [PubMed]

131. Zhao, H.; Ding, Y.; Tie, B.; Sun, Z.F.; Jiang, J.Y.; Zhao, J.; Lin, X.; Cui, S. miRNA expression pattern associated with prognosis in elderly patients with advanced OPSC and OCC. *Int. J. Oncol.* **2013**, *43*, 839–849. [CrossRef] [PubMed]

132. Calura, E.; Fruscio, R.; Paracchini, L.; Bignotti, E.; Ravaggi, A.; Martini, P.; Sales, G.; Beltrame, L.; Clivio, L.; Ceppi, L.; et al. miRNA landscape in stage i epithelial ovarian cancer defines the histotype specificities. *Clin. Cancer Res.* **2013**, *19*, 4114–4123. [CrossRef] [PubMed]

133. Suryawanshi, S.; Vlad, A.M.; Lin, H.M.; Mantia-Smaldone, G.; Laskey, R.; Lee, M.; Lin, Y.; Donnellan, N.; Klein-Patel, M.; Lee, T.; et al. Plasma microRNAs as novel biomarkers for endometriosis and endometriosis-associated ovarian cancer. *Clin. Cancer Res.* **2013**, *19*, 1213–1224. [CrossRef] [PubMed]

134. Liu, S.; Gao, S.; Wang, X.Y.; Wang, D.B. Expression of miR-126 and Crk in endometriosis: miR-126 may affect the progression of endometriosis by regulating Crk expression. *Arch. Gynecol. Obstet.* **2012**, *285*, 1065–1072. [CrossRef] [PubMed]

135. Ebrahimi, F.; Gopalan, V.; Smith, R.A.; Lam, A.K. miR-126 in human cancers: Clinical roles and current perspectives. *Exp. Mol. Pathol.* **2014**, *96*, 98–107. [CrossRef] [PubMed]

136. Sestito, R.; Cianfrocca, R.; Rosano, L.; Tocci, P.; Semprucci, E.; Di Castro, V.; Caprara, V.; Ferrandina, G.; Sacconi, A.; Blandino, G.; et al. miR-30a inhibits endothelin a receptor and chemoresistance in ovarian carcinoma. *Oncotarget* **2016**, *7*, 4009–4023. [CrossRef] [PubMed]

137. Bai, L.; Wang, H.; Wang, A.H.; Zhang, L.Y.; Bai, J. microRNA-532 and microRNA-3064 inhibit cell proliferation and invasion by acting as direct regulators of human telomerase reverse transcriptase in ovarian cancer. *PLoS ONE* **2017**, *12*, e0173912. [CrossRef] [PubMed]

138. Humphries, B.; Yang, C. The microRNA-200 family: Small molecules with novel roles in cancer development, progression and therapy. *Oncotarget* **2015**, *6*, 6472–6498. [CrossRef] [PubMed]

139. Greaves, E.; Critchley, H.O.D.; Horne, A.W.; Saunders, P.T.K. Relevant human tissue resources and laboratory models for use in endometriosis research. *Acta. Obstet. Gynecol. Scand.* **2017**, *96*, 644–658. [CrossRef] [PubMed]

140. King, C.M.; Barbara, C.; Prentice, A.; Brenton, J.D.; Charnock-Jones, D.S. Models of endometriosis and their utility in studying progression to ovarian clear cell carcinoma. *J. Pathol.* **2016**, *238*, 185–196. [CrossRef] [PubMed]

141. Cancer Genome Atlas Research Network. Integrated genomic analyses of ovarian carcinoma. *Nature* **2011**, *474*, 609–615. [CrossRef] [PubMed]

142. Hardy, S.; Kitamura, M.; HarrisStansil, T.; Dai, Y.M.; Phipps, M.L. Construction of adenovirus vectors through Cre-lox recombination. *J. Virol.* **1997**, *71*, 1842–1849. [PubMed]

143. Mullany, L.K.; Fan, H.Y.; Liu, Z.; White, L.D.; Marshall, A.; Gunaratne, P.; Anderson, M.L.; Creighton, C.J.; Xin, L.; Deavers, M.; et al. Molecular and functional characteristics of ovarian surface epithelial cells transformed by KrasG12D and loss of Pten in a mouse model in vivo. *Oncogene* **2011**, *30*, 3522–3536. [CrossRef] [PubMed]

144. Jamin, S.P.; Arango, N.A.; Mishina, Y.; Hanks, M.C.; Behringer, R.R. Requirement of bmpr1a for mullerian duct regression during male sexual development. *Nat. Genet.* **2002**, *32*, 408–410. [CrossRef] [PubMed]

145. Fan, H.Y.; Shimada, M.; Liu, Z.; Cahill, N.; Noma, N.; Wu, Y.; Gossen, J.; Richards, J.S. Selective expression of KrasG12D in granulosa cells of the mouse ovary causes defects in follicle development and ovulation. *Development* **2008**, *135*, 2127–2137. [CrossRef] [PubMed]

146. Wu, R.; Zhai, Y.; Kuick, R.; Karnezis, A.N.; Garcia, P.; Naseem, A.; Hu, T.C.; Fearon, E.R.; Cho, K.R. Impact of oviductal versus ovarian epithelial cell of origin on ovarian endometrioid carcinoma phenotype in the mouse. *J. Pathol.* **2016**, *240*, 341–351. [CrossRef] [PubMed]

147. Russo, A.; Czarnecki, A.A.; Dean, M.; Modi, D.A.; Lantvit, D.D.; Hardy, L.; Baligod, S.; Davis, D.A.; Wei, J.J.; Burdette, J.E. Pten loss in the fallopian tube induces hyperplasia and ovarian tumor formation. *Oncogene* **2018**, *37*, 1976–1990. [CrossRef] [PubMed]

148. Soyal, S.M.; Mukherjee, A.; Lee, K.Y.S.; Li, J.; Li, H.; DeMayo, F.J.; Lydon, J.P. Cre-mediated recombination in cell lineages that express the progesterone receptor. *Genesis* **2005**, *41*, 58–66. [CrossRef] [PubMed]

149. Wu, R.; Zhai, Y.; Fearon, E.R.; Cho, K.R. Diverse mechanisms of beta-catenin deregulation in ovarian endometrioid adenocarcinomas. *Cancer Res.* **2001**, *61*, 8247–8255. [PubMed]

150. Saegusa, M.; Okayasu, I. Frequent nuclear beta-catenin accumulation and associated mutations in endometrioid-type endometrial and ovarian carcinomas with squamous differentiation. *J. Pathol.* **2001**, *194*, 59–67. [CrossRef] [PubMed]

151. Palacios, J.; Gamallo, C. Mutations in the beta-catenin gene (CTNNB1) in endometrioid ovarian carcinomas. *Cancer Res.* **1998**, *58*, 1344–1347. [PubMed]

152. Gamallo, C.; Palacios, J.; Moreno, G.; Calvo de Mora, J.; Suarez, A.; Armas, A. Beta-catenin expression pattern in stage I and II ovarian carcinomas: Relationship with beta-catenin gene mutations, clinicopathological features, and clinical outcome. *Am. J. Pathol.* **1999**, *155*, 527–536. [CrossRef]

153. Wright, K.; Wilson, P.; Morland, S.; Campbell, I.; Walsh, M.; Hurst, T.; Ward, B.; Cummings, M.; Chenevix-Trench, G. Beta-catenin mutation and expression analysis in ovarian cancer: Exon 3 mutations and nuclear translocation in 16% of endometrioid tumours. *Int. J. Cancer* **1999**, *82*, 625–629. [CrossRef]

154. Dharmaraj, N.; Chapela, P.J.; Morgado, M.; Hawkins, S.M.; Lessey, B.A.; Young, S.L.; Carson, D.D. Expression of the transmembrane mucins, MUC1, MUC4 and MUC16, in normal endometrium and in endometriosis. *Hum. Reprod. (Oxf. Engl.)* **2014**, *29*, 1730–1738. [CrossRef] [PubMed]

155. Campbell, I.G.; Russell, S.E.; Choong, D.Y.; Montgomery, K.G.; Ciavarella, M.L.; Hooi, C.S.; Cristiano, B.E.; Pearson, R.B.; Phillips, W.A. Mutation of the PIK3CA gene in ovarian and breast cancer. *Cancer Res.* **2004**, *64*, 7678–7681. [CrossRef] [PubMed]
156. Kurman, R.J.; Shih, I.-M. Molecular pathogenesis and extraovarian origin of epithelial ovarian cancer—Shifting the paradigm. *Hum. Pathol.* **2011**, *42*, 918–931. [CrossRef] [PubMed]
157. Chandler, R.L.; Damrauer, J.S.; Raab, J.R.; Schisler, J.C.; Wilkerson, M.D.; Didion, J.P.; Starmer, J.; Serber, D.; Yee, D.; Xiong, J. Coexistent ARID1A–PIK3CA mutations promote ovarian clear-cell tumorigenesis through pro-tumorigenic inflammatory cytokine signalling. *Nat. Commun.* **2015**, *6*, 6118. [CrossRef] [PubMed]
158. Guan, B.; Rahmanto, Y.S.; Wu, R.C.; Wang, Y.; Wang, Z.; Wang, T.L.; Shih Ie, M. Roles of deletion of ARID1A, a tumor suppressor, in mouse ovarian tumorigenesis. *J. Natl. Cancer Inst.* **2014**, *106*. [CrossRef] [PubMed]
159. Wang, X.; Khatri, S.; Broaddus, R.; Wang, Z.; Hawkins, S.M. Deletion of ARID1A in reproductive tract mesenchymal cells reduces fertility in female mice. *Biol. Reprod.* **2016**, *94*, 93. [CrossRef] [PubMed]
160. Kim, T.H.; Yoo, J.Y.; Wang, Z.; Lydon, J.P.; Khatri, S.; Hawkins, S.M.; Leach, R.E.; Fazleabas, A.T.; Young, S.L.; Lessey, B.A.; et al. Arid1a is essential for endometrial function during early pregnancy. *PLoS Genet.* **2015**, *11*, e1005537. [CrossRef] [PubMed]
161. Wu, R.; Hendrix-Lucas, N.; Kuick, R.; Zhai, Y.; Schwartz, D.R.; Akyol, A.; Hanash, S.; Misek, D.E.; Katabuchi, H.; Williams, B.O.; et al. Mouse model of human ovarian endometrioid adenocarcinoma based on somatic defects in the Wnt/beta-catenin and PI3K/Pten signaling pathways. *Cancer Cell* **2007**, *11*, 321–333. [CrossRef] [PubMed]
162. Dinulescu, D.M.; Ince, T.A.; Quade, B.J.; Shafer, S.A.; Crowley, D.; Jacks, T. Role of K-ras and Pten in the development of mouse models of endometriosis and endometrioid ovarian cancer. *Nat. Med.* **2005**, *11*, 63–70. [CrossRef] [PubMed]
163. Fan, H.-Y.; Liu, Z.; Paquet, M.; Wang, J.; Lydon, J.P.; DeMayo, F.J.; Richards, J.S. Cell type–specific targeted mutations of Kras and Pten document proliferation arrest in granulosa cells versus oncogenic insult to ovarian surface epithelial cells. *Cancer Res.* **2009**, *69*, 6463–6472. [CrossRef] [PubMed]
164. Lague, M.N.; Paquet, M.; Fan, H.Y.; Kaartinen, M.J.; Chu, S.; Jamin, S.P.; Behringer, R.R.; Fuller, P.J.; Mitchell, A.; Dore, M.; et al. Synergistic effects of Pten loss and Wnt/CTNNB1 signaling pathway activation in ovarian granulosa cell tumor development and progression. *Carcinogenesis* **2008**, *29*, 2062–2072. [CrossRef] [PubMed]
165. Tanwar, P.S.; Zhang, L.; Kaneko-Tarui, T.; Curley, M.D.; Taketo, M.M.; Rani, P.; Roberts, D.J.; Teixeira, J.M. Mammalian target of rapamycin is a therapeutic target for murine ovarian endometrioid adenocarcinomas with dysregulated Wnt/β-catenin and Pten. *PLoS ONE* **2011**, *6*, e20715. [CrossRef] [PubMed]
166. Van der Horst, P.H.; van der Zee, M.; Heijmans-Antonissen, C.; Jia, Y.; DeMayo, F.J.; Lydon, J.P.; van Deurzen, C.H.; Ewing, P.C.; Burger, C.W.; Blok, L.J. A mouse model for endometrioid ovarian cancer arising from the distal oviduct. *Int. J. Cancer* **2014**, *135*, 1028–1037. [CrossRef] [PubMed]
167. Wu, R.; Baker, S.J.; Hu, T.C.; Norman, K.M.; Fearon, E.R.; Cho, K.R. Type I to type II ovarian carcinoma progression: Mutant Trp53 or PIK3CA confers a more aggressive tumor phenotype in a mouse model of ovarian cancer. *Am. J. Pathol.* **2013**, *182*, 1391–1399. [CrossRef] [PubMed]
168. Budiu, R.A.; Diaconu, I.; Chrissluis, R.; Dricu, A.; Edwards, R.P.; Vlad, A.M. A conditional mouse model for human muc1-positive endometriosis shows the presence of anti-muc1 antibodies and foxp3+ regulatory t cells. *Dis. Model Mech.* **2009**, *2*, 593–603. [CrossRef] [PubMed]
169. Cousins, F.L.; Murray, A.; Esnal, A.; Gibson, D.A.; Critchley, H.O.; Saunders, P.T. Evidence from a mouse model that epithelial cell migration and mesenchymal-epithelial transition contribute to rapid restoration of uterine tissue integrity during menstruation. *PLoS ONE* **2014**, *9*, e86378. [CrossRef] [PubMed]
170. Brasted, M.; White, C.A.; Kennedy, T.G.; Salamonsen, L.A. Mimicking the events of menstruation in the murine uterus. *Biol. Reprod.* **2003**, *69*, 1273–1280. [CrossRef] [PubMed]
171. Cheng, C.W.; Bielby, H.; Licence, D.; Smith, S.K.; Print, C.G.; Charnock-Jones, D.S. Quantitative cellular and molecular analysis of the effect of progesterone withdrawal in a murine model of decidualization. *Biol. Reprod.* **2007**, *76*, 871–883. [CrossRef] [PubMed]
172. Cheng, C.W.; Licence, D.; Cook, E.; Luo, F.; Arends, M.J.; Smith, S.K.; Print, C.G.; Charnock-Jones, D.S. Activation of mutated K-ras in donor endometrial epithelium and stroma promotes lesion growth in an intact immunocompetent murine model of endometriosis. *J. Pathol.* **2011**, *224*, 261–269. [CrossRef] [PubMed]

173. Greaves, E.; Cousins, F.L.; Murray, A.; Esnal-Zufiaurre, A.; Fassbender, A.; Horne, A.W.; Saunders, P.T. A novel mouse model of endometriosis mimics human phenotype and reveals insights into the inflammatory contribution of shed endometrium. *Am. J. Pathol.* **2014**, *184*, 1930–1939. [CrossRef] [PubMed]

174. Chandler, R.L.; Raab, J.R.; Vernon, M.; Magnuson, T.; Schisler, J.C. Global gene expression profiling of a mouse model of ovarian clear cell carcinoma caused by ARID1A and PIK3CA mutations implicates a role for inflammatory cytokine signaling. *Genom. Data* **2015**, *5*, 329–332. [CrossRef] [PubMed]

175. Harada, N.; Tamai, Y.; Ishikawa, T.; Sauer, B.; Takaku, K.; Oshima, M.; Taketo, M.M. Intestinal polyposis in mice with a dominant stable mutation of the beta-catenin gene. *EMBO J.* **1999**, *18*, 5931–5942. [CrossRef] [PubMed]

176. Uehara, S.; Abe, H.; Hoshiai, H.; Yajima, A.; Suzuki, M. Establishment and characterization of ovarian endometrioid carcinoma cell line. *Gynecol. Oncol.* **1984**, *17*, 314–325. [CrossRef]

177. Gorai, I.; Nakazawa, T.; Miyagi, E.; Hirahara, F.; Nagashima, Y.; Minaguchi, H. Establishment and characterization of two human ovarian clear cell adenocarcinoma lines from metastatic lesions with different properties. *Gynecol. Oncol.* **1995**, *57*, 33–46. [CrossRef] [PubMed]

178. Domcke, S.; Sinha, R.; Levine, D.A.; Sander, C.; Schultz, N. Evaluating cell lines as tumour models by comparison of genomic profiles. *Nat. Commun.* **2013**, *4*, 2126. [CrossRef] [PubMed]

179. Anglesio, M.S.; Wiegand, K.C.; Melnyk, N.; Chow, C.; Salamanca, C.; Prentice, L.M.; Senz, J.; Yang, W.; Spillman, M.A.; Cochrane, D.R.; et al. Type-specific cell line models for type-specific ovarian cancer research. *PLoS ONE* **2013**, *8*, e72162. [CrossRef]

180. Beaufort, C.M.; Helmijr, J.C.; Piskorz, A.M.; Hoogstraat, M.; Ruigrok-Ritstier, K.; Besselink, N.; Murtaza, M.; van, I.W.F.; Heine, A.A.; Smid, M.; et al. Ovarian cancer cell line panel (OCCP): Clinical importance of in vitro morphological subtypes. *PLoS ONE* **2014**, *9*, e103988. [CrossRef] [PubMed]

181. Ince, T.A.; Sousa, A.D.; Jones, M.A.; Harrell, J.C.; Agoston, E.S.; Krohn, M.; Selfors, L.M.; Liu, W.; Chen, K.; Yong, M.; et al. Characterization of twenty-five ovarian tumour cell lines that phenocopy primary tumours. *Nat. Commun.* **2015**, *6*, 7419. [CrossRef] [PubMed]

182. Blayney, J.K.; Davison, T.; McCabe, N.; Walker, S.; Keating, K.; Delaney, T.; Greenan, C.; Williams, A.R.; McCluggage, W.G.; Capes-Davis, A.; et al. Prior knowledge transfer across transcriptional data sets and technologies using compositional statistics yields new mislabelled ovarian cell line. *Nucleic Acids Res.* **2016**, *44*, e137. [CrossRef] [PubMed]

183. Zeitvogel, A.; Baumann, R.; Starzinski-Powitz, A. Identification of an invasive, n-cadherin-expressing epithelial cell type in endometriosis using a new cell culture model. *Am. J. Pathol.* **2001**, *159*, 1839–1852. [CrossRef]

184. Brueggmann, D.; Templeman, C.; Starzinski-Powitz, A.; Rao, N.P.; Gayther, S.A.; Lawrenson, K. Novel three-dimensional in vitro models of ovarian endometriosis. *J. Ovarian Res.* **2014**, *7*, 17. [CrossRef] [PubMed]

185. Bono, Y.; Kyo, S.; Takakura, M.; Maida, Y.; Mizumoto, Y.; Nakamura, M.; Nomura, K.; Kiyono, T.; Inoue, M. Creation of immortalised epithelial cells from ovarian endometrioma. *Br. J. Cancer* **2012**, *106*, 1205–1213. [CrossRef] [PubMed]

186. Ohta, I.; Gorai, I.; Miyamoto, Y.; Yang, J.; Zheng, J.H.; Kawata, N.; Hirahara, F.; Shirotake, S. Cyclophosphamide and 5-fluorouracil act synergistically in ovarian clear cell adenocarcinoma cells. *Cancer Lett.* **2001**, *162*, 39–48. [CrossRef]

187. Provencher, D.M.; Lounis, H.; Champoux, L.; Tetrault, M.; Manderson, E.N.; Wang, J.C.; Eydoux, P.; Savoie, R.; Tonin, P.N.; Mes-Masson, A.M. Characterization of four novel epithelial ovarian cancer cell lines. *In Vitro Cell Dev. Biol. Anim.* **2000**, *36*, 357–361. [CrossRef]

188. Nozawa, S.; Tsukazaki, K.; Sakayori, M.; Jeng, C.H.; Iizuka, R. Establishment of a human ovarian clear cell carcinoma cell line (RMG-I) and its single cell cloning-with special reference to the stem cell of the tumor. *Hum. Cell* **1988**, *1*, 426–435. [PubMed]

189. Wong, W.S.; Wong, Y.F.; Ng, Y.T.; Huang, P.D.; Chew, E.C.; Ho, T.H.; Chang, M.Z. Establishment and characterization of a new human cell line derived from ovarian clear cell carcinoma. *Gynecol. Oncol.* **1990**, *38*, 37–45. [CrossRef]

190. Yamada, K.; Tachibana, T.; Hashimoto, H.; Suzuki, K.; Yanagida, S.; Endoh, H.; Kimura, E.; Yasuda, M.; Tanaka, T.; Ishikawa, H. Establishment and characterization of cell lines derived from serous adenocarcinoma (JHOS-2) and clear cell adenocarcinoma (JHOC-5, JHOC-6) of human ovary. *Hum. Cell* **1999**, *12*, 131–138. [PubMed]

191. Lau, D.H.; Lewis, A.D.; Ehsan, M.N.; Sikic, B.I. Multifactorial mechanisms associated with broad cross-resistance of ovarian carcinoma cells selected by cyanomorpholino doxorubicin. *Cancer Res.* **1991**, *51*, 5181–5187. [PubMed]

192. Yanagibashi, T.; Gorai, I.; Nakazawa, T.; Miyagi, E.; Hirahara, F.; Kitamura, H.; Minaguchi, H. Complexity of expression of the intermediate filaments of six new human ovarian carcinoma cell lines: New expression of cytokeratin 20. *Br. J. Cancer* **1997**, *76*, 829–835. [CrossRef] [PubMed]

193. Stordal, B.; Timms, K.; Farrelly, A.; Gallagher, D.; Busschots, S.; Renaud, M.; Thery, J.; Williams, D.; Potter, J.; Tran, T.; et al. Brca1/2 mutation analysis in 41 ovarian cell lines reveals only one functionally deleterious brca1 mutation. *Mol. Oncol.* **2013**, *7*, 567–579. [CrossRef] [PubMed]

194. Benard, J.; Da Silva, J.; De Blois, M.C.; Boyer, P.; Duvillard, P.; Chiric, E.; Riou, G. Characterization of a human ovarian adenocarcinoma line, IGROV1, in tissue culture and in nude mice. *Cancer Res.* **1985**, *45*, 4970–4979. [PubMed]

195. Hills, C.A.; Kelland, L.R.; Abel, G.; Siracky, J.; Wilson, A.P.; Harrap, K.R. Biological properties of ten human ovarian carcinoma cell lines: Calibration in vitro against four platinum complexes. *Br. J. Cancer* **1989**, *59*, 527–534. [CrossRef] [PubMed]

196. Van den Berg-Bakker, C.A.; Hagemeijer, A.; Franken-Postma, E.M.; Smit, V.T.; Kuppen, P.J.; van Ravenswaay Claasen, H.H.; Cornelisse, C.J.; Schrier, P.I. Establishment and characterization of 7 ovarian carcinoma cell lines and one granulosa tumor cell line: Growth features and cytogenetics. *Int. J. Cancer* **1993**, *53*, 613–620. [CrossRef] [PubMed]

197. Eva, A.; Robbins, K.C.; Andersen, P.R.; Srinivasan, A.; Tronick, S.R.; Reddy, E.P.; Ellmore, N.W.; Galen, A.T.; Lautenberger, J.A.; Papas, T.S.; et al. Cellular genes analogous to retroviral onc genes are transcribed in human tumour cells. *Nature* **1982**, *295*, 116–119. [CrossRef] [PubMed]

198. Buick, R.N.; Pullano, R.; Trent, J.M. Comparative properties of five human ovarian adenocarcinoma cell lines. *Cancer Res.* **1985**, *45*, 3668–3676. [PubMed]

199. Fogh, J. MSKCC. Available online: http://www.mskcc.org (accessed on 14 June 2018).

200. Han, S.J.; Hawkins, S.M.; Begum, K.; Jung, S.Y.; Kovanci, E.; Qin, J.; Lydon, J.P.; DeMayo, F.J.; O'Malley, B.W. A new isoform of steroid receptor coactivator-1 is crucial for pathogenic progression of endometriosis. *Nat. Med.* **2012**, *18*, 1102–1111. [CrossRef] [PubMed]

201. Komiyama, S.; Aoki, D.; Katsuki, Y.; Nozawa, S. Proliferative activity of early ovarian clear cell adenocarcinoma depends on association with endometriosis. *Eur. J. Obstet. Gynecol. Reprod. Biol.* **2006**, *127*, 130–136. [CrossRef] [PubMed]

202. Lee, J.M.; Mhawech-Fauceglia, P.; Lee, N.; Parsanian, L.C.; Lin, Y.G.; Gayther, S.A.; Lawrenson, K. A three-dimensional microenvironment alters protein expression and chemosensitivity of epithelial ovarian cancer cells in vitro. *Lab. Investig.* **2013**, *93*, 528–542. [PubMed]

203. Lal-Nag, M.; McGee, L.; Guha, R.; Lengyel, E.; Kenny, H.A.; Ferrer, M. A high-throughput screening model of the tumor microenvironment for ovarian cancer cell growth. *SLAS Discov.* **2017**, *22*, 494–506. [CrossRef] [PubMed]

204. Chowanadisai, W.; Messerli, S.M.; Miller, D.H.; Medina, J.E.; Hamilton, J.W.; Messerli, M.A.; Brodsky, A.S. Cisplatin resistant spheroids model clinically relevant survival mechanisms in ovarian tumors. *PLoS ONE* **2016**, *11*, e0151089. [CrossRef] [PubMed]

205. Tanenbaum, L.M.; Mantzavinou, A.; Subramanyam, K.S.; Del Carmen, M.G.; Cima, M.J. Ovarian cancer spheroid shrinkage following continuous exposure to cisplatin is a function of spheroid diameter. *Gynecol. Oncol.* **2017**, *146*, 161–169. [CrossRef] [PubMed]

206. Arnold, J.T.; Kaufman, D.G.; Seppala, M.; Lessey, B.A. Endometrial stromal cells regulate epithelial cell growth in vitro: A new co-culture model. *Hum. Reprod. (Oxf. Engl.)* **2001**, *16*, 836–845. [CrossRef]

207. Mori, M.; Ito, F.; Shi, L.; Wang, Y.; Ishida, C.; Hattori, Y.; Niwa, M.; Hirayama, T.; Nagasawa, H.; Iwase, A.; et al. Ovarian endometriosis-associated stromal cells reveal persistently high affinity for iron. *Redox Biol.* **2015**, *6*, 578–586. [CrossRef] [PubMed]

208. Chan, R.W.S.; Lee, C.L.; Ng, E.H.Y.; Yeung, W.S.B. Co-culture with macrophages enhances the clonogenic and invasion activity of endometriotic stromal cells. *Cell Prolif.* **2017**, *50*. [CrossRef] [PubMed]

209. Turco, M.Y.; Gardner, L.; Hughes, J.; Cindrova-Davies, T.; Gomez, M.J.; Farrell, L.; Hollinshead, M.;

Marsh, S.G.E.; Brosens, J.J.; Critchley, H.O.; et al. Long-term, hormone-responsive organoid cultures of human endometrium in a chemically defined medium. *Nat. Cell Biol.* **2017**, *19*, 568–577. [CrossRef] [PubMed]

210. Boretto, M.; Cox, B.; Noben, M.; Hendriks, N.; Fassbender, A.; Roose, H.; Amant, F.; Timmerman, D.; Tomassetti, C.; Vanhie, A.; et al. Development of organoids from mouse and human endometrium showing endometrial epithelium physiology and long-term expandability. *Development* **2017**, *144*, 1775–1786. [CrossRef] [PubMed]

211. Practice bulletin No. 114: Management of endometriosis. *Obstet. Gynecol.* **2010**, *116*, 223–236.

212. Shakiba, K.; Bena, J.F.; McGill, K.M.; Minger, J.; Falcone, T. Surgical treatment of endometriosis: A 7-year follow-up on the requirement for further surgery. *Obstet. Gynecol.* **2008**, *111*, 1285–1292. [CrossRef] [PubMed]

213. Yeung, T.L.; Sheng, J.; Leung, C.S.; Li, F.; Kim, J.; Ho, S.Y.; Matzuk, M.M.; Lu, K.H.; Wong, S.T.C.; Mok, S.C. Systematic identification of druggable epithelial-stromal crosstalk signaling networks in ovarian cancer. *J. Natl. Cancer Inst.* **2018**. [CrossRef] [PubMed]

7

The Impact of Mesothelin in the Ovarian Cancer Tumor Microenvironment

Tyvette S. Hilliard

Department of Chemistry and Biochemistry, Harper Cancer Research Institute, University of Notre Dame, Notre Dame, IN 46617, USA; thilliar@nd.edu

Abstract: Ovarian cancer is the deadliest gynecological disease among U.S. women. Poor 5-year survival rates (<30%) are due to presentation of most women at diagnosis with advanced stage disease with widely disseminated intraperitoneal metastasis. However, when diagnosed before metastatic propagation the overall 5-year survival rate is >90%. Metastasizing tumor cells grow rapidly and aggressively attach to the mesothelium of all organs within the peritoneal cavity, including the parietal peritoneum and the omentum, producing secondary lesions. In this review, the involvement of mesothelin (MSLN) in the tumor microenvironment is discussed. MSLN, a 40kDa glycoprotein that is overexpressed in many cancers including ovarian and mesotheliomas is suggested to play a role in cell survival, proliferation, tumor progression, and adherence. However, the biological function of MSLN is not fully understood as MSLN knockout mice do not present with an abnormal phenotype. Conversely, MSLN has been shown to bind to the ovarian cancer antigen, CA-125, and thought to play a role in the peritoneal diffusion of ovarian tumor cells. Although the cancer-specific expression of MSLN makes it a potential therapeutic target, more studies are needed to validate the role of MSLN in tumor metastasis.

Keywords: ovarian cancer; mesothelin; CA125; tumor microenvironment

1. Introduction

Ovarian cancer is the fifth leading cause of cancer death in U.S. women, making it the most lethal gynecological malignancy. The American Cancer Society estimates that about 22,240 new cases of ovarian cancer will be diagnosed in the United States in 2018, of which 14,070 (>60%) women will die of the disease [1]. The overall 5-year survival rate of women diagnosed with ovarian cancer is 47% and for women diagnosed with advanced stage disease, presenting with intraperitoneal metastasis, the 5-year survival rate is only 29% [1,2]. Ovarian cancer is a heterogeneous disease composed of seven histological subtypes: high-grade serous, low-grade serous, mucinous, endometrioid, clear cell, carcinosarcoma, and Brenner tumors [3]. Approximately 90% of ovarian cancers are classified as malignant epithelial ovarian carcinomas (EOCs), of which high-grade serous carcinomas (HGSC) account for 70% of tumor types [4–7]. Early signs or symptoms of ovarian cancer are often subtle and nonspecific which are frequently ignored or treated with medicine to relieve discomfort. In 50–80% of high-grade serous carcinomas, the most frequent genetic change is a p53 mutation found in tumors of all stages [8–10]. Mutations in BRCA1 and BRCA2, tumor suppressor genes, are found in about 50% and 70% of ovarian cancer patients with a family history of ovarian cancer, but 95% of ovarian cancer cases are sporadic [11–13].

The major cause of death is due to therapy-resistant metastasis from the primary tumor to the peritoneum [14–18]. The lack of successful eradication of the disease can be owing to the various complex overlapping signaling networks, together with the peritoneal tumor microenvironment composed of mesothelial cells, the submesothelial matrix, and adipose. Unlike other cancers, ovarian cancer uniquely metastasizes by the detachment of tumor cells, either single or multicellular aggregates, from the primary ovarian/fallopian tube tumor instead of the classically studied pattern of hematogenous metastasis (Figure 1A,B) [15,16,18,19]. Recent studies have challenged this mode of metastasis, suggesting that hematogenous spread of ovarian cancer may play a larger role in ovarian cancer cell metastasis; however, for the purpose of this review, ovarian cancer metastasis will be discussed as direct shedding of tumor cells [20,21]. This distinctive process bypasses several steps of intra- and extravasation before metastasis to other organs [19]. These detached cells undergo epithelial to mesenchymal transition before detaching, resulting in the loss of E-cadherin, a glycoprotein located at cellular junctions, and an invasive phenotype [22]. The metastatic cells disseminate throughout the peritoneal cavity, facilitated by natural fluid flow and preferentially attach to the mesothelium that covers all the organs in the peritoneal cavity including the omentum, abdominal peritoneum and the contralateral ovary (Figure 1C,D) [14,23,24]. Proliferation of disseminated tumor cells on the omentum eventually results in the obstruction of the bowel and stomach [25,26]. It is unknown if the primary tumor prepares secondary metastatic sites, including the omentum and peritoneum, for colonization, a process that has been implicated in other cancers [19].

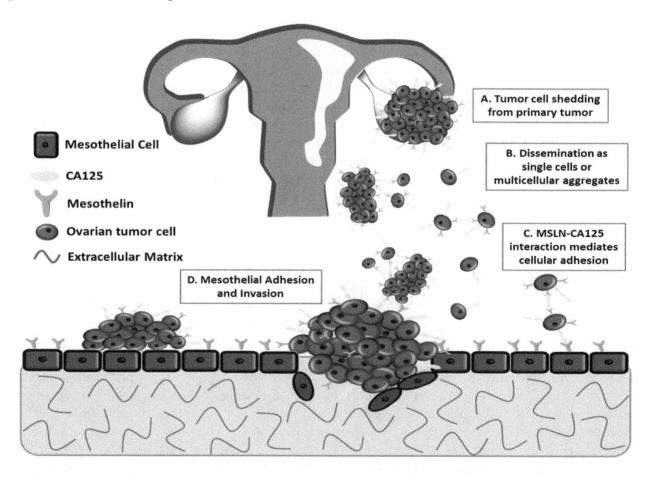

Figure 1. Model for peritoneal metastasis of ovarian tumors. Ovarian cancer metastasis is unique as tumor cells shed from the primary tumor and spread throughout the peritoneal cavity. MSLN:CA125 interaction mediates heterotypic and homotypic cellular adhesion.

Currently, there are no simple screening tests available to detect ovarian cancer. However, available diagnostic testing includes pelvic examinations, transvaginal ultrasonography and serum measurements of cancer antigen-125 (CA125) [27]. Identification of additional screening strategies to accurately diagnose patients in early stages are of great need. Moreover, mesothelin, a glycoprotein expressed in mesothelial cells and overexpressed in EOCs, could be useful as both a screening biomarker as well as a therapeutic target [28]. Understanding the interaction of the tumor and mesothelium and regulating the molecules that modify the metastatic tumor microenvironment is of great importance for the development of future therapeutics.

2. CA125

CA125, a repeating peptide epitope of the mucin 16 (MUC16), is a large membrane-bound cell surface mucin, discovered in 1981 by a monoclonal antibody OC125 developed from mice immunized with human ovarian cancer cells [29]. CA125 is a heavily glycosylated type I transmembrane protein belonging to the family of tethered mucins containing both O-linked and N-linked oligosaccharides [30]. CA125 is overexpressed in many tumors of epithelial origin suggesting that it plays an important role in tumorigenesis [30,31]. CA125 is commonly used as a biomarker to monitor ovarian cancer disease progression and relapse as it is highly expressed in ovarian carcinomas yet minimally expressed in normal ovarian tissues [32–34]. CA125/MUC16 has been shown to inhibit cytolytic responses of human natural killer cells in ovarian cancer, therefore acting as a suppressor of the immune response directed against the ovarian tumors [35,36]. CA125 has been shown to promote cancer cell proliferation [37]. Although the role of CA125 is mainly studied in ovarian cancer, recent studies have shown that CA125 is also highly expressed in other cancers including peritoneal mesotheliomas, pancreatic, and colorectal cancer, implicating a mesothelial cell interaction [38–40].

3. Mesothelial Cells

All organs of the abdominal cavity are covered by the mesothelium, a monolayer of mesothelial cells covering a basement membrane composed of fibronectin, collagen I and IV and laminin [41,42]. Mesothelial cells are flattened squamous-like cells derived from the mesoderm and possess both epithelial and mesenchymal characteristics [43,44]. Mesothelial cells have well-developed cell–cell junction complexes, including tight junctions, that are critical for cell surface polarity and the formation and maintenance of a semi-permeable diffusion barrier. The mesothelium functions to provide a protective barrier as well as a frictionless interface for the free movement of organs and tissues [45]. The mesothelium also plays an important role in contributing to the homeostasis of the peritoneal cavity, fluid and cell transport, tissue repair, initiation and resolution of inflammation and possibly tumor dissemination [46,47]. In the tumor microenvironment, mesothelial cells are preconditioned by the cancer cell secretome to induce the expression of multiple pro-inflammatory factors [48]. Mesothelial cells are implicated in both epithelial-to-mesenchymal transition (EMT) and mesothelial-to-mesenchymal transition (MMT), an EMT-like process [49–51]. EMT is the biological process by which epithelial cells lose cell–cell adhesion and gain migratory properties and MMT is a biologic process in which mesothelial cells of the peritoneal cavity acquire a fibroblast-like phenotype, with increased migratory capabilities [50,52]. Mesothelial cells, expressing mesothelin, line the peritoneal wall and all the organs of the peritoneal cavity that is susceptible to ovarian cancer metastasis.

4. Mesothelin

Mesothelin (MSLN), first identified in 1992 [53], is synthesized as a 70 kDa precursor that is proteolytically cleaved at Arg295, resulting in an approximately 30 kDa fragment called megakaryocyte potentiating factor (MPF) and the 40 kDa MSLN membrane-bound fragment (Figure 2) [54,55]. Both MSLN and MPF are biologically active; however, the exact function remains unknown [56]. MSLN is a glycosylphosphatidylinositol (GPI)-anchored membrane glycoprotein that is physiologically expressed at the cell surface of mesothelial cells lining the pleura, pericardium, and peritoneum [57,58]. Composed of 16 exons spanning 7733 bp, the human MSLN gene occupies approximately 8 kb located at chromosome 16 p 13.3. Alternative splicing results in the predominant variant 1 encoded by MSLN1, variant 2 (24 bp insert), and variant 3 (82 bp insert) [55,57,59,60].

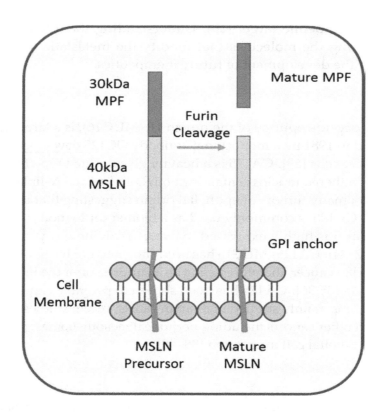

Figure 2. Structure of mesothelin (MSLN). The 70 kDa MSLN precursor protein is proteolytically cleaved to release the 30 kDa N-terminal megakaryocyte potentiating factor (MPF) and is displayed as mature MSLN on the cell surface.

Although many prediction programs have attempted to predict the three-dimensional structure of the MSLN precursor and mature MSLN, the structure still remains unknown [61]. MSLN1 was found by Hellstrom et al. to be primarily expressed at the cell surface and was also released into body fluids of patients of several tumor types. Soluble MSLN results from a cleavage of variants 1 at the C-terminal domain [60]. An 18-bp enhancer sequence, CanScript, located −65 to −46 bp 5′ of one of three transcriptional start sites in the promoter region of the *MSLN* gene, was identified in cancer cell lines with aberrant overexpression of MSLN. The CanScript sequence enhancer consists of two functionally putative binding motifs: the conventional MCAT element and a SP1-like element [62]. All eight nucleotides in the MCAT element were shown to be essential for its function; conversely, the SP1-like element was shown to have two mutations suggesting, that the cancer-specific expression of MSLN is thought to occur through the binding of an unknown transcription factor. Transcription factors such as KLF6 and YAP1 have been investigated but binding of these factors are not adequate for MSLN overexpression in certain cancer types [63]. Nonetheless, the essential transcriptional factor that regulates the MSLN overexpression in human cancers has not been identified.

MSLN is normally expressed in mesothelial cells in trace amounts. In contrast, MSLN is highly expressed in human cancers including 70% of ovarian cancers [54,64–66], mesotheliomas [54], and pancreatic adenocarcinoma [67,68] and therefore identified as a tumor-associated marker. The biological function of MSLN is not fully understood as MSLN knockout mice do not present with an abnormal phenotype, suggesting that MSLN is a non-essential protein [58]. Furthermore, MSLN is reported to play a role in cell adhesion [69], tumor progression [65,70–73], and chemoresistance [73–76]. Specifically, MSLN has been shown to have oncogenic properties by increasing ovarian cancer invasion by inducing MMP-7 through MAPK/ERK and JNK pathways and by inducing drug resistance through PI3K/AKT and MAPK/ERK signaling pathways [65,74]. Albeit, mechanisms that regulate MSLN cell-surface expression are not well understood.

5. MSLN and CA125

CA125, the ovarian cancer antigen/biomarker, has been identified as a MSLN ligand and could potentially mediate cell adhesion [69]. Rump et al. demonstrated MSLN–CA125 interaction mediates heterotypic cellular adhesion (Figure 1C) of the human ovarian cancer cell line, OVCAR3, expressing CA125 to a MSLN expressing endothelial-like cell line [69]. Additionally, Gubbels et al. established that MSLN binds to CA125 in a specific and N-linked glycan-dependent manner, thus CA125-expressing ovarian tumor cells could bind specifically to the mesothelin-expressing peritoneal lining (Figure 1D) [77]. The N-linked oligosaccharides of CA125 are necessary for the binding to MSLN with MSLN having a strong affinity to CA125 with an apparent dissociation constant (K_d) of 5 nM [77–79]. Consequently, MSLN:CA125-dependent cell attachment may play an important role in the peritoneal implantation of ovarian tumor cells [54,80]. The MSLN:CA125 role in cell attachment is supported by work from Bruney et al., demonstrating the overexpression of membrane type 1 matrix metalloproteinase (MT1-MMP) in human ovarian cancer cells (OVCA433-MT)-decreased cell surface expression of CA125/MUC16, subsequently increasing CA125/MUC16 ectodomain shedding, resulting in the release of CA125 from the cell surface. Additionally, there was decreased adhesion of OVCA433-MT to human mesothelial cells (LP9) and to intact peritoneal explants, suggesting the importance of MSLN:CA125 initial adhesion of [81]. After initial attachment of ovarian cancer cells to the peritoneal mesothelium, the co-overexpression of both MSLN and CA125 can lead to recruitment of other ovarian cancer cells being sloughed off from the primary site (Figure 1B,C) [82]. Therefore, the tumor load at secondary sites could be a combination of excessive proliferation and adhesion of circulating single or multicellular aggregates in peritoneal ascites fluid [77,83]. Conversely, the exact function of MSLN in tumor progression remains unclear [84]; however, understanding the importance of CA125:mesothelin binding may lead to novel therapies to control ovarian peritoneal metastasis.

6. Targeting MSLN

Clarifying the function of MSLN will enhance its clinical application in ovarian cancer, including early detection, chemo-response, prognosis and therapeutic targeting. Several features of MSLN make it a useful candidate for cancer therapy, including that it is well-internalized, enabling it to be a good target for immunotoxins [85]. Additionally, MSLN is actively shed from the cell surface generating a pool of antigens in ascites or blood circulation allowing for the quantification of circulating serum MSLN levels potentially used for diagnosis of ovarian cancer patients [28,86–88]. The use of MSLN as a plasma biomarker has been investigated by several groups using blood ELISA tests and demonstrated that serum MSLN levels decrease after surgical therapy and, therefore, may be useful in monitoring treatment response in MSLN expression cancers [86,89]. Pools of antigens, from shed MSLN, in the tumor interstitial space will unavoidably interact with a targeting agent during tumor dissemination [60,85,87]. The first identified sheddase, TNF-α converting enzyme (TACE) was shown to mediate MSLN shedding. TACE is a transmembrane glycoprotein, known for its role in releasing EGFR ligands from the cell surface, therefore regulating the activation of the EGFR pathway [60,90]. Tumor targeting is a complex process and, furthermore, modulation of MSLN shedding could have an influence on drug kinetics in both circulation and tumor tissue. However, shedding is not the only way MSLN could be modulated. The expression levels of MSLN could potentially be regulated similarly to other antigens by trogocytosis [91] or antigen masking [92]; however, the role of these antigens remains to be elucidated. Furthermore, MSLN is expressed in dispensable mesothelial cells so the risk of non-specific toxicity is decreased.

6.1. Molecular Imaging for the Detection of MSLN

Mesothelin has recently been investigated as a target for molecular imaging probes. These probes are designed to guide antibody-based treatments that can be used to assess tumor uptake, response to treatment and the distribution in primary tumors and secondary sites. Prantner et al. identified and characterized an antimesothelin nanobody (NbG3a) used for in vitro diagnostic applications [93]. Further studies from the same group established the potential use of NbG3a for a novel molecular imaging probe with promising results for human imaging and therapeutic applications [94]. Terwisscha van Scheltinga et al. investigated the use of an antibody–drug conjugate (anti-mesothelin antibody-monomethyl auristatin E) coupled to molecular imaging with ^{89}Zr immuno-positive emission tomography (PET). Using this technique, quantitative immuno-PET measurement of relative antibody uptake was determined to correlate with tumor growth inhibition [95]. Furthermore, non-antibody protein scaffolds have successfully been engineered to bind to mesothelin with high affinity [96]. Unlike antibodies that are large in size and have slow clearance from circulation, non-antibody protein scaffolds have demonstrated specific binding to identify tumors expressing the molecular target in murine models [97–99] and have demonstrated promising results in both preclinical and clinical evaluations [100]. The use of these techniques demonstrates the translational potential of MSLN.

6.2. Clinical Trials

There are many clinical trials testing MSLN-targeting agents using strategies such as antibody-based immunotoxins such as SS1P, consisting of an anti-MLSN Fv obtained from a phage display library of immunized mice with recombinant MSLN fused to a truncated form of the Pseudomonas Exotoxin PE38 that mediates cell death. The mechanism of action of an immunotoxin is threefold. First, the immunotoxin binds to cell-bound MSLN; second, this complex is internalized by endocytosis, undergoes retrograde transport to the endoplasmic reticulum and the PE portion is translocated to the cytosol; and third, the PE catalyzes ADP-ribosylation of the elongation factor-2, halting protein synthesis and activating apoptosis [85,101]. There have been two Phase I clinical trials with different modes of administration using either continuous infusion or as bolus intravenous infusions in mesotheliomas, ovarian, and pancreatic cancers. Continuous infusion was well tolerated and showed modest clinical activity; however, there was advantage seen over bolus dosing [102,103]. Additionally, there is a high affinity chimeric antibody, amatuximab (MORAb-009), with high affinity and specificity for mesothelin that is under investigation in clinical trials. Amatuximab works by inducing antibody-dependent cellular cytoxicity [104]. It was observed that upon treatment with amatuximab, patients had an increase in CA125 levels suggesting that amatuximab interferes with the MSLN:CA125 interaction [105]. A tumor vaccine CRS-207 utilizing a live attenuated strain of bacterium Listeria monocytogenes (Lm) expressing human MSLN has shown good tolerance and MSLN-specific T-cell response in a phase I study of safety clinical trial. This phase I study not only demonstrated that vaccines are safe and tolerable but also showed that a tumor antigen-modified Lm can induce tumor antigen-specific T-cell responses in patients with advanced cancer, suggesting that further evaluation of Lm vaccine as a candidate biomarker of improved clinical outcomes is needed [106]. A two-part phase I/II trial is underway using combination therapy with CRS-207, epacadostat, and pembrolizumab (keytruda) in patients with platinum-resistant ovarian, fallopian tube, and peritoneal cancers using different combinations of the three treatments (ClinicalTrials.gov Identifier NCT02575807). Antibody–drug conjugates is another strategy used to target MSLN. An ongoing phase I clinical trial with anetumab ravtansine (BAY94-9343) to determine the safety and maximum tolerated dose for patients with advanced solid tumors including ovarian carcinoma and mesothelioma opened in 2011 (ClinicalTrials.gov Identifier NCT01439152). Anetumab ravtansine consists of the fully human anti-MSLN IgG1 linked to a potent tubulin-binding drug, DM4. In preclinical trials, anetumab ravtansine inhibited both subcutaneous and orthotopic tumor growth in xenograft models of ovarian, pancreatic, and mesothelioma cancers [107]. In patients with recurrent MSLN-expressing platinum-resistant recurrent ovarian, fallopian tube or primary peritoneal cancer, a phase Ib clinical trial to determine the maximum tolerated dose of anetumab ravtansine that could be safely combined with pegylated liposomal doxorubicin is underway (ClinicalTrials.gov Identifier NCT02751918). Several ongoing clinical trials are utilizing anti-MSLN CAR-modified T cells as MSLN targeting agent. The T cells are obtained by apheresis and introduced to a temporary gene which will cause them to make a new type of antibody that will attach to MSLN. Once attached, the cells will become activated and stimulate the host immune system to attack the MSLN-expressing cells [108]. The above clinical trials have confirmed that targeting MSLN could be beneficial in improving existing therapeutic options for patients diagnosed with a MSLN-expressing cancer, including ovarian cancer.

7. Conclusions

Ovarian cancer is the deadliest gynecological malignancy among U.S. women and is often diagnosed at a late stage when the disease has metastasized into the peritoneal cavity. Mesothelin, a glycoprotein normally expressed in mesothelial cells, is highly expressed in several cancers including ovarian, pancreatic, and mesotheliomas. It has been shown that MSLN binds to the ovarian cancer biomarker CA125 and this interaction plays a role in the peritoneal metastasis of ovarian cancer. The differential expression of mesothelin in normal and cancer tissues makes it a promising candidate for targeted therapeutics. Several candidate immunotherapies targeting MSLN are in ongoing clinical trials. New strategies to disrupt the MSLN:CA125 interaction are emerging. Although MSLN is implicated in many cancers, the role of MSLN is still poorly understood warranting further investigation and clinical trial studies. Future advances in ovarian cancer therapy depend on novel treatment mechanisms in combination with current chemotherapeutic approaches that will result in cytotoxicity, inhibition of metastasis and angiogenesis, and increasing the immunological detection of tumors. Further mechanistic studies on MSLN are needed to validate the potential role of MSLN in tumor metastasis that possibly will provide insight for effective MSLN-targeting therapies for several cancers.

Acknowledgments: I would like to thank members of the Stack lab at the University of Notre Dame for help with editing this manuscript.

References

1. Siegel, R.L.; Miller, K.D.; Jemal, A. Cancer statistics, 2018. *CA Cancer J. Clin.* **2018**, *68*, 7–30. [CrossRef] [PubMed]
2. Peres, L.C.; Cushing-Haugen, K.L.; Kobel, M.; Harris, H.R.; Berchuck, A.; Rossing, M.A.; Schildkraut, J.M.; Doherty, J.A. Invasive epithelial ovarian cancer survival by histotype and disease stage. *J. Natl. Cancer Inst.* **2018**. [CrossRef] [PubMed]
3. Meinhold-Heerlein, I.; Fotopoulou, C.; Harter, P.; Kurzeder, C.; Mustea, A.; Wimberger, P.; Hauptmann, S.; Sehouli, J. The new who classification of ovarian, fallopian tube, and primary peritoneal cancer and its clinical implications. *Arch. Gynecol. Obstet.* **2016**, *293*, 695–700. [CrossRef] [PubMed]
4. Auersperg, N.; Wong, A.S.; Choi, K.C.; Kang, S.K.; Leung, P.C. Ovarian surface epithelium: Biology, endocrinology, and pathology. *Endocr. Rev.* **2001**, *22*, 255–288. [CrossRef] [PubMed]
5. Choi, J. Ovarian epithelial cancer: Etiology and pathogenesis. *Biowave* **2008**, *10*, 32.
6. Auersperg, N. The origin of ovarian cancers–hypotheses and controversies. *Front. Biosci. (Sch. Ed.)* **2013**, *5*, 709–719. [CrossRef]
7. Mutch, D.G.; Prat, J. 2014 FIGO staging for ovarian, fallopian tube and peritoneal cancer. *Gynecol. Oncol.* **2014**, *133*, 401–404. [CrossRef] [PubMed]
8. Kohler, M.F.; Marks, J.R.; Wiseman, R.W.; Jacobs, I.J.; Davidoff, A.M.; Clarke-Pearson, D.L.; Soper, J.T.; Bast, R.C., Jr.; Berchuck, A. Spectrum of mutation and frequency of allelic deletion of the p53 gene in ovarian cancer. *J. Natl. Cancer Inst.* **1993**, *85*, 1513–1519. [CrossRef] [PubMed]
9. Singer, G.; Stohr, R.; Cope, L.; Dehari, R.; Hartmann, A.; Cao, D.F.; Wang, T.L.; Kurman, R.J.; Shih, I.M. Patterns of p53 mutations separate ovarian serous borderline tumors and low- and high-grade carcinomas and provide support for a new model of ovarian carcinogenesis: A mutational analysis with immunohistochemical correlation. *Am. J. Surg. Pathol.* **2005**, *29*, 218–224. [CrossRef] [PubMed]
10. Milner, B.J.; Allan, L.A.; Eccles, D.M.; Kitchener, H.C.; Leonard, R.C.; Kelly, K.F.; Parkin, D.E.; Haites, N.E. P53 mutation is a common genetic event in ovarian carcinoma. *Cancer Res.* **1993**, *53*, 2128–2132. [PubMed]

11. Struewing, J.P.; Hartge, P.; Wacholder, S.; Baker, S.M.; Berlin, M.; McAdams, M.; Timmerman, M.M.; Brody, L.C.; Tucker, M.A. The risk of cancer associated with specific mutations of brca1 and brca2 among ashkenazi jews. *N. Engl. J. Med.* **1997**, *336*, 1401–1408. [CrossRef] [PubMed]

12. Antoniou, A.; Pharoah, P.D.; Narod, S.; Risch, H.A.; Eyfjord, J.E.; Hopper, J.L.; Loman, N.; Olsson, H.; Johannsson, O.; Borg, A.; et al. Average risks of breast and ovarian cancer associated with BRCA1 or BRCA2 mutations detected in case series unselected for family history: A combined analysis of 22 studies. *Am. J. Hum. Genet.* **2003**, *72*, 1117–1130. [CrossRef] [PubMed]

13. Mavaddat, N.; Peock, S.; Frost, D.; Ellis, S.; Platte, R.; Fineberg, E.; Evans, D.G.; Izatt, L.; Eeles, R.A.; Adlard, J.; et al. Cancer risks for BRCA1 and BRCA2 mutation carriers: Results from prospective analysis of embrace. *J. Natl. Cancer Inst.* **2013**, *105*, 812–822. [CrossRef] [PubMed]

14. Tan, D.S.; Agarwal, R.; Kaye, S.B. Mechanisms of transcoelomic metastasis in ovarian cancer. *Lancet Oncol.* **2006**, *7*, 925–934. [CrossRef]

15. Burleson, K.M.; Casey, R.C.; Skubitz, K.M.; Pambuccian, S.E.; Oegema, T.R., Jr.; Skubitz, A.P. Ovarian carcinoma ascites spheroids adhere to extracellular matrix components and mesothelial cell monolayers. *Gynecol. Oncol.* **2004**, *93*, 170–181. [CrossRef] [PubMed]

16. Burleson, K.M.; Hansen, L.K.; Skubitz, A.P. Ovarian carcinoma spheroids disaggregate on type i collagen and invade live human mesothelial cell monolayers. *Clin. Exp. Metastasis* **2004**, *21*, 685–697. [CrossRef] [PubMed]

17. Carmignani, C.P.; Sugarbaker, T.A.; Bromley, C.M.; Sugarbaker, P.H. Intraperitoneal cancer dissemination: Mechanisms of the patterns of spread. *Cancer Metastasis Rev.* **2003**, *22*, 465–472. [CrossRef] [PubMed]

18. Buy, J.N.; Moss, A.A.; Ghossain, M.A.; Sciot, C.; Malbec, L.; Vadrot, D.; Paniel, B.J.; Decroix, Y. Peritoneal implants from ovarian tumors: Ct findings. *Radiology* **1988**, *169*, 691–694. [CrossRef] [PubMed]

19. Gupta, G.P.; Massague, J. Cancer metastasis: Building a framework. *Cell* **2006**, *127*, 679–695. [CrossRef] [PubMed]

20. Pradeep, S.; Kim, S.W.; Wu, S.Y.; Nishimura, M.; Chaluvally-Raghavan, P.; Miyake, T.; Pecot, C.V.; Kim, S.J.; Choi, H.J.; Bischoff, F.Z.; et al. Hematogenous metastasis of ovarian cancer: Rethinking mode of spread. *Cancer Cell* **2014**, *26*, 77–91. [CrossRef] [PubMed]

21. Coffman, L.G.; Burgos-Ojeda, D.; Wu, R.; Cho, K.; Bai, S.; Buckanovich, R.J. New models of hematogenous ovarian cancer metastasis demonstrate preferential spread to the ovary and a requirement for the ovary for abdominal dissemination. *Transl. Res.* **2016**, *175*, 92–102. [CrossRef] [PubMed]

22. Kalluri, R.; Weinberg, R.A. The basics of epithelial-mesenchymal transition. *J. Clin. Investig.* **2009**, *119*, 1420–1428. [CrossRef] [PubMed]

23. Meyers, M.A.; Oliphant, M.; Berne, A.S.; Feldberg, M.A. The peritoneal ligaments and mesenteries: Pathways of intraabdominal spread of disease. *Radiology* **1987**, *163*, 593–604. [CrossRef] [PubMed]

24. Coakley, F.V.; Hricak, H. Imaging of peritoneal and mesenteric disease: Key concepts for the clinical radiologist. *Clin. Radiol.* **1999**, *54*, 563–574. [CrossRef]

25. White, E.A.; Kenny, H.A.; Lengyel, E. Three-dimensional modeling of ovarian cancer. *Adv. Drug Deliv. Rev.* **2014**, *79–80*, 184–192. [CrossRef] [PubMed]

26. Lengyel, E. Ovarian cancer development and metastasis. *Am. J. Pathol.* **2010**, *177*, 1053–1064. [CrossRef] [PubMed]

27. Cannistra, S.A. Cancer of the ovary. *N. Engl. J. Med.* **2004**, *351*, 2519–2529. [CrossRef] [PubMed]

28. Scholler, N.; Fu, N.; Yang, Y.; Ye, Z.; Goodman, G.E.; Hellstrom, K.E.; Hellstrom, I. Soluble member(s) of the mesothelin/megakaryocyte potentiating factor family are detectable in sera from patients with ovarian carcinoma. *Proc. Natl. Acad. Sci. USA* **1999**, *96*, 11531–11536. [CrossRef] [PubMed]

29. Bast, R.C., Jr.; Feeney, M.; Lazarus, H.; Nadler, L.M.; Colvin, R.B.; Knapp, R.C. Reactivity of a monoclonal antibody with human ovarian carcinoma. *J. Clin. Investig.* **1981**, *68*, 1331–1337. [CrossRef] [PubMed]

30. O'Brien, T.J.; Beard, J.B.; Underwood, L.J.; Shigemasa, K. The ca 125 gene: A newly discovered extension of the glycosylated N-terminal domain doubles the size of this extracellular superstructure. *Tumour Biol.* **2002**, *23*, 154–169. [PubMed]

31. Yin, B.W.; Lloyd, K.O. Molecular cloning of the ca125 ovarian cancer antigen: Identification as a new mucin, muc16. *J. Biol. Chem.* **2001**, *276*, 27371–27375. [CrossRef] [PubMed]

32. Gubbels, J.A.; Claussen, N.; Kapur, A.K.; Connor, J.P.; Patankar, M.S. The detection, treatment, and biology of epithelial ovarian cancer. *J. Ovarian Res.* **2010**, *3*, 8. [CrossRef] [PubMed]

33. Bast, R.C., Jr.; Klug, T.L.; St John, E.; Jenison, E.; Niloff, J.M.; Lazarus, H.; Berkowitz, R.S.; Leavitt, T.; Griffiths, C.T.; Parker, L.; et al. A radioimmunoassay using a monoclonal antibody to monitor the course of epithelial ovarian cancer. *N. Engl. J. Med.* **1983**, *309*, 883–887. [CrossRef] [PubMed]

34. Yin, B.W.; Dnistrian, A.; Lloyd, K.O. Ovarian cancer antigen ca125 is encoded by the muc16 mucin gene. *Int. J. Cancer* **2002**, *98*, 737–740. [CrossRef] [PubMed]

35. Patankar, M.S.; Jing, Y.; Morrison, J.C.; Belisle, J.A.; Lattanzio, F.A.; Deng, Y.; Wong, N.K.; Morris, H.R.; Dell, A.; Clark, G.F. Potent suppression of natural killer cell response mediated by the ovarian tumor marker ca125. *Gynecol. Oncol.* **2005**, *99*, 704–713. [CrossRef] [PubMed]

36. Senapati, S.; Das, S.; Batra, S.K. Mucin-interacting proteins: From function to therapeutics. *Trends Biochem. Sci.* **2010**, *35*, 236–245. [CrossRef] [PubMed]

37. Reinartz, S.; Failer, S.; Schuell, T.; Wagner, U. Ca125 (muc16) gene silencing suppresses growth properties of ovarian and breast cancer cells. *Eur. J. Cancer* **2012**, *48*, 1558–1569. [CrossRef] [PubMed]

38. Streppel, M.M.; Vincent, A.; Mukherjee, R.; Campbell, N.R.; Chen, S.H.; Konstantopoulos, K.; Goggins, M.G.; Van Seuningen, I.; Maitra, A.; Montgomery, E.A. Mucin 16 (cancer antigen 125) expression in human tissues and cell lines and correlation with clinical outcome in adenocarcinomas of the pancreas, esophagus, stomach, and colon. *Hum. Pathol.* **2012**, *43*, 1755–1763. [CrossRef] [PubMed]

39. Shimizu, A.; Hirono, S.; Tani, M.; Kawai, M.; Okada, K.; Miyazawa, M.; Kitahata, Y.; Nakamura, Y.; Noda, T.; Yokoyama, S.; et al. Coexpression of muc16 and mesothelin is related to the invasion process in pancreatic ductal adenocarcinoma. *Cancer Sci.* **2012**, *103*, 739–746. [CrossRef] [PubMed]

40. Baratti, D.; Kusamura, S.; Martinetti, A.; Seregni, E.; Oliva, D.G.; Laterza, B.; Deraco, M. Circulating ca125 in patients with peritoneal mesothelioma treated with cytoreductive surgery and intraperitoneal hyperthermic perfusion. *Ann. Surg. Oncol.* **2007**, *14*, 500–508. [CrossRef] [PubMed]

41. Yeung, T.L.; Leung, C.S.; Yip, K.P.; Au Yeung, C.L.; Wong, S.T.; Mok, S.C. Cellular and molecular processes in ovarian cancer metastasis. *Am. J. Physiol. Cell Physiol.* **2015**, *309*, C444–C456. [CrossRef] [PubMed]

42. Kenny, H.A.; Chiang, C.Y.; White, E.A.; Schryver, E.M.; Habis, M.; Romero, I.L.; Ladanyi, A.; Penicka, C.V.; George, J.; Matlin, K.; et al. Mesothelial cells promote early ovarian cancer metastasis through fibronectin secretion. *J. Clin. Investig.* **2014**, *124*, 4614–4628. [CrossRef] [PubMed]

43. Van Baal, J.O.; Van de Vijver, K.K.; Nieuwland, R.; van Noorden, C.J.; van Driel, W.J.; Sturk, A.; Kenter, G.G.; Rikkert, L.G.; Lok, C.A. The histophysiology and pathophysiology of the peritoneum. *Tissue Cell* **2017**, *49*, 95–105. [CrossRef] [PubMed]

44. Ferrandez-Izquierdo, A.; Navarro-Fos, S.; Gonzalez-Devesa, M.; Gil-Benso, R.; Llombart-Bosch, A. Immunocytochemical typification of mesothelial cells in effusions: In vivo and in vitro models. *Diagn. Cytopathol.* **1994**, *10*, 256–262. [CrossRef] [PubMed]

45. Mutsaers, S.E. The mesothelial cell. *Int. J. Biochem. Cell Biol.* **2004**, *36*, 9–16. [CrossRef]

46. Roth, J. Ultrahistochemical demonstration of saccharide components of complex carbohydrates at the alveolar cell surface and at the mesothelial cell surface of the pleura visceralis of mice by means of concanavalin A. *Exp. Pathol. (Jena)* **1973**, *8*, 157–167. [PubMed]

47. Yung, S.; Chan, T.M. Pathophysiology of the peritoneal membrane during peritoneal dialysis: The role of hyaluronan. *J. Biomed. Biotechnol.* **2011**, *2011*, 180594. [CrossRef] [PubMed]

48. Ren, J.; Xiao, Y.J.; Singh, L.S.; Zhao, X.; Zhao, Z.; Feng, L.; Rose, T.M.; Prestwich, G.D.; Xu, Y. Lysophosphatidic acid is constitutively produced by human peritoneal mesothelial cells and enhances adhesion, migration, and invasion of ovarian cancer cells. *Cancer Res.* **2006**, *66*, 3006–3014. [CrossRef] [PubMed]

49. Du, J.; Sun, B.; Zhao, X.; Gu, Q.; Dong, X.; Mo, J.; Sun, T.; Wang, J.; Sun, R.; Liu, Y. Hypoxia promotes vasculogenic mimicry formation by inducing epithelial-mesenchymal transition in ovarian carcinoma. *Gynecol. Oncol.* **2014**, *133*, 575–583. [CrossRef] [PubMed]

50. Yanez-Mo, M.; Lara-Pezzi, E.; Selgas, R.; Ramirez-Huesca, M.; Dominguez-Jimenez, C.; Jimenez-Heffernan, J.A.; Aguilera, A.; Sanchez-Tomero, J.A.; Bajo, M.A.; Alvarez, V.; et al. Peritoneal dialysis and epithelial-to-mesenchymal transition of mesothelial cells. *N. Engl. J. Med.* **2003**, *348*, 403–413. [CrossRef] [PubMed]

51. Sandoval, P.; Jimenez-Heffernan, J.A.; Rynne-Vidal, A.; Perez-Lozano, M.L.; Gilsanz, A.; Ruiz-Carpio, V.; Reyes, R.; Garcia-Bordas, J.; Stamatakis, K.; Dotor, J.; et al. Carcinoma-associated fibroblasts derive from mesothelial cells via mesothelial-to-mesenchymal transition in peritoneal metastasis. *J. Pathol.* **2013**, *231*, 517–531. [CrossRef] [PubMed]

52. Rynne-Vidal, A.; Au-Yeung, C.L.; Jimenez-Heffernan, J.A.; Perez-Lozano, M.L.; Cremades-Jimeno, L.; Barcena, C.; Cristobal-Garcia, I.; Fernandez-Chacon, C.; Yeung, T.L.; Mok, S.C.; et al. Mesothelial-to-mesenchymal transition as a possible therapeutic target in peritoneal metastasis of ovarian cancer. *J. Pathol.* **2017**, *242*, 140–151. [CrossRef] [PubMed]

53. Chang, K.; Pastan, I.; Willingham, M.C. Isolation and characterization of a monoclonal antibody, k1, reactive with ovarian cancers and normal mesothelium. *Int. J. Cancer* **1992**, *50*, 373–381. [CrossRef] [PubMed]

54. Chang, K.; Pastan, I. Molecular cloning of mesothelin, a differentiation antigen present on mesothelium, mesotheliomas, and ovarian cancers. *Proc. Natl. Acad. Sci. USA* **1996**, *93*, 136–140. [CrossRef] [PubMed]

55. Hassan, R.; Bera, T.; Pastan, I. Mesothelin: A new target for immunotherapy. *Clin. Cancer Res. Off. J. Am. Assoc. Cancer Res.* **2004**, *10*, 3937–3942. [CrossRef] [PubMed]

56. Yamaguchi, N.; Yamamura, Y.; Konishi, E.; Ueda, K.; Kojima, T.; Hattori, K.; Oheda, M.; Imai, N.; Taniguchi, Y.; Tamura, M.; et al. Characterization, molecular cloning and expression of megakaryocyte potentiating factor. *Stem Cells* **1996**, *14*, 62–74. [CrossRef] [PubMed]

57. Scholler, N. Mesothelin. In *Encyclopedia of Cancer*; Schwab, M., Ed.; Springer: Berlin/Heidelberg, Germany, 2011; pp. 2241–2245.

58. Bera, T.K.; Pastan, I. Mesothelin is not required for normal mouse development or reproduction. *Mol. Cell. Biol.* **2000**, *20*, 2902–2906. [CrossRef] [PubMed]

59. Muminova, Z.E.; Strong, T.V.; Shaw, D.R. Characterization of human mesothelin transcripts in ovarian and pancreatic cancer. *BMC Cancer* **2004**, *4*, 19. [CrossRef] [PubMed]

60. Hellstrom, I.; Raycraft, J.; Kanan, S.; Sardesai, N.Y.; Verch, T.; Yang, Y.; Hellstrom, K.E. Mesothelin variant 1 is released from tumor cells as a diagnostic marker. *Cancer Epidemiol. Biomark. Prev.* **2006**, *15*, 1014–1020. [CrossRef] [PubMed]

61. Sathyanarayana, B.K.; Hahn, Y.; Patankar, M.S.; Pastan, I.; Lee, B. Mesothelin, stereocilin, and otoancorin are predicted to have superhelical structures with arm-type repeats. *BMC Struct. Biol.* **2009**, *9*, 1. [CrossRef] [PubMed]

62. Hucl, T.; Brody, J.R.; Gallmeier, E.; Iacobuzio-Donahue, C.A.; Farrance, I.K.; Kern, S.E. High cancer-specific expression of mesothelin (MSLN) is attributable to an upstream enhancer containing a transcription enhancer factor dependent mcat motif. *Cancer Res.* **2007**, *67*, 9055–9065. [CrossRef] [PubMed]

63. Ren, Y.R.; Patel, K.; Paun, B.C.; Kern, S.E. Structural analysis of the cancer-specific promoter in mesothelin and in other genes overexpressed in cancers. *J. Biol. Chem.* **2011**, *286*, 11960–11969. [CrossRef] [PubMed]

64. Hassan, R.; Kreitman, R.J.; Pastan, I.; Willingham, M.C. Localization of mesothelin in epithelial ovarian cancer. *Appl. Immunohistochem. Mol. Morphol.* **2005**, *13*, 243–247. [CrossRef] [PubMed]

65. Chang, M.C.; Chen, C.A.; Chen, P.J.; Chiang, Y.C.; Chen, Y.L.; Mao, T.L.; Lin, H.W.; Lin Chiang, W.H.; Cheng, W.F. Mesothelin enhances invasion of ovarian cancer by inducing mmp-7 through Mapk/Erk and Jnk pathways. *Biochem. J.* **2012**, *442*, 293–302. [CrossRef] [PubMed]

66. Yen, M.J.; Hsu, C.Y.; Mao, T.L.; Wu, T.C.; Roden, R.; Wang, T.L.; Shih Ie, M. Diffuse mesothelin expression correlates with prolonged patient survival in ovarian serous carcinoma. *Clin. Cancer Res. Off. J. Am. Assoc. Cancer Res.* **2006**, *12*, 827–831. [CrossRef] [PubMed]

67. Wang, K.; Bodempudi, V.; Liu, Z.; Borrego-Diaz, E.; Yamoutpoor, F.; Meyer, A.; Woo, R.A.; Pan, W.; Dudek, A.Z.; Olyaee, M.S.; et al. Inhibition of mesothelin as a novel strategy for targeting cancer cells. *PLoS ONE* **2012**, *7*, e33214. [CrossRef] [PubMed]

68. Argani, P.; Iacobuzio-Donahue, C.; Ryu, B.; Rosty, C.; Goggins, M.; Wilentz, R.E.; Murugesan, S.R.; Leach, S.D.; Jaffee, E.; Yeo, C.J.; et al. Mesothelin is overexpressed in the vast majority of ductal adenocarcinomas of the pancreas: Identification of a new pancreatic cancer marker by serial analysis of gene expression (sage). *Clin. Cancer Res. Off. J. Am. Assoc. Cancer Res.* **2001**, *7*, 3862–3868.

69. Rump, A.; Morikawa, Y.; Tanaka, M.; Minami, S.; Umesaki, N.; Takeuchi, M.; Miyajima, A. Binding of ovarian cancer antigen ca125/muc16 to mesothelin mediates cell adhesion. *J. Biol. Chem.* **2004**, *279*, 9190–9198. [CrossRef] [PubMed]

70. Li, M.; Bharadwaj, U.; Zhang, R.; Zhang, S.; Mu, H.; Fisher, W.E.; Brunicardi, F.C.; Chen, C.; Yao, Q. Mesothelin is a malignant factor and therapeutic vaccine target for pancreatic cancer. *Mol. Cancer Ther.* **2008**, *7*, 286–296. [CrossRef] [PubMed]

71. Bharadwaj, U.; Li, M.; Chen, C.; Yao, Q. Mesothelin-induced pancreatic cancer cell proliferation involves alteration of cyclin e via activation of signal transducer and activator of transcription protein 3.

Mol. Cancer Res. **2008**, *6*, 1755–1765. [CrossRef] [PubMed]

72. Bharadwaj, U.; Marin-Muller, C.; Li, M.; Chen, C.; Yao, Q. Mesothelin overexpression promotes autocrine il-6/sil-6r trans-signaling to stimulate pancreatic cancer cell proliferation. *Carcinogenesis* **2011**, *32*, 1013–1024. [CrossRef] [PubMed]

73. Bharadwaj, U.; Marin-Muller, C.; Li, M.; Chen, C.; Yao, Q. Mesothelin confers pancreatic cancer cell resistance to tnf-alpha-induced apoptosis through akt/pi3k/nf-kappab activation and il-6/mcl-1 overexpression. *Mol. Cancer* **2011**, *10*, 106. [CrossRef] [PubMed]

74. Chang, M.C.; Chen, C.A.; Hsieh, C.Y.; Lee, C.N.; Su, Y.N.; Hu, Y.H.; Cheng, W.F. Mesothelin inhibits paclitaxel-induced apoptosis through the pi3k pathway. *Biochem. J.* **2009**, *424*, 449–458. [CrossRef] [PubMed]

75. Cheng, W.F.; Huang, C.Y.; Chang, M.C.; Hu, Y.H.; Chiang, Y.C.; Chen, Y.L.; Hsieh, C.Y.; Chen, C.A. High mesothelin correlates with chemoresistance and poor survival in epithelial ovarian carcinoma. *Br. J. Cancer* **2009**, *100*, 1144–1153. [CrossRef] [PubMed]

76. Uehara, N.; Matsuoka, Y.; Tsubura, A. Mesothelin promotes anchorage-independent growth and prevents anoikis via extracellular signal-regulated kinase signaling pathway in human breast cancer cells. *Mol. Cancer Res.* **2008**, *6*, 186–193. [CrossRef] [PubMed]

77. Gubbels, J.A.; Belisle, J.; Onda, M.; Rancourt, C.; Migneault, M.; Ho, M.; Bera, T.K.; Connor, J.; Sathyanarayana, B.K.; Lee, B.; et al. Mesothelin-muc16 binding is a high affinity, n-glycan dependent interaction that facilitates peritoneal metastasis of ovarian tumors. *Mol. Cancer* **2006**, *5*, 50. [CrossRef] [PubMed]

78. Kui Wong, N.; Easton, R.L.; Panico, M.; Sutton-Smith, M.; Morrison, J.C.; Lattanzio, F.A.; Morris, H.R.; Clark, G.F.; Dell, A.; Patankar, M.S. Characterization of the oligosaccharides associated with the human ovarian tumor marker ca125. *J. Biol. Chem.* **2003**, *278*, 28619–28634. [CrossRef] [PubMed]

79. Kaneko, O.; Gong, L.; Zhang, J.; Hansen, J.K.; Hassan, R.; Lee, B.; Ho, M. A binding domain on mesothelin for ca125/muc16. *J. Biol. Chem.* **2009**, *284*, 3739–3749. [CrossRef] [PubMed]

80. Scholler, N.; Garvik, B.; Hayden-Ledbetter, M.; Kline, T.; Urban, N. Development of a ca125-mesothelin cell adhesion assay as a screening tool for biologics discovery. *Cancer Lett.* **2007**, *247*, 130–136. [CrossRef] [PubMed]

81. Bruney, L.; Conley, K.C.; Moss, N.M.; Liu, Y.; Stack, M.S. Membrane-type i matrix metalloproteinase-dependent ectodomain shedding of mucin16/ca-125 on ovarian cancer cells modulates adhesion and invasion of peritoneal mesothelium. *Biol. Chem.* **2014**, *395*, 1221–1231. [CrossRef] [PubMed]

82. Tang, Z.; Qian, M.; Ho, M. The role of mesothelin in tumor progression and targeted therapy. *Anticancer Agents Med. Chem.* **2013**, *13*, 276–280. [CrossRef] [PubMed]

83. Bast, R.C., Jr.; Badgwell, D.; Lu, Z.; Marquez, R.; Rosen, D.; Liu, J.; Baggerly, K.A.; Atkinson, E.N.; Skates, S.; Zhang, Z.; et al. New tumor markers: Ca125 and beyond. *Int. J. Gynecol. Cancer* **2005**, *15*, 274–281. [CrossRef] [PubMed]

84. Hilliard, T.; Iwamoto, K.; Loughran, E.; Liu, Y.; Yang, J.; Asem, M.; Tarwater, L.; Klymenko, Y.; Johnson, J.; Shi, Z.; et al. Mesothelin expression increases ovarian cancer metastasis in the peritoneal microenvironment. *Cancer Lett.* **2018**, in press.

85. Pastan, I.; Zhang, Y. Modulating mesothelin shedding to improve therapy. *Oncotarget* **2012**, *3*, 114–115. [CrossRef] [PubMed]

86. Hassan, R.; Remaley, A.T.; Sampson, M.L.; Zhang, J.; Cox, D.D.; Pingpank, J.; Alexander, R.; Willingham, M.; Pastan, I.; Onda, M. Detection and quantitation of serum mesothelin, a tumor marker for patients with mesothelioma and ovarian cancer. *Clin. Cancer Res. Off. J. Am. Assoc. Cancer Res.* **2006**, *12*, 447–453. [CrossRef] [PubMed]

87. Ho, M.; Onda, M.; Wang, Q.C.; Hassan, R.; Pastan, I.; Lively, M.O. Mesothelin is shed from tumor cells. *Cancer Epidemiol. Biomark. Prev.* **2006**, *15*, 1751. [CrossRef] [PubMed]

88. Huang, C.Y.; Cheng, W.F.; Lee, C.N.; Su, Y.N.; Chien, S.C.; Tzeng, Y.L.; Hsieh, C.Y.; Chen, C.A. Serum mesothelin in epithelial ovarian carcinoma: A new screening marker and prognostic factor. *Anticancer Res.* **2006**, *26*, 4721–4728. [PubMed]

89. McIntosh, M.W.; Drescher, C.; Karlan, B.; Scholler, N.; Urban, N.; Hellstrom, K.E.; Hellstrom, I. Combining ca 125 and smr serum markers for diagnosis and early detection of ovarian carcinoma. *Gynecol. Oncol.* **2004**, *95*, 9–15. [CrossRef] [PubMed]

90. Zhang, Y.; Chertov, O.; Zhang, J.; Hassan, R.; Pastan, I. Cytotoxic activity of immunotoxin ss1p is modulated by tace-dependent mesothelin shedding. *Cancer Res.* **2011**, *71*, 5915–5922. [CrossRef] [PubMed]

91. Pham, T.; Mero, P.; Booth, J.W. Dynamics of macrophage trogocytosis of rituximab-coated b cells. *PLoS ONE* **2011**, *6*, e14498. [CrossRef] [PubMed]

92. Nagy, P.; Friedlander, E.; Tanner, M.; Kapanen, A.I.; Carraway, K.L.; Isola, J.; Jovin, T.M. Decreased accessibility and lack of activation of erbb2 in jimt-1, a herceptin-resistant, muc4-expressing breast cancer cell line. *Cancer Res.* **2005**, *65*, 473–482. [PubMed]

93. Prantner, A.M.; Turini, M.; Kerfelec, B.; Joshi, S.; Baty, D.; Chames, P.; Scholler, N. Anti-mesothelin nanobodies for both conventional and nanoparticle-based biomedical applications. *J. Biomed. Nanotechnol.* **2015**, *11*, 1201–1212. [CrossRef] [PubMed]

94. Prantner, A.M.; Yin, C.; Kamat, K.; Sharma, K.; Lowenthal, A.C.; Madrid, P.B.; Scholler, N. Molecular imaging of mesothelin-expressing ovarian cancer with a human and mouse cross-reactive nanobody. *Mol. Pharm.* **2018**, *15*, 1403–1411. [CrossRef] [PubMed]

95. Terwisscha van Scheltinga, A.G.; Ogasawara, A.; Pacheco, G.; Vanderbilt, A.N.; Tinianow, J.N.; Gupta, N.; Li, D.; Firestein, R.; Marik, J.; Scales, S.J.; et al. Preclinical efficacy of an antibody-drug conjugate targeting mesothelin correlates with quantitative 89zr-immunopet. *Mol. Cancer Ther.* **2017**, *16*, 134–142. [CrossRef] [PubMed]

96. Sirois, A.R.; Deny, D.A.; Baierl, S.R.; George, K.S.; Moore, S.J. Fn3 proteins engineered to recognize tumor biomarker mesothelin internalize upon binding. *PLoS ONE* **2018**, *13*, e0197029. [CrossRef] [PubMed]

97. Hackel, B.J.; Kimura, R.H.; Gambhir, S.S. Use of (64)cu-labeled fibronectin domain with egfr-overexpressing tumor xenograft: Molecular imaging. *Radiology* **2012**, *263*, 179–188. [CrossRef] [PubMed]

98. Abou-Elkacem, L.; Wilson, K.E.; Johnson, S.M.; Chowdhury, S.M.; Bachawal, S.; Hackel, B.J.; Tian, L.; Willmann, J.K. Ultrasound molecular imaging of the breast cancer neovasculature using engineered fibronectin scaffold ligands: A novel class of targeted contrast ultrasound agent. *Theranostics* **2016**, *6*, 1740–1752. [CrossRef] [PubMed]

99. Park, S.H.; Park, S.; Kim, D.Y.; Pyo, A.; Kimura, R.H.; Sathirachinda, A.; Choy, H.E.; Min, J.J.; Gambhir, S.S.; Hong, Y. Isolation and characterization of a monobody with a fibronectin domain iii scaffold that specifically binds epha2. *PLoS ONE* **2015**, *10*, e0132976. [CrossRef] [PubMed]

100. Miao, Z.; Levi, J.; Cheng, Z. Protein scaffold-based molecular probes for cancer molecular imaging. *Amino Acids* **2011**, *41*, 1037–1047. [CrossRef] [PubMed]

101. Alewine, C.; Hassan, R.; Pastan, I. Advances in anticancer immunotoxin therapy. *Oncologist* **2015**, *20*, 176–185. [CrossRef] [PubMed]

102. Kreitman, R.J.; Hassan, R.; Fitzgerald, D.J.; Pastan, I. Phase i trial of continuous infusion anti-mesothelin recombinant immunotoxin ss1p. *Clin. Cancer Res. Off. J. Am. Assoc. Cancer Res.* **2009**, *15*, 5274–5279. [CrossRef] [PubMed]

103. Hassan, R.; Bullock, S.; Premkumar, A.; Kreitman, R.J.; Kindler, H.; Willingham, M.C.; Pastan, I. Phase i study of ss1p, a recombinant anti-mesothelin immunotoxin given as a bolus i.V. Infusion to patients with mesothelin-expressing mesothelioma, ovarian, and pancreatic cancers. *Clin. Cancer Res. Off. J. Am. Assoc. Cancer Res.* **2007**, *13*, 5144–5149. [CrossRef] [PubMed]

104. Hassan, R.; Schweizer, C.; Lu, K.F.; Schuler, B.; Remaley, A.T.; Weil, S.C.; Pastan, I. Inhibition of mesothelin-ca-125 interaction in patients with mesothelioma by the anti-mesothelin monoclonal antibody morab-009: Implications for cancer therapy. *Lung Cancer* **2010**, *68*, 455–459. [CrossRef] [PubMed]

105. Hassan, R.; Cohen, S.J.; Phillips, M.; Pastan, I.; Sharon, E.; Kelly, R.J.; Schweizer, C.; Weil, S.; Laheru, D. Phase i clinical trial of the chimeric anti-mesothelin monoclonal antibody morab-009 in patients with mesothelin-expressing cancers. *Clin. Cancer Res. Off. J. Am. Assoc. Cancer Res.* **2010**, *16*, 6132–6138. [CrossRef] [PubMed]

106. Le, D.T.; Brockstedt, D.G.; Nir-Paz, R.; Hampl, J.; Mathur, S.; Nemunaitis, J.; Sterman, D.H.; Hassan, R.; Lutz, E.; Moyer, B.; et al. A live-attenuated listeria vaccine (anz-100) and a live-attenuated listeria vaccine expressing mesothelin (crs-207) for advanced cancers: Phase i studies of safety and immune induction. *Clin. Cancer Res. Off. J. Am. Assoc. Cancer Res.* **2012** *18*, 858–868. [CrossRef] [PubMed]

107. Golfier, S.; Kopitz, C.; Kahnert, A.; Heisler, I.; Schatz, C.A.; Stelte-Ludwig, B.; Mayer-Bartschmid, A.; Unterschemmann, K.; Bruder, S.; Linden, L.; et al. Anetumab ravtansine: A novel mesothelin-targeting

antibody-drug conjugate cures tumors with heterogeneous target expression favored by bystander effect. *Mol. Cancer Ther.* **2014**, *13*, 1537–1548. [CrossRef] [PubMed]

108. Beatty, G.L.; Haas, A.R.; Maus, M.V.; Torigian, D.A.; Soulen, M.C.; Plesa, G.; Chew, A.; Zhao, Y.; Levine, B.L.; Albelda, S.M.; et al. Mesothelin-specific chimeric antigen receptor mrna-engineered t cells induce anti-tumor activity in solid malignancies. *Cancer Immunol. Res.* **2014**, *2*, 112–120. [CrossRef] [PubMed]

8

Can Stemness and Chemoresistance be Therapeutically Targeted via Signaling Pathways in Ovarian Cancer?

Lynn Roy [1,2] **and Karen D. Cowden Dahl** [1,2,3,4,*]

1   Harper Cancer Research Institute, South Bend, IN 46617, USA; lmroy@iupui.edu
2   Department of Biochemistry and Molecular Biology, Indiana University School of Medicine-South Bend, South Bend, IN 46617, USA
3   Department of Chemistry and Biochemistry, University of Notre Dame, Notre Dame, IN 46617, USA
4   Indiana University Melvin and Bren Simon Cancer Center, Indianapolis, IN 46202, USA
*   Correspondence: kcowdend@iupui.edu

Abstract: Ovarian cancer is the most lethal gynecological malignancy. Poor overall survival, particularly for patients with high grade serous (HGS) ovarian cancer, is often attributed to late stage at diagnosis and relapse following chemotherapy. HGS ovarian cancer is a heterogenous disease in that few genes are consistently mutated between patients. Additionally, HGS ovarian cancer is characterized by high genomic instability. For these reasons, personalized approaches may be necessary for effective treatment and cure. Understanding the molecular mechanisms that contribute to tumor metastasis and chemoresistance are essential to improve survival rates. One favored model for tumor metastasis and chemoresistance is the cancer stem cell (CSC) model. CSCs are cells with enhanced self-renewal properties that are enriched following chemotherapy. Elimination of this cell population is thought to be a mechanism to increase therapeutic response. Therefore, accurate identification of stem cell populations that are most clinically relevant is necessary. While many CSC identifiers (ALDH, OCT4, CD133, and side population) have been established, it is still not clear which population(s) will be most beneficial to target in patients. Therefore, there is a critical need to characterize CSCs with reliable markers and find their weaknesses that will make the CSCs amenable to therapy. Many signaling pathways are implicated for their roles in CSC initiation and maintenance. Therapeutically targeting pathways needed for CSC initiation or maintenance may be an effective way of treating HGS ovarian cancer patients. In conclusion, the prognosis for HGS ovarian cancer may be improved by combining CSC phenotyping with targeted therapies for pathways involved in CSC maintenance.

Keywords: ovarian cancer; cancer stem cells; signaling; chemoresistance; metastasis

1. Introduction

In the United States, ovarian cancer is the fifth leading cause of cancer death in women [1]. The American Cancer Society (ACS) estimates that this year approximately 22,240 women will be newly diagnosed with ovarian cancer, and ~14,075 women will die as a result of the disease, making it the most lethal gynecologic malignancy (ACS Facts and Figures 2018). The vagueness of symptoms (bloating, abdominal/pelvic pain, difficulty eating/feeling of fullness, and frequent urination) and the lack of early detection methods contribute to the majority of patients (70–75%) receiving diagnoses in advanced stages (stage III or stage IV) when the cancer has metastasized throughout the peritoneal cavity [1,2]. The five-year survival rate for women with advanced-stage ovarian cancer is ~25% [3,4].

There are several major ovarian cancer subtypes. Additionally, there is mutational and gene expression heterogeneity within each subgenre. Mutational and gene expression heterogeneity is also found in different subpopulations within a single tumor. Patients with the same pathological diagnosis, such as high grade serous (HGS) carcinoma, often vary greatly with respect to gene expression and specific genetic mutations [3,5,6]. The lack of consistent mutations or mis-expressed genes makes developing novel targeted therapeutics difficult. The current standard of care is a "one size fits all" approach consisting of aggressive debulking surgery to resect visible tumor followed by platinum and taxane combination chemotherapy [1,7–9]. Residual tumor implants measuring less than 1 cm are considered indicative of optimal debulking [1]. Debulking surgery performed by a gynecological oncologist improves the chance of survival; however, many patients are not treated by gynecological oncologists [1,7,8]. Therefore, in some cases, chemotherapy prior to surgery is equally effective as primary debulking [4]. Chemotherapy treatment is initially effective in 70–80% of patients [2,10,11]. However, recurrence of the disease will occur in the majority of patients (80–90%) within 5 years, and the tumors often acquire resistance to the chemotherapeutics [1,9,11]. The presence of microscopic tumors left behind during surgical debulking and the limitations of current chemotherapeutics contribute to the likelihood of relapse. The presence or enrichment of cancer stem cells (CSCs), which are defined as tumor cells that survive and/or accumulate after chemotherapy, have activation of self-renewing signaling pathways, and exhibit increased tumor-initiating properties, may contribute to relapse [11–13]. We will discuss how CSC properties contribute to chemoresistance and how investigating these properties may lead to novel therapeutics to eliminate ovarian cancer and prevent relapse.

2. Histologic Types of Ovarian Cancer

Ovarian tumors are divided into three types: epithelial (60%), germ cell (30%), and specialized stromal cells tumors (8%) [3,14]. Epithelial tumors comprise the majority of malignant ovarian tumors (80–90%) [10,14]. Within the epithelial tumors there are four major subtypes: serous, endometrioid, clear cell, and mucinous [5,15,16]. Serous tumors are the most common of the epithelial subtypes and comprise two-thirds of all cases [2,3,5,15]. Historically, serous ovarian cancer is classified according to three different three-tiered systems based on morphology/histology. The three systems are the FIGO (the International Federation of Gynecology and Obstetrics) system based on architectural features, the World Health Organization system based on architectural and cytological features, and the Shimizu/Silverberg system based on architectural features, degree of atypical cytological features, and mitotic index, with the most common system being the FIGO system [17]. Within the FIGO system, serous ovarian carcinomas are classified as low grade (Grade 1), intermediate grade (Grade 2), and high grade (Grade 3) [16]. Historically, low grade and high grade serous ovarian tumors were considered to be different grades of the same tumor [5]. However, molecular and genetic studies suggest that it is likely low grade and HGS tumors are distinct diseases with different genetic mutations and different prognoses [5,15,18]. A newer two-tier system combines the current histopathological classification system with molecular genetic findings and clinical features. In this system, ovarian tumors are designated as Type I or Type II [17,19] (Figure 1).

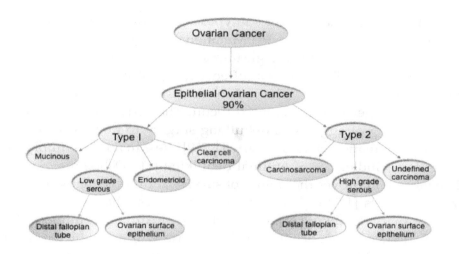

Figure 1. Classification of the Epithelial Ovarian Cancer histological subtype according to the two tier system. Type I tumors include endometroid, clear cell carcinoma, mucinous, and low grade serous. Type II tumors are mostly comprised of high grade serous but also include carcinosarcoma and undefined carcinomas [5,15,18,20].

Low grade serous, mucinous, endometrioid, and clear cell carcinomas fall within the Type I classification [5]. These tumors arise from endometrial tissue, fallopian tube tissue, germ cells, and transitional epithelium [5,14,15,18,21,22]. Type I tumors grow more slowly (are indolent) and are considered to be more genetically stable [5,14,20]. Type II tumors typically have a higher disease volume throughout the peritoneal cavity and a higher incidence of ascites than Type I tumors [20]. They appear to follow a stepwise pattern from a benign precursor to a malignancy with genetic changes in specific cell signaling pathways [2]. Type I tumors are predominantly of non-serous type [10]. Low grade serous ovarian cancer accounts for approximately 5–10% of all serous ovarian cancers [2,10,16]. The most common pathway disrupted in low grade serous ovarian cancer is the mitogen-activated protein kinase (MAPK) pathway [5,6,16,17]. Specifically, activating mutations in BRAF and KRAS are common [2,10,23]. An active MAPK pathway is found in 80% of low grade serous tumors as well as in 78% of their putative precursor lesions (borderline tumors) [16]. Other genes/pathways that are commonly altered in Type I tumors include PTEN, PI3K, ARID1A, Wnt/β-catenin, and ERRB2 [2,6,15,18,20,24,25] (Figure 2).

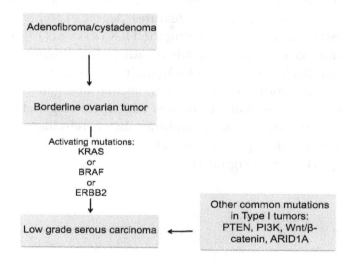

Figure 2. Pathway for Type I tumor formation. Type I tumors appear to form in a stepwise manner from benign precursor lesions. Progression from a borderline ovarian tumors to low grade serous carcinoma commonly includes activating mutations in one of the following members of the MAPK pathway: KRAS, BRAF, or ERBB2.

Prognosis for early-stage tumors is good with a >80% 5-year survival rate with chemotherapy [9]. When dividing all ovarian tumors between stages, Type I tumors are heavily represented in stage I/II (clear cell, 26%; endometrioid, 27%; mucinous, 8%). Only about 36% of early stage tumors are serous [18]. Treatment options for Type I ovarian tumors are identical to those used for Type II tumors and include debulking surgery followed by chemotherapy [17,18]. The response of Type I tumors to chemotherapy is poor due to the relative insensitivity to drug regimens and lack of targeted therapies [7,26]. Low grade serous ovarian tumors have a low response rate to platinum-based therapies with 4% showing a complete response, none with a partial response, 88% with stable disease, and 8% with progression [27]. Another study demonstrated that low grade serous tumors are less responsive than HGS tumors to both paclitaxel (69% vs. 14%) and carboplatin (50% vs. 17%) [27,28]. Type I tumors account for only 10% of ovarian cancer deaths [20]. The poor response of Type I tumors to therapy and the chemoresistance that arises in Type II tumors highlight the need for novel treatment strategies.

HGS tumors comprise 75% of all Type II tumors [3]. HGS neoplasms are typically aggressive and develop rapidly (high mitotic activity) [5,18,20]. Previously, it was thought that HGS ovarian cancer was derived from the ovarian surface epithelium or from cortical inclusion cysts [18,29]. Recent molecular and mouse studies suggest that these tumors likely arise from the epithelium of the distal fallopian tube and that serous tubal intra-epithelial carcinoma (STIC) lesions are the precursors to HGS ovarian cancer [29–31]. One study examined histological sections from fallopian tubes of ovarian cancer patients for evidence of STIC lesions. STIC lesions were identified in 61% of the fallopian tubes from HGS patients with 92% of the lesions being in the fimbriated end of the fallopian tube [32]. Kroeger et al. compiled a list of 15 studies showing that approximately 50–60% of HGS tumors are associated with STIC lesions in the fimbriated end of the fallopian tube [3]. Furthermore, in a molecular profiling analysis, HGS tumors with and without STIC lesions exhibited molecular profiles similar to fallopian tube epithelium [29]. To establish if HGS ovarian cancer can be recapitulated in the mouse, transgenic mouse models have been developed. Dicer and PTEN were conditionally deleted in the reproductive tract using anti-Müllerian hormone receptor type 2-directed Cre (*Amhr2-Cre*) [33]. These mice exhibited abnormal proliferation in the stromal compartment of the fallopian tube [33]. Primary and metastatic tumors that developed in the mice were histologically serous carcinoma, and they shared a similar gene expression profile with human HGS tumors [33]. In another model, Pax8-Cre was used to drive the deletion of *Brca/Pten/Tp53* in the fallopian tube. These mice developed STIC lesions and serous carcinomas [31]. Interestingly, loss of PTEN alone in the fallopian tube (via Pax-8-Cre) was sufficient to generate endometrioid and serous borderline tumors [34]. This raises the possibility of fallopian tube origins for some Type I tumors and non-HGS tumors. While it is possible that a portion of HGS tumors arise from the ovarian surface epithelium, it is likely that a major site of origin for HGS tumors is the fallopian tube [30,35].

Unlike Type I tumors, there is a significant amount of genetic instability within the Type II subgroup, and few genes are consistently mutated [5,14]. The main exception is that in Type II tumors, TP53 mutations are common (both inactivating and gain of function) [36,37]. TP53 mutations are rare in Type I tumors [6]. Type II tumors often exhibit active DNA damage repair mechanisms (e.g., PARP) [3,20]. Overexpression of oncogenes ERRB2 (20–67%) and AKT (12–30%) also occur in some cases [6]. Other common mutations in Type II tumors are BRCA1 or BRCA2. Epithelial ovarian cancer is sporadic in 90% of cases with the remaining 10% being hereditary [2]. In 90–95% of hereditary Type II ovarian tumors, there are germline mutations in BRCA1 or BRCA2 [2]. Importantly, BRCA1 and BRCA2 are often mutated or inactivated in spontaneous ovarian cancer. BRCA1 and BRCA2 mutations are detected in around 5–9% and 3–4% of spontaneous ovarian cancer, respectively [38–42]. Loss of BRCA function through other means, particularly promoter methylation, is common in ovarian cancer (particularly when mutations are not present) [43,44]. Therefore, the p53 and BRCA1/2 pathways are highly implicated in development of HGS ovarian cancer.

Most Type II tumors are found in advanced stages of the disease, which leads to a poor overall prognosis. While Type II tumors respond well to chemotherapy (70–80%) initially, almost all patients relapse and Type II tumors result in 90% of all deaths from ovarian cancer [20]. The advanced stage of disease and development of chemoresistance with Type II tumors results in high mortality. A contributing factor to tumor metastasis and chemoresistance is the presence or enrichment of tumor-initiating/cancer stem cells (CSCs) [45]. Devising new treatments that eliminate this cell demographic is of particular interest for HGS ovarian cancer.

3. Definition of Ovarian Cancer Stem Cells

Heterogeneity is a common feature in ovarian cancer tumors. Different models are proposed to explain tumor heterogeneity. In the stochastic or clonal model, tumors arise from a group of homogeneous cells (clonal). Tumor heterogeneity then occurs through random (stochastic) events within this population. Any of the cells within this population can be tumor initiating provided they possess the necessary genetic mutations, epigenetic changes, and a receptive microenvironment [46–50]. The second model (CSC model) recapitulates the stem cell hierarchy found in development of tissues like the hematopoietic system. In this model, tumors are made of groups of heterogeneous cells that all arise from precursor cells with stem-like properties. These "stem-like" precursors differentiate and/or acquire different mutations that lead to diverse activation of pathways. The resultant cells have unique phenotypes and a hierarchical pattern of inheritance from the initiating CSCs [47,49–52] (Figure 3).

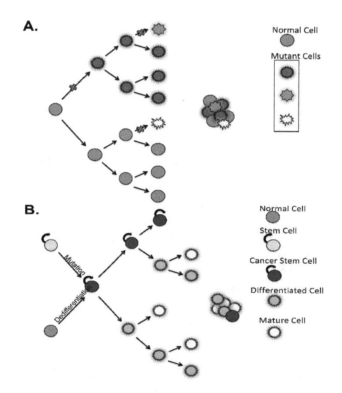

Figure 3. Models of tumor development and heterogeneity. (**A**) The clonal evolution model for tumor initiation. A genetic event occurs in a cell giving rise to a mutant cell population. Any cell is capable of becoming a tumor cell if there is an initiating genetic event. Tumor heterogeneity is due to propagation of cells carrying mutations that are the result of multiple genetic events. (**B**) The cancer stem cell model for tumor initiation. Either a normal stem cell has a genetic event resulting in a cancer stem cell capable of indefinite self-renewal and/or differentiation or a differentiated cell has a genetic event that activates a stem like program within the cell resulting in a cancer stem cell. Tumor cells have a hierarchical inheritance pattern from their cancer stem cell but develop different phenotypes as they acquire further mutations as they differentiate resulting in tumor heterogeneity.

Normal stem cells divide asymmetrically, allowing for self-renewal. One daughter cell retains all the characteristics and programing of the parent cell while the other daughter cell differentiates or acquires new properties [53]. To maintain their undifferentiated state and the ability to self-renew, stem cells reside in a "stem cell niche" comprising various stromal cells, vascular support, and soluble factors that provide a permissive environment [49,54]. CSCs display self-renewal characteristics and retain the ability to produce cells that are highly proliferative and invasive [47,53]. Other characteristics of CSCs include significant DNA repair capability and resistance to therapy [49,53]. In fact, ovarian CSCs (CD133$^+$ and Sca1$^+$) persisted following chemotherapy in a mouse model of ovarian cancer and in cells treated with carboplatin in vitro [45,55]. Moreover, these cells express stem cell markers and maintain tumor initiating potential [45]. Additionally, in vitro studies demonstrated that treatment of ovarian cancer cells with chemotherapy enriches the stem cell pool [56–58]. These studies imply that CSCs are protected from chemotherapy and may be initiators of tumor relapse.

4. Stem Cell Identification in Ovarian Cancer

In 2005, Bapat et al. described the first example of a putative ovarian CSC. A single cell was taken from the ascites of an ovarian cancer patient. Once propagated, the cell was able to form anchorage-independent spheroids in culture and was able to seed tumors in mice via serial transplantation over several generations, illustrating the stem-like capabilities of the cell [59]. Since this initial study, many other investigations have been conducted to identify and validate ovarian CSCS. Identification of CSCs relies on the presence of markers (cell surface and intracellular) that are unique to this particular subset of tumor cells [46,47,50]. In ovarian cancer, a variety of markers are used to denote the presence of CSCs. Cells isolated based on these markers can be tested for "stemness" in vitro via spheroid forming assays, resistance to chemotherapeutics, and in vivo with limiting dilution assays (LDAs) to examine the tumorgenicity of the sample [52]. In the LDA, mice are injected with a defined number of cells from a mixed population of cells or cells isolated that express the stem cell markers. The population that is more stem-like will initiate tumors from significantly fewer cells [60]. Table 1 contains a list of some putative ovarian CSC markers.

Table 1. Putative Ovarian Cancer Stem Cell Markers.

Marker	Type of Protein	Suspected Role in Stem Cells	References
CD24	Cell surface transmembrane glycoprotein	Stem gene expression, tumor initiation, chemoresistance, stem cell maintenance	[46,53,61,62]
CD44	Cell surface transmembrane glycoprotein (hyaluronic acid receptor)	Chemoresistance, tumor initiation, stem gene expression, spheroid formation	[13,46,53,61–67]
cKit/CD117	Tyrosine kinase receptor	Chemoresistance, stem cell maintenance, tumor initiation	[11,53,59,61,68,69]
PROM1/CD133	Cell surface transmembrane glycoprotein	Tumor initiation, chemoresistance, spheroid formation, high cell proliferation	[13,46,53,61,62,70–76]
ALDH1	Cytosolic aldehyde dehydrogenase enzyme	Tumor initiation, chemoresistance, spheroid formation	[46,53,61,75,77,78]
ROR1	Tyrosine kinase receptor	Spheroid formation, tumor initiation, proliferation	[79,80]
SOX2	Transcription factor	Stem cell maintenance, self-renewal	[8,81–84]
NANOG	Transcription factor	Stem cell maintenance, self-renewal, chemoresistance	[8,53,61,66,81–83]
POU5F1/OCT4	Transcription factor	Tumor initiation, chemoresistance	[8,53,61,81–83]
MYC	Transcription factor	Tumor initiation, chemoresistance	[85,86]
EpCAM	Cell surface membrane glycoprotein	Tumor initiation, spheroid formation, proliferation	[13,46,53,61,62]
MDR1/ABCB1	ATP binding cassette transporter	Chemoresistance	[46,49,53,61,66,87–91]
ABCG2	ATP binding cassette transporter	Chemoresistance	[46,49,53,61,87,88,90,91]

4.1. Side Population

One way in which ovarian CSCs are identified is by their ability to efflux DNA-binding dyes such as Hoechst 33342 and Rhodamine 123 resulting in a side population (SP) using flow cytometry. The ability to efflux these dyes identifies a CSC population that overexpress ATP binding cassette transporters such as MDR1/ABCB1 and ABCG2 that can efflux chemotherapeutic agents [46,49,61,87,88]. This SP demonstrates stem cell properties including the ability to repopulate tumors in an LDA and resistance to chemotherapy. Expression of ABCB1 and ABCG2 correlates with resistance to cisplatin and paclitaxel in ovarian cancer cell lines (2008, KF28, TU-OM-1, OVCAR3, SKOV3) and in cells from patient and mouse ascites [89–91]. However, the SP of cells is heterogeneous and can display different combinations of other stem cell markers, so it may be unknown which cells within this population is most "stem-like" or which population(s) are reconstituting the tumor [53].

4.2. Cell Surface Markers

Cell surface makers are essential in the identification of CSCs for multiple tumor types. When Bapat et al. first described ovarian CSCs, CD117 was demonstrated to be a cell surface marker for the ovarian CSCs [59]. Human serous ovarian cancer patient-derived xenografts (PDXs) showed that CD117$^+$ cells isolated from the xenografts were able to recapitulate a tumor with only 10,000 cells; this was a 100-fold increase in tumor initiating capability compared with the CD117$^-$ cells [68]. CD117$^+$ cells were also successful at generating tumors when serially transplanted [68]. Other ovarian CSC surface markers include CD24, CD44, EpCAM, and CD133 [13,46,53,61,62]. One of the most commonly reported ovarian CSC markers is CD133. CD133 expression correlates with poor prognosis in ovarian cancer and increased chemoresistance [70–72]. In cell lines, CD133 promotes a number of stem characteristics. CD133$^+$ and CD133$^-$ cells were single cell isolated and expanded from A2780 and PEO1 cell lines [73]. The CD133$^-$ cells only produced CD133$^-$ cells while CD133$^+$ cells divided asymmetrically to produce both CD133$^+$ and CD133$^-$ cells, suggesting that the CD133$^+$ cells retain stem cell properties [73]. CD133$^+$ cells exhibit increased resistance to cisplatin and were more tumorigenic in xenograft and serial transplantation studies [73,74]. Another one of the common CSC markers is CD44. CD44 is the hyaluronate receptor and is important in adhesion. In ovarian cancer, CD44 correlates with chemoresistance and tumor progression [63–65]. One function of CD44 is to activate Stat3 [66]. CD44 is commonly used as a stem cell marker in combination with CD117, MyD88, E-cadherin/CD34, and CD24/EpCAM. Each of these CD44$^+$ cell populations has been demonstrated to have stem-like properties (reviewed in Klemba et al.) [67]. In conclusion, there are multiple surface markers used to identify CSCs in ovarian cancer. Some investigations use these surface markers alone or in combination with other markers. However, we are still uncertain if there is a definitive ovarian CSC marker/population, if multiple CSC populations co-exist, or if CSC identity varies by patient.

4.3. ALDH Activity

In addition to cell surface markers, CSCs often are identified using the expression of the enzyme aldehyde dehydrogenase 1 (ALDH1) and its activity. The enzymatic activity of ALDH1 is used to identify and define CSCs in cancer types including breast, colon, liver, and ovarian [46]. Several studies suggest that ALDH1 expression correlates with poor prognosis. In one study of ovarian cancer patients, ALDH1A1 expression was found in 72.9% of tumors, and this expression correlated with decreased progression-free survival (6.05 vs. 13.81 months) [77]. A second study demonstrated that patients with high ALDH1 expression (by immunohistochemistry in >50% of the tumor section) exhibited poorer prognosis [78]. Cell lines with high ALDH1 exhibited increased chemoresistance and tumorgenicity [78]. Silva et al. examined 13 primary human ovarian tumors and 5 ascites samples for various putative CSC markers. ALDH1 was expressed in all cases [75]. Ovarian cancer cell lines were then examined for these CSC markers. Each of the cell lines examined (A2008, SKOV3, HEY-1, A2780, OVCAR8, OVCAR3, and OVCAR432) had a subpopulation of cells with ALDH1 expression [75]. Conversely, knockdown of ALDH1A1 in an orthotopic mouse model (from both taxane- and platinum-resistant cell lines) sensitized the tumors to treatment, resulting in reduced tumor growth [77]. The expression and activity of ALDH1 alone or in combination with cell surface stem cell markers is a popular and accepted method for identifying ovarian CSCs.

4.4. Transcription Factors

Pluripotency transcription factors necessary for normal stem cell maintenance are commonly expressed in ovarian CSCs [53,81–83]. In addition to being markers for ovarian CSCs, transcription factors such as OCT4, SOX2, and NANOG are expressed during development and are essential for normal stem cell maintenance and proliferation [62,66,84,92–95]. Aberrant expression of stem cell genes in differentiated cells, progenitor cells, or stem cell populations can lead to enhanced self-renewal and proliferative capability [96]. Expression of stem cell transcription factors not only provides evidence for the CSC model of tumor development, it also explains in part how stem cell properties of self-renewal and asymmetric division are maintained in CSCs. By comparing normal stem cell populations to CSCs we can gain insight into tumor initiation and regulation of the CSC phenotype. In embryonic stem cells (ESCs) the pluripotency transcription factors form a protein interaction network [83]. Many of these interactions are critical for stem cell functions. In addition, expression of pluripotency factors and protein–protein interactions are retained in CSCs. Among these factors is ARID3B. ARID3B and its paralog ARID3A are expressed in ESCs in a complex with NANOG, OCT4, and NAC1 [83]. ARID3B is overexpressed in serous ovarian cancer and its expression in the nucleus correlates with relapse following chemotherapy [58,97]. ARID3B increases expression of stem cell markers [76]. In particular, ARID3B induces expression of the stem cell marker Prom1 (CD133) [58]. ARID3B additionally increases the pool of CD133+ cells, suggesting that it has a role in promoting a stem cell phenotype [58,76]. In fact, ARID3A and ARID3B co-localize with CD133 in ovarian cancer tumor sections. Additionally, ARID3B is enriched in ovarian cancer ascites sorted for CD133+ cells (Figure 4). These data suggest that ARID3B+ cells are found in a stem cell niche (Figure 4). Future studies on pluripotency factors common in ovarian CSCs including OCT4, MYC, and ARID3B will provide clarity for how cancer stemness is maintained [85,86].

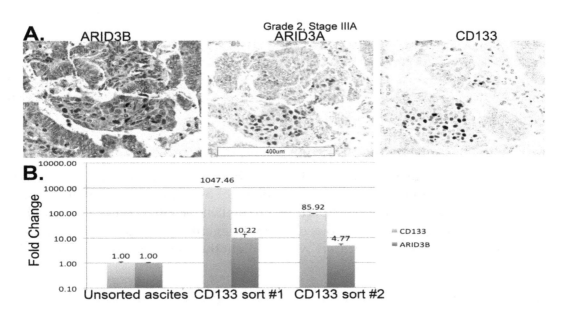

Figure 4. ARID3B expression correlates with CD133-stem cell niche. (**A**) IHC shows nuclear ARID3A and ARID3B co-localize with CD133+ regions in serial HGSOC sections. (**B**) HGSOC patient ascites was sorted for CD133+ cells. RT-qPCR was conducted for Prom1(CD133) and ARID3B on unsorted and independent sorts [98].

Different stem cell markers may confer different selective advantages to different pools of "CSCs". Patients may have more than one pool of stem cells and different patients may have CSCs with different phenotypes. An example is included in Figure 5. To enrich for CSCs, OVCA429 and Kuramochi cells were untreated or treated with cisplatin and paclitaxel and then cultured on nonadherent plates in stem cell media [56]. Flow cytometry was performed for CD117 (gene = CKIT) and CD133. OVCA429 cells have a clear CD117$^+$CD133$^-$ population of CSCs that is enriched following chemotherapy treatment. Following chemotherapy treatment, multiple cell populations are expanded in Kuramochi cells including CD133$^+$/CD117$^-$, CD133$^+$/CD117$^+$, and CD117$^+$/CD133$^-$. These experiments suggest that different stem cell pools may be more prevalent in an individual cell type or patient tumor. Importantly, each of the CSC markers may have its own each unique function. The kinase activity of CD117 may provide a survival advantage over CD117$^-$ cells [69]. However, CD133$^+$ cells may have an adhesion or metastatic advantage over cells lacking CD133 [76]. Although we can detect cell-to-cell variation in the expression of markers, we do not know if these different CSC lineages arise from common progenitors. CSC lineage tracing to define the hierarchy of cells in a stem cell population has not been conducted for all putative ovarian CSC subtypes. Additionally, LDAs need to be conducted to verify stem cell potential for each putative ovarian CSC population. In order for studies of CSCs to be translational, we will need to define how the different CSC populations pertain to patient prognosis, relapse, and response to therapy. Moving forward, we need to establish the clinical significance of different ovarian CSC marker profiles [47,52,53,61,99]. Comparing survival and relapse potential for patients based on these different marker profiles is essential for us to develop effective treatments for the clinically relevant ovarian CSC populations.

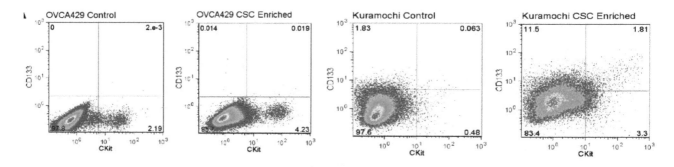

Figure 5. Flow cytometry for the stem cell markers CD117 and CD133 on ovarian cancer cells before and after CSC enrichment. Untreated OVCA429 and Kuramochi cells or cells enriched for CSCs (by treatment with cisplatin and paclitaxel followed by culturing CSCs in stem cell media on ultra low adhesion plates) [56] were stained for stem cell markers CD117 (cKIT is the gene that encodes CD117) (X-axis) and CD133 (Y-axis).

5. Pathways That Promote Stemness and Chemoresistance in HGSOC

We chose to focus on the major pathways that drive both stemness and chemoresistance in HGS ovarian cancer. These properties of highly metastatic HGS ovarian cancer are inextricably linked. Understanding the pathways that are most pertinent to metastatic HGS ovarian cancer will provide us with putative targets to develop efficacious therapeutic agents. As there are numerous pathways involved in stemness and chemoresistance, we will highlight the ones that have a clear role in ovarian cancer and are potentially targetable.

5.1. PI3K/PTEN/AKT Signaling

Aberrant PI3K/PTEN/AKT signaling often results from genomic alterations in many cancers including clear cell ovarian cancer. In HGS carcinoma, there are few mutations in the components of the PI3K/PTEN/AKT pathway, but by immunohistochemistry (IHC) about half of the HGS tumors have evidence of pathway activation [100,101]. A meta-analysis of the literature reports that both univariate and multivariate analysis show that high expression of activated AKT (pAKT) is associated with poor progression-free survival and poor overall survival [102]. Due to mutations in many parts of the PI3K/PTEN/AKT pathway, activated AKT signaling is highly relevant for ovarian cancer development and progression.

The PI3K/PTEN/AKT pathway is also implicated in ovarian CSCs. PI3K/PTEN/AKT signaling regulates enrichment of CSCs, maintenance of a CSC phenotype, and chemoresistance [103–106]. Spheroids derived from SKOV3 and HO8910 cell lines expressed elevated phosphorylated AKT1 and decreased expression of PTEN [103]. The spheroids exhibited increased resistance to paclitaxel [103]. Conversely, inhibiting AKT1 activation decreased spheroid formation and migration [104]. Knockdown of AKT1 via siRNA resulted in the loss of CSC marker expression (OCT4, SOX2, ALDH1, and ABCG2) as well as loss of spheroid formation and paclitaxel resistance [104]. These studies demonstrate the importance of the PI3K/PTEN/AKT pathway in CSC formation, maintenance, and chemoresistance to paclitaxel.

The PI3K/PTEN/AKT pathway also regulates cisplatin resistance in ovarian cancer. In cisplatin-resistant A2780 cells (A2780-CP), AKT regulates the expression of PPM1D [105]. PPM1D inhibits the DNA damage and apoptotic response after DNA damage occurs [105]. Downregulation of AKT activity results in loss of PPM1D stability and increases its degradation [105]. Loss of PPM1D increases the response of the A2780-CP cells to cisplatin [105].

The PI3K/PTEN/AKT signaling pathway promotes the enrichment of ovarian CSC populations and regulates ovarian CSC chemoresistance, thus making it an ideal target for therapeutics to eliminate ovarian CSCs. There are currently PI3K/PTEN/AKT inhibitors such as BKM120, Everdimus, and Perifosine that are being used to treat cancer patients [100]. Future efforts to stratify patients that are likely to benefit from PI3K/PTEN/AKT inhibition will be needed for this therapy to be effective in ovarian cancer patients.

5.2. Jak2/STAT3

Proliferation, survival, and differentiation are all regulated by the Jak2/STAT3 pathway in several solid tumors [107]. In ovarian cancer, the Jak/STAT pathway is constitutively active in most cases [108]. Jak/STAT is implicated for having a key role in the development of HGS ovarian cancer. Activation of STAT3 via phosphorylation at Tyr705 and the loss of the STAT3 inhibitor PIAS3 may serve as a tumor-initiating event in the distal fallopian tube for the formation of HGS ovarian cancer [109]. Phosphorylated STAT3 is expressed in 86% of ovarian tumors examined (from different histotypes) and constitutive pSTAT3 expression is expressed in 63% of the HGS tumors examined [110]. Phosphorylated, nuclear STAT3 is associated with poor prognosis [110]. In tissue microarrays (TMAs), patients whose tumors had high nuclear pSTAT3 staining (>10% nuclei stained) had poorer survival rates than women with low nuclear pSTAT3 staining (<10% nuclei stained) [110]. These patient findings implicate the Jak/STAT pathway as being highly important for ovarian cancer initiation and progression.

The Jak/STAT pathway also regulates ovarian CSCs. CD24$^+$ ovarian CSCs require Jak2/STAT3 signaling for growth and metastasis [111]. Primary tumors generated in the Apc^-; $Pten^-$; $Trp53^-$ (transgenic mouse model in which APC, PTEN, and Trp53 are conditionally deleted in the ovarian surface epithelium) were collected, dissociated, and sorted via fluorescence-activated cell sorting (FACS) using stem cell markers [111]. LDAs confirmed that the CD24$^+$ cells isolated were a CSC population [111]. This population of cells expressed elevated pSTAT3 and stem cell marker NANOG, which is required for stem cell renewal [111]. CD24$^+$ cells were injected into mice and the mice were then treated with cisplatin or with cisplatin+TG101209, a Jak2 inhibitor [111]. The mice treated with cisplatin+TG101209 showed significantly increased survival and almost no metastases (1 out of 14) [111].

Other studies show a role for the Jak/STAT pathway in ovarian CSC maintenance and chemoresistance. Abubaker et al. collected tumor cells from patient ascites or the HEY8 ovarian cancer cell line and treated them with paclitaxel [108]. Treatment with paclitaxel induced the expression of CSC markers CD117, OCT4, and EpCAM in ascites and HEY8 cells [108]. In both the paclitaxel-treated ascites and HEY8 cells, the Jak2/STAT3 pathway was activated [108]. This suggests that the Jak2/STAT3 pathway regulates the expression of stem-like genes necessary for CSC maintenance. Moreover, paclitaxel-treated cells were also treated with the Jak2-specific small molecule inhibitor (CYT387), which resulted in inhibition of the Jak2/STAT3 pathway activation, loss of stem cell marker expression, and increased sensitivity of the cells to paclitaxel treatment [108]. When paclitaxel-treated and paclitaxel+CYT387-treated cells were injected into mice, the mice injected with the paclitaxel+CYT387-treated cells showed a reduced tumor burden and enhanced sensitivity to paclitaxel [108]. These studies demonstrate that in models of ovarian cancer, Jak2 inhibitors are effective at reducing stem cell characteristics and inhibiting tumor growth. These inhibitors also increase survival and response to therapy. Because the Jak/STAT pathway promotes stemness and chemoresistance in the CSC population, it is a viable target for therapies aimed at reducing ovarian CSC populations.

5.3. NFκB

The NFκB pathway plays a role in normal cellular processes such as survival, proliferation, and apoptosis. In cancer the NFκB pathway is implicated in invasion and metastasis. However, the pathway is also involved in CSC maintenance [112]. In ovarian cancer, both the canonical and noncanonical NFκB pathways are active. A CD44$^+$ ovarian CSC population isolated from patient ascites exhibited constitutive NFκB pathway activation via a luciferase reporter assay, formed spheroids in culture, and formed tumors when injected into mice [13]. Another study showed that CD44$^+$ CSCs from SKOV3 cells (that also express NANOG, SOX2, and OCT4) exhibited increased expression of NFκB pathway members RelA, RelB, and IKKα [113]. Inhibition of the NFκB pathway with a dominant-negative form of IκBα resulted in a decrease in the CD44$^+$ CSC population with a reduction from 65.3% CD44$^+$ cells to just 27.7% [113]. These data suggest that NFκB signaling regulates expression of stemness genes.

The NFκB pathway is also involved in ovarian CSC chemoresistance. CD44$^+$ ovarian CSCs from patient ascites have constitutively active NFkB [13]. When treated with TNFα, the CD44$^+$ cells showed increased NFκB activity and cytokine production as well as resistance to TNFα-induced apoptosis [13]. The resistance to apoptotic pathway activation suggests a mechanism for ovarian CSC survival when treated with chemotherapeutics. Treatment of ovarian CSCs with Eriocalyxin B (EriB) inhibits the NFκB pathway and induces cell death in ovarian CSCs [114]. EriB inhibited the TNFα-induced NFκB activity and cytokine production and sensitized the cells to TNFα- and FasL-induced cell death [114]. This suggests that inhibition of the canonical NFκB pathway could sensitize ovarian CSCs to therapy [114].

While many studies focused on the canonical NFκB pathway, the noncanonical pathway is also active in promoting stemness and chemoresistance in ovarian cancer. RelB in particular is important for ovarian CSC regulation. RelB is overexpressed in ovarian CSC populations including CD44$^+$ SKOV3 cells and ALDH$^+$/CD133$^+$ OV90 and ACI23 cell lines [113,115]. In the OV90 and ACI23 cells, ALDH1 activity and expression of RelB both increase with carboplatin treatment [115]. This suggests a role for the noncanonical NFκB pathway and RelB in promoting stemness and chemoresistance. Knockdown of RelB with shRNA reduced the number of ALDH$^+$/CD133$^+$ CSCs in vitro in both cell lines and in xenografts by 50% [115]. The RelB knockdown decreased expression of other stem cell markers (NANOG and CD44) and increased sensitivity to carboplatin [115]. In addition, ACI23 and OV90 cells, when stably transfected with inducible shRNA for RelB, showed reduced spheroid formation and reduced tumorgenicity [115]. The noncanonical pathway through RelB promotes tumor growth as well as the expression of stemness genes [115]. RelB also regulates chemoresistance in ovarian CSCs [115]. Thus, both the canonical and noncanonical NFκB pathways are excellent targets for therapeutics to reduce the CSC population.

5.4. Notch

Notch signaling has a role in multiple cellular processes. Notch is a critical component in regulating progenitor cell maintenance, differentiation, cell proliferation, and apoptosis. Notch is also important for cell–cell communication [116,117]. In HGS ovarian cancer, Notch3 expression is amplified/overexpressed [118]. By analyzing 31 fresh HGS ovarian cancer samples, Notch3 amplification correlated with protein expression [118]. Notch3 was overexpressed more often in high grade tumors (66%) than in low grade tumors (33%) [118]. Further, according to The Cancer Genome Atlas (TCGA), Notch3 is amplified in 17% of HGS tumors. The most highly expressed Notch3 ligand in ovarian serous carcinoma is Jagged 1, which is predominantly expressed in the mesothelial cells within the tumor microenvironment, suggesting a role for Notch3/Jagged 1 signaling in cell adhesion and proliferation [119].

In the majority of patients with recurrent HGS ovarian cancer, Notch3 is overexpressed [120]. Tumors from patients with either primary disease or recurrent disease were examined for Notch3 overexpression and survival [120]. In the group with primary disease, there was no difference in survival between those with Notch3 overexpression and those without [120]. Those in the group with recurrent disease did show a difference. Those expressing high Notch3 levels had decreased overall survival (22 vs. 37 months) and decreased progression-free survival (3 vs. 8 months) suggesting that Notch3 expression is a factor in the recurrence of ovarian cancer as well as a prognostic indicator in recurrent disease [120].

Chemoresistance is a hallmark of CSCs and disease recurrence/relapse, and Notch3 expression affects the expression of stemness factors as well as chemoresistance. The transcription factor OCT4 promotes self-renewal of ovarian CSCs while SOX2 is required for their maintenance [84,92]. Overexpression of Notch3 in ovarian cancer cell lines (IOSE-80pc and MPSC1) enhances expression of stem cell markers (NANOG, OCT4, and SOX2) and increases expression of the ABCB1 transporter protein [120]. The ABCB1 transporter increases chemoresistance in these ovarian CSCs and NANOG promotes the epithelial to mesenchymal transition (EMT) in ovarian cancer [121]. To demonstrate the role of Notch3 on chemoresistance, Nocth3 was knocked down in OVCAR3 cells using shRNA resulting in reduced IC_{50} compared to control cells [120]. These studies all implicate Notch3 signaling in ovarian CSC chemoresistance.

Other Notch signaling molecules are also implicated in stemness and chemoresistance including Jagged 1 and downstream signaling molecules. Downregulation of Jagged 1 in SKOV3TRip2 cells via siRNA increased sensitivity of cells to docetaxel [122]. In ovarian cancer cells isolated for the SP, Notch pathway genes (FPTG, ST3GAL6, and ADAM19), stem cell markers NANOG and OCT4, and three ABC transporter genes (ABCG2 [both lines], ABCC4 [SKOV3 only], and ABCB1 [A224 only]) were induced [95]. Collectively, the data suggest that Notch signaling is involved in promoting stemness and chemoresistance, and expression of Notch3 in particular may serve as a prognostic indicator for patients with recurrent disease. Notch signaling is an attractive target for therapeutics aimed at ovarian CSCs. Currently, there are experimental γ-secretase inhibitors, γ-secretase modifiers, Notch soluble decoys, and negative regulatory region monoclonal antibodies that are already being developed [116].

5.5. Wnt

Wnt signaling is particularly important during development where it regulates cell fate determination during embryogenesis including the cardiovascular system, central nervous system, and craniofacial development [116,123]. In adults, Wnt signaling is critical for self-renewal in tissues (e.g., bone growth plate, hair follicles, colon, etc.) [116,124,125]. The major processes regulated by noncanonical Wnt signaling include cell polarity and motility; however, Wnt also plays a role in maintaining stem cells, quiescence, and chemoresistance [126]. Wnt signaling is complex and many components of Wnt signaling are implicated in ovarian CSCs and chemoresistance (Figure 6).

A.

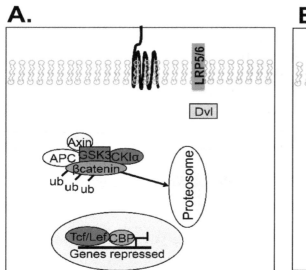

B.

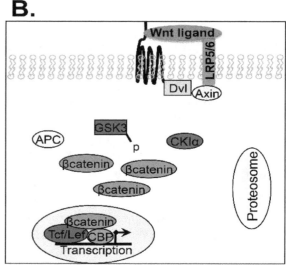

Figure 6. Wnt Signaling Cascade. (**A**) Basal state without the presence of Wnt ligand activation. β-catenin is ubiquitinated and sent to the proteosome for destruction. (**B**) Activation of the Wnt pathway via binding of a Wnt ligand to the Frizzled receptor and LRP5/6 resulting in recruitment of Disheveled (Dvl) and axin to the cell membrane. β-catenin is released from the destruction complex and translocates to the nucleus to act as a co-transcription factor.

With regards to ovarian cancer, Wnt signaling is involved in normal development of the ovarian and fallopian tube stem cells. Wnt signaling also has functions in tumor development. LGR5 is a stem cell marker for ovarian stem cells and LGR6 is a stem cell marker for the fallopian tube, and expression of either one is a sign of elevated Wnt signaling [127–129]. LGR5 and LGR6 are expressed in HGS tumors [127]. LGR5⁺ cell-driven lineage tracing was performed in mice, illustrating the importance of LGR5 and Wnt signaling in embryonic and adult ovarian stem cells for homeostasis and regenerative repair and self-renewal [130]. Since the fimbria of the fallopian tube are implicated as a site of origin in HGS tumors, fallopian tube stems cells also must be examined [129]. Using a Tcf-eGFP reporter and confocal microscopy on fallopian tube organoid cultures, active Wnt signaling was needed for the expression of stem cell factors to support organoid growth [129]. Understanding how abnormal regulation of Wnt signaling drives initiation or maintenance of ovarian CSCs is critical.

Disregulation of Wnt signaling is frequently involved in the development of cancer [123,131]. In ovarian cancer, aberrant Wnt signaling differs by histotype. Wnt signaling stabilization and subsequent nuclear translocation of β-catenin leads to activation of Wnt target genes including those involved in stemness. β-catenin is frequently mutated at GSK3β phosphorylation sites that allow β-catenin to be ubiquinated and degraded in the absence of Wnt signaling (54%) resulting in nuclear localization in approximately 70% of cases of low grade endometrioid ovarian carcinomas [132]. Activating mutations of proteins in the Wnt pathway are rare in serous ovarian carcinomas [132]. However, there is evidence of nuclear β-catenin in HGS [132]. With regards to the noncanonical Wnt pathway, Wnt5A was highly expressed in a collection of 583 ovarian tumors and it is found in the ascites [126,132]. Receptor tyrosine kinase-like orphan receptor 1 (ROR1) (a pseudokinase and receptor for Wnt5A) is expressed in ovarian cancer and is correlated with poor outcomes [79]. Survival analysis showed that patients with high expression of ROR1 had significantly reduced progression-free survival and overall survival [79]. Cells isolated from ROR1⁺ patient-derived xenografts exhibited stem-like qualities including ALDH1 expression, ability to form spheroids, and increased tumorgenicity [80]. These data suggest that ROR1 is a potential CSC marker for ovarian cancer and that noncanonical Wnt signaling is a component of ovarian cancer stemness.

In ovarian CSCs, Wnt signaling helps promote both stemness and chemoresistance. The CSC marker/receptor tyrosine kinase, CD117, is upregulated in ovarian CSCs. Many factors contribute to acquisition of CD117 expression including the hypoxic microenvironment of the stem cell niche [106]. CD117 leads to activation of AKT and the phosphorylation of GSK3β and nuclear expression of β-catenin [106]. β-catenin activity induces expression of ABCG2, a drug transporter which increases cisplatin and paclitaxel resistance [106]. Therefore, the hypoxic niche supports stemness by activation of Wnt target genes.

Wnt signaling in ovarian cancer CSCs is complex. Collectively, the patient studies combined with cell culture and animal models suggest that multiple Wnt signaling pathways contribute to stemness and chemoresistance in ovarian cancer. A number of potential molecules in the Wnt pathways may be viable targets for therapeutic intervention. Wnt inhibitors such as compounds that target Disheveled (NSC668036 and FJ9), Frizzled receptor antibody, Thiazolidinedione (target β-catenin reverse transport), and Sulindac (unknown action but potentially effects β-catenin proteasomal degradation) are being examined for use in cancer treatment [116]. Deciphering the cross-talk between Wnt and other pathways in addition to more sophisticated assessment of the contribution of particular Wnt molecules and pathways will enable development of future Wnt-targeted drugs that can be used in ovarian cancer treatment.

5.6. Hedgehog

During embryogenesis, Hedgehog signaling (Hh) regulates tissue polarity as well as patterning and stem cell maintenance [116]. In cancer, the Hh pathway is dysregulated in one of two ways: (1) constitutive expression of endogenous ligand (e.g., Sonic hedgehog [Shh]) or (2) mutations of proteins within the pathway (Patched, SMO, SUFU) [133]. We will explore the ways Hedgehog signaling has emerged as an important regulator of proliferation, chemoresistance, and stemness in ovarian cancer [133,134].

Overexpression of Gli1 (a transcription factor activated by Hh signaling) as well as PTCH (Hh receptor) is correlated with poor prognosis and survival in patients [133]. Eighty cases of epithelial ovarian tumor were examined by IHC [133]. All cases expressed PTCH, though PTCH was highly expressed in 34.1% of cases [133]. Gli1 expression varied by histotype of the tumor with high Gli1 expression being most common in serous tumors [133]. High expression of either Gli1 or PTCH correlated with poor survival compared to those patients with low expression [133]. These data suggest that Gli1 and/or PTCH expression may be prognostic indicators for ovarian cancer patients. Gli1 antagonists such as HPI 1–4 that are currently being developed as well as drugs targeting PTCH may be useful therapies for ovarian cancer patients with activated Hh signaling.

In ovarian cancer, Gli1 appears to be a critical contributor. Gli1 is a regulator of proliferation and tumor growth in ovarian cancer. Gli1 is elevated in several ovarian cancer cell lines (OVCAR5, OV-202, and OV-167) compared with normal ovarian surface epithelium [135]. Inhibition of the Hh pathway with cyclopamine resulted in Gli1 decreasing in a dose-dependent manner (60–80%) [135]. The decrease in Gli1 mRNA and protein correlated with a decrease in proliferation in all three cancer lines [135]. In addition to the in vitro results, a mouse xenograft model using OVCAR5 cells found that cyclopamine significantly inhibited tumor growth [135]. In agreement with these findings, exogenous expression of Gli1 in ovarian cancer cell lines SKOV3, OVCAR3, and OVCA433 increased cell proliferation 2-fold and increased invasiveness 200–500% over control; whereas knockdown of Gli1 with siRNA suppressed proliferation and invasiveness (40–60%) [133]. These studies suggest that Gli1 is an important regulator of proliferation and tumor growth in ovarian cancer.

The Hh pathway regulates stemness in ovarian cancer. In one study, ES2, SKOV3, and TOV112D cells were treated with recombinant Shh and Ihh, both Hh pathway agonists [134]. In all three cell lines, spheroid formation increased significantly [134]. When treated with cyclopamine, there was significant impairment of spheroid formation [134]. This demonstrates a role for the Hh pathway in maintaining stemness in ovarian cancer.

Gli1 also is implicated in chemoresistance in ovarian cancer cells. Gli1 has an interesting role in the DNA damage response following cisplatin treatment [136]. In cisplatin-resistant A2780 cells

(A2780-CP), cells with anti-Gli1 shRNA or a scrambled shRNA were treated with cisplatin and then DNA repair was assessed [136]. After 12 h the control cells had repaired 78% of the DNA adducts compared to 33% in cells treated with anti-Gli1 shRNA [136]. In addition to impairing the cell's ability to repair the cisplatin adducts, pretreatment with the anti-Gli1 shRNA sensitized the cells to cisplatin resulting, in a shift of the IC_{50} from 30 μM to 5 μM [136]. This suggests that Gli1 regulates DNA adduct repair and sensitivity to cisplatin in ovarian cancer. Additionally, Gli1, SMO, and PTCH are overexpressed in borderline and malignant ovarian cancer [137]. Moreover, Gli1 and SMO were highly overexpressed in platinum-resistant ovarian cancer [137]. Both cell culture and patient studies suggest an important role for Gli1 and Hh signaling in ovarian cancer chemoresistance.

While Hh signaling is studied in regard to other cancer types, Hh signaling in ovarian cancer is relatively understudied. Current findings suggest that Gli1 has an important role in ovarian cancer stemness, tumorigenicity, and chemoresistance. Further studies on the role of Hh signaling in ovarian cancer will allow for personalized medicine approaches for those patients with active Hh. Future therapy options could include the Hh inhibitor GDC-0449 that is currently in clinical trials for use in ovarian cancer [138].

5.7. Developing Therapeutics Targeting Ovarian Cancer Stem Cells

There are multiple pathways involved in promoting a stem cell phenotype and chemoresistance in ovarian cancer. Each pathway has the potential to be therapeutically targeted. However, a major challenge is defining which population of cells needs to be targeted with pathway inhibitors.

If a therapeutic goal is to eliminate the CSC population, more studies are needed to define CSC populations, markers, and critical pathways that are required for stem cell maintenance (Table 2: Summary of targetable genes).

Table 2. Summary of targetable genes.

Pathway	Gene	Potential Therapeutics in Trials
PI3K/PTEN/AKT	AKT1 PTEN PPMID	BKM120, Everdimus, Perifosine
Jak/STAT	STAT3 JAK2	
NFκB	RelA RelB IKK IκBα TNFα	
Notch	Notch3 Jagged1	γ-secretase inhibitors, γ-secretase modifiers, Notch soluble decoys, negative regulatory region monoclonal antibodies
Wnt	β-catenin Wnt5A Disheveled Frizzled	NSC668036, FJ9, Frizzled receptor antibodies, Thiazoldinedone, Suldinac
Hedgehog	Patched Gli1	HPI-1, HPI-2, HPI-3, HPI-4, GDC-0449

6. Future Studies

Ovarian CSCs in HGS ovarian cancer are an attractive target for therapeutics in order to prevent relapse following chemotherapy. Prior to targeting these insidious cells, a number of issues should be considered. One complication in treating patients with HGS ovarian cancer is the amount of heterogeneity found within the tumors. Additionally, HGS is characterized by genomic instability rather than specific driving mutations. This level of heterogeneity makes identifying drug targets that help a wide population of HGS ovarian cancer patients difficult. More phenotypic, genetic, and epigenetic studies of patient CSCs need to be conducted to assess which CSC populations are the most critical ones to target. Hierarchical lineage tracing efforts will allow us to decipher if different CSC populations arise from a common progenitor cell. Detailing the mechanisms that are required for CSC maintenance is critical. Delineating the role of the microenvironment in CSC maintenance is also important. Do these varying marker profiles denote differing niches for the CSCs and, therefore, different survival and renewal pathways that are active in different populations of CSCs? Are different CSC subpopulations present at different times during cancer progression? These questions underscore the need for personalized medicine in the treatment of ovarian cancer. Three potential targets for new therapeutics include stem cell markers, stem cell signaling pathways needed for renewal and/or survival, and the stem cell niche. Careful studies examining the contribution of CSC subpopulations and signaling pathways to CSC survival and maintenance will lead to directed therapeutic target design.

Author Contributions: L.R. contributed to the conceptualization, data curation, writing—original draft preparation, and writing—review and editing. K.D.C.D. contributed to conceptualization and writing—review and editing.

Acknowledgments: We would like to acknowledge Elizabeth Fisher for her help in gathering sources, Paige Dausinas for proofreading, and Jeffrey Kurkewich for the flow cytometry data. We would also like to acknowledge the Department of Defense Ovarian Cancer Research Program (W81XWH-15-1-0071) and the Indiana CTSI Research Enhancement Grant for their support of KDCD.

References

1. Schorge, J.O.; McCann, C.; Del Carmen, M.G. Surgical debulking of ovarian cancer: What difference does it make? *Rev. Obstet. Gynecol.* **2010**, *3*, 111–117. [PubMed]
2. Lalwani, N.; Prasad, S.R.; Vikram, R.; Shanbhogue, A.K.; Huettner, P.C.; Fasih, N. Histologic, molecular, and cytogenetic features of ovarian cancers: Implications for diagnosis and treatment. *Radiographics* **2011**, *31*, 625–646. [CrossRef] [PubMed]
3. Kroeger, P.T., Jr.; Drapkin, R. Pathogenesis and heterogeneity of ovarian cancer. *Curr. Opin. Obstet. Gynecol.* **2017**, *29*, 26–34. [CrossRef] [PubMed]
4. Kehoe, S.; Hook, J.; Nankivell, M.; Jayson, G.C.; Kitchener, H.; Lopes, T.; Luesley, D.; Perren, T.; Bannoo, S.; Mascarenhas, M.; et al. Primary chemotherapy versus primary surgery for newly diagnosed advanced ovarian cancer (chorus): An open-label, randomised, controlled, non-inferiority trial. *Lancet* **2015**, *386*, 249–257. [CrossRef]
5. Rojas, V.; Hirshfield, K.M.; Ganesan, S.; Rodriguez-Rodriguez, L. Molecular characterization of epithelial ovarian cancer: Implications for diagnosis and treatment. *Int. J. Mol. Sci.* **2016**, *17*, 2113. [CrossRef] [PubMed]
6. Koshiyama, M.; Matsumura, N.; Konishi, I. Recent concepts of ovarian carcinogenesis: Type I and type II. *Biomed. Res. Int.* **2014**, *2014*. [CrossRef] [PubMed]
7. Kommoss, S.; Gilks, C.B.; du Bois, A.; Kommoss, F. Ovarian carcinoma diagnosis: The clinical impact of 15 years of change. *Br. J. Cancer* **2016**, *115*, 993–999. [CrossRef] [PubMed]
8. Ottevanger, P.B. Ovarian cancer stem cells more questions than answers. *Semin. Cancer Biol.* **2017**, *44*, 67–71. [CrossRef] [PubMed]
9. Ozols, R.F. Treatment goals in ovarian cancer. *Int. J. Gynecol. Cancer* **2005**, *15*, 3–11. [CrossRef] [PubMed]
10. Gilks, C.B.; Prat, J. Ovarian carcinoma pathology and genetics: Recent advances. *Hum. Pathol.* **2009**, *40*, 1213–1223. [CrossRef] [PubMed]
11. Zhang, S.; Balch, C.; Chan, M.W.; Lai, H.C.; Matei, D.; Schilder, J.M.; Yan, P.S.; Huang, T.H.; Nephew, K.P. Identification and characterization of ovarian cancer-initiating cells from primary human tumors. *Cancer Res.* **2008**, *68*, 4311–4320. [CrossRef] [PubMed]
12. Steg, A.D.; Bevis, K.S.; Katre, A.A.; Ziebarth, A.; Dobbin, Z.C.; Alvarez, R.D.; Zhang, K.; Conner, M.; Landen, C.N. Stem cell pathways contribute to clinical chemoresistance in ovarian cancer. *Clin. Cancer Res.* **2012**, *18*, 869–881. [CrossRef] [PubMed]

13. Alvero, A.B.; Chen, R.; Fu, H.H.; Montagna, M.; Schwartz, P.E.; Rutherford, T.; Silasi, D.A.; Steffensen, K.D.; Waldstrom, M.; Visintin, I.; et al. Molecular phenotyping of human ovarian cancer stem cells unravels the mechanisms for repair and chemoresistance. *Cell Cycle* **2009**, *8*, 158–166. [CrossRef] [PubMed]

14. Devouassoux-Shisheboran, M.; Genestie, C. Pathobiology of ovarian carcinomas. *Chin. J. Cancer* **2015**, *34*, 50–55. [CrossRef] [PubMed]

15. Ramalingam, P. Morphologic, immunophenotypic, and molecular features of epithelial ovarian cancer. *Oncology* **2016**, *30*, 166–176. [PubMed]

16. Kaldawy, A.; Segev, Y.; Lavie, O.; Auslender, R.; Sopik, V.; Narod, S.A. Low-grade serous ovarian cancer: A review. *Gynecol. Oncol.* **2016**, *143*, 433–438. [CrossRef] [PubMed]

17. Diaz-Padilla, I.; Malpica, A.L.; Minig, L.; Chiva, L.M.; Gershenson, D.M.; Gonzalez-Martin, A. Ovarian low-grade serous carcinoma: A comprehensive update. *Gynecol. Oncol.* **2012**, *126*, 279–285. [CrossRef] [PubMed]

18. McCluggage, W.G. Morphological subtypes of ovarian carcinoma: A review with emphasis on new developments and pathogenesis. *Pathology* **2011**, *43*, 420–432. [CrossRef] [PubMed]

19. Malpica, A.; Deavers, M.T.; Lu, K.; Bodurka, D.C.; Atkinson, E.N.; Gershenson, D.M.; Silva, E.G. Grading ovarian serous carcinoma using a two-tier system. *Am. J. Surg. Pathol.* **2004**, *28*, 496–504. [CrossRef] [PubMed]

20. Kurman, R.J.; Shih, I.M. The dualistic model of ovarian carcinogenesis: Revisited, revised, and expanded. *Am. J. Pathol.* **2016**, *186*, 733–747. [CrossRef] [PubMed]

21. Moss, E.L.; Evans, T.; Pearmain, P.; Askew, S.; Singh, K.; Chan, K.K.; Ganesan, R.; Hirschowitz, L. Should all cases of high-grade serous ovarian, tubal, and primary peritoneal carcinomas be reclassified as tubo-ovarian serous carcinoma? *Int. J. Gynecol. Cancer* **2015**, *25*, 1201–1207. [CrossRef] [PubMed]

22. Soslow, R.A. Histologic subtypes of ovarian carcinoma: An overview. *Int. J. Gynecol. Pathol.* **2008**, *27*, 161–174. [CrossRef] [PubMed]

23. O'Neill, C.J.; McBride, H.A.; Connolly, L.E.; Deavers, M.T.; Malpica, A.; McCluggage, W.G. High-grade ovarian serous carcinoma exhibits significantly higher p16 expression than low-grade serous carcinoma and serous borderline tumour. *Histopathology* **2007**, *50*, 773–779. [CrossRef] [PubMed]

24. Jones, S.; Wang, T.L.; Shih, I.M.; Mao, T.L.; Nakayama, K.; Roden, R.; Glas, R.; Slamon, D.; Diaz, L.A., Jr.; Vogelstein, B.; et al. Frequent mutations of chromatin remodeling gene arid1a in ovarian clear cell carcinoma. *Science* **2010**, *330*, 228–231. [CrossRef] [PubMed]

25. Huang, H.N.; Lin, M.C.; Huang, W.C.; Chiang, Y.C.; Kuo, K.T. Loss of arid1a expression and its relationship with PI3K-Akt pathway alterations and ZNF217 amplification in ovarian clear cell carcinoma. *Mod. Pathol.* **2014**, *27*, 983–990. [CrossRef] [PubMed]

26. Gershenson, D.M.; Sun, C.C.; Bodurka, D.; Coleman, R.L.; Lu, K.H.; Sood, A.K.; Deavers, M.; Malpica, A.L.; Kavanagh, J.J. Recurrent low-grade serous ovarian carcinoma is relatively chemoresistant. *Gynecol. Oncol.* **2009**, *114*, 48–52. [CrossRef] [PubMed]

27. Schmeler, K.M.; Sun, C.C.; Bodurka, D.C.; Deavers, M.T.; Malpica, A.; Coleman, R.L.; Ramirez, P.T.; Gershenson, D.M. Neoadjuvant chemotherapy for low-grade serous carcinoma of the ovary or peritoneum. *Gynecol. Oncol.* **2008**, *108*, 510–514. [CrossRef] [PubMed]

28. Santillan, A.; Kim, Y.W.; Zahurak, M.L.; Gardner, G.J.; Giuntoli, R.L., 2nd; Shih, I.M.; Bristow, R.E. Differences of chemoresistance assay between invasive micropapillary/low-grade serous ovarian carcinoma and high-grade serous ovarian carcinoma. *Int. J. Gynecol. Cancer* **2007**, *17*, 601–606. [CrossRef] [PubMed]

29. Ducie, J.; Dao, F.; Considine, M.; Olvera, N.; Shaw, P.A.; Kurman, R.J.; Shih, I.M.; Soslow, R.A.; Cope, L.; Levine, D.A. Molecular analysis of high-grade serous ovarian carcinoma with and without associated serous tubal intra-epithelial carcinoma. *Nat. Commun.* **2017**, *8*, 990. [CrossRef] [PubMed]

30. Kessler, M.; Fotopoulou, C.; Meyer, T. The molecular fingerprint of high grade serous ovarian cancer reflects its fallopian tube origin. *Int. J. Mol. Sci.* **2013**, *14*, 6571–6596. [CrossRef] [PubMed]

31. Perets, R.; Wyant, G.A.; Muto, K.W.; Bijron, J.G.; Poole, B.B.; Chin, K.T.; Chen, J.Y.; Ohman, A.W.; Stepule, C.D.; Kwak, S.; et al. Transformation of the fallopian tube secretory epithelium leads to high-grade serous ovarian cancer in BRCA; TP53; PTEN models. *Cancer Cell* **2013**, *24*, 751–765. [CrossRef] [PubMed]

32. Przybycin, C.G.; Kurman, R.J.; Ronnett, B.M.; Shih, I.M.; Vang, R. Are all pelvic (nonuterine) serous carcinomas of tubal origin? *Am. J. Surg. Pathol.* **2010**, *34*, 1407–1416. [CrossRef] [PubMed]

33. Kim, J.; Coffey, D.M.; Creighton, C.J.; Yu, Z.; Hawkins, S.M.; Matzuk, M.M. High-grade serous ovarian cancer arises from fallopian tube in a mouse model. *Proc. Natl. Acad. Sci. USA* **2012**, *109*, 3921–3926. [CrossRef] [PubMed]

34. Russo, A.; Czarnecki, A.A.; Dean, M.; Modi, D.A.; Lantvit, D.D.; Hardy, L.; Baligod, S.; Davis, D.A.; Wei, J.J.; Burdette, J.E. Pten loss in the fallopian tube induces hyperplasia and ovarian tumor formation. *Oncogene* **2018**, *37*, 1976–1990. [CrossRef] [PubMed]

35. Kim, J.; Coffey, D.M.; Ma, L.; Matzuk, M.M. The ovary is an alternative site of origin for high-grade serous ovarian cancer in mice. *Endocrinology* **2015**, *156*, 1975–1981. [CrossRef] [PubMed]

36. Ahmed, A.A.; Etemadmoghadam, D.; Temple, J.; Lynch, A.G.; Riad, M.; Sharma, R.; Stewart, C.; Fereday, S.; Caldas, C.; Defazio, A.; et al. Driver mutations in TP53 are ubiquitous in high grade serous carcinoma of the ovary. *J. Pathol.* **2010**, *221*, 49–56. [CrossRef] [PubMed]

37. Mullany, L.K.; Wong, K.K.; Marciano, D.C.; Katsonis, P.; King-Crane, E.R.; Ren, Y.A.; Lichtarge, O.; Richards, J.S. Specific TP53 mutants overrepresented in ovarian cancer impact CNV, TP53 activity, responses to nutlin-3a, and cell survival. *Neoplasia* **2015**, *17*, 789–803. [CrossRef] [PubMed]

38. Merajver, S.D.; Pham, T.M.; Caduff, R.F.; Chen, M.; Poy, E.L.; Cooney, K.A.; Weber, B.L.; Collins, F.S.; Johnston, C.; Frank, T.S. Somatic mutations in the BRCA1 gene in sporadic ovarian tumours. *Nat. Genet.* **1995**, *9*, 439–443. [CrossRef] [PubMed]

39. Berchuck, A.; Heron, K.A.; Carney, M.E.; Lancaster, J.M.; Fraser, E.G.; Vinson, V.L.; Deffenbaugh, A.M.; Miron, A.; Marks, J.R.; Futreal, P.A.; et al. Frequency of germline and somatic BRCA1 mutations in ovarian cancer. *Clin. Cancer Res.* **1998**, *4*, 2433–2437. [PubMed]

40. Hennessy, B.T.; Timms, K.M.; Carey, M.S.; Gutin, A.; Meyer, L.A.; Flake, D.D., 2nd; Abkevich, V.; Potter, J.; Pruss, D.; Glenn, P.; et al. Somatic mutations in BRCA1 and BRCA2 could expand the number of patients that benefit from poly (ADP ribose) polymerase inhibitors in ovarian cancer. *J. Clin. Oncol.* **2010**, *28*, 3570–3576. [CrossRef] [PubMed]

41. Foster, K.A.; Harrington, P.; Kerr, J.; Russell, P.; DiCioccio, R.A.; Scott, I.V.; Jacobs, I.; Chenevix-Trench, G.; Ponder, B.A.; Gayther, S.A. Somatic and germline mutations of the BRCA2 gene in sporadic ovarian cancer. *Cancer Res.* **1996**, *56*, 3622–3625. [PubMed]

42. Hilton, J.L.; Geisler, J.P.; Rathe, J.A.; Hattermann-Zogg, M.A.; DeYoung, B.; Buller, R.E. Inactivation of BRCA1 and BRCA2 in ovarian cancer. *J. Natl. Cancer Inst.* **2002**, *94*, 1396–1406. [CrossRef] [PubMed]

43. Geisler, J.P.; Hatterman-Zogg, M.A.; Rathe, J.A.; Buller, R.E. Frequency of BRCA1 dysfunction in ovarian cancer. *J. Natl. Cancer Inst.* **2002**, *94*, 61–67. [CrossRef] [PubMed]

44. Rzepecka, I.K.; Szafron, L.; Stys, A.; Bujko, M.; Plisiecka-Halasa, J.; Madry, R.; Osuch, B.; Markowska, J.; Bidzinski, M.; Kupryjanczyk, J. High frequency of allelic loss at the BRCA1 locus in ovarian cancers: Clinicopathologic and molecular associations. *Cancer Genet.* **2012**, *205*, 94–100. [CrossRef] [PubMed]

45. Kulkarni-Datar, K.; Orsulic, S.; Foster, R.; Rueda, B.R. Ovarian tumor initiating cell populations persist following paclitaxel and carboplatin chemotherapy treatment in vivo. *Cancer Lett.* **2013**, *339*, 237–246. [CrossRef] [PubMed]

46. Foster, R.; Buckanovich, R.J.; Rueda, B.R. Ovarian cancer stem cells: Working towards the root of stemness. *Cancer Lett.* **2013**, *338*, 147–157. [CrossRef] [PubMed]

47. Clevers, H. The cancer stem cell: Premises, promises and challenges. *Nat. Med.* **2011**, *17*, 313–319. [CrossRef] [PubMed]

48. Nowell, P.C. The clonal evolution of tumor cell populations. *Science* **1976**, *194*, 23–28. [CrossRef] [PubMed]

49. Prieto-Vila, M.; Takahashi, R.U.; Usuba, W.; Kohama, I.; Ochiya, T. Drug resistance driven by cancer stem cells and their niche. *Int. J. Mol. Sci.* **2017**, *18*, 2574. [CrossRef] [PubMed]

50. Abdullah, L.N.; Chow, E.K. Mechanisms of chemoresistance in cancer stem cells. *Clin. Transl. Med.* **2013**, *2*, 3. [CrossRef] [PubMed]

51. Burgos-Ojeda, D.; Rueda, B.R.; Buckanovich, R.J. Ovarian cancer stem cell markers: Prognostic and therapeutic implications. *Cancer Lett.* **2012**, *322*, 1–7. [CrossRef] [PubMed]

52. Visvader, J.E.; Lindeman, G.J. Cancer stem cells in solid tumours: Accumulating evidence and unresolved questions. *Nat. Rev. Cancer* **2008**, *8*, 755–768. [CrossRef] [PubMed]

53. Ahmed, N.; Abubaker, K.; Findlay, J.; Quinn, M. Cancerous ovarian stem cells: Obscure targets for therapy but relevant to chemoresistance. *J. Cell. Biochem.* **2013**, *114*, 21–34. [CrossRef] [PubMed]

54. Borovski, T.; De Sousa, E.M.F.; Vermeulen, L.; Medema, J.P. Cancer stem cell niche: The place to be. *Cancer Res.* **2011**, *71*, 634–639. [CrossRef] [PubMed]

55. Starbuck, K.; Al-Alem, L.; Eavarone, D.A.; Hernandez, S.F.; Bellio, C.; Prendergast, J.M.; Stein, J.; Dransfield, D.T.; Zarrella, B.; Growdon, W.B.; et al. Treatment of ovarian cancer by targeting the tumor stem cell-associated carbohydrate antigen, sialyl-thomsen-nouveau. *Oncotarget* **2018**, *9*, 23289–23305. [CrossRef] [PubMed]

56. Cole, J.M.; Joseph, S.; Sudhahar, C.G.; Cowden Dahl, K.D. Enrichment for chemoresistant ovarian cancer stem cells from human cell lines. *J. Vis. Exp.* **2014**, 51891. [CrossRef] [PubMed]

57. Ma, L.; Lai, D.; Liu, T.; Cheng, W.; Guo, L. Cancer stem-like cells can be isolated with drug selection in human ovarian cancer cell line SKOV3. *Acta Biochim. Biophys. Sin.* **2010**, *42*, 593–602. [CrossRef] [PubMed]

58. Roy, L.; Samyesudhas, S.J.; Carrasco, M.; Li, J.; Joseph, S.; Dahl, R.; Cowden Dahl, K.D. Arid3b increases ovarian tumor burden and is associated with a cancer stem cell gene signature. *Oncotarget* **2014**, *5*, 8355–8366. [CrossRef] [PubMed]

59. Bapat, S.A.; Mali, A.M.; Koppikar, C.B.; Kurrey, N.K. Stem and progenitor-like cells contribute to the aggressive behavior of human epithelial ovarian cancer. *Cancer Res.* **2005**, *65*, 3025–3029. [CrossRef] [PubMed]

60. Agro, L.; O'Brien, C. In vitro and in vivo limiting dilution assay for colorectal cancer. *Bio-protocol* **2015**, *5*, 1–11. [CrossRef] [PubMed]

61. Ahmed, N.; Abubaker, K.; Findlay, J.K. Ovarian cancer stem cells: Molecular concepts and relevance as therapeutic targets. *Mol. Aspects Med.* **2014**, *39*, 110–125. [CrossRef] [PubMed]

62. Gao, M.Q.; Choi, Y.P.; Kang, S.; Youn, J.H.; Cho, N.H. CD24+ cells from hierarchically organized ovarian cancer are enriched in cancer stem cells. *Oncogene* **2010**, *29*, 2672–2680. [CrossRef] [PubMed]

63. Zhao, L.; Gu, C.; Huang, K.; Zhang, Z.; Ye, M.; Fan, W.; Han, W.; Meng, Y. The prognostic value and clinicopathological significance of CD44 expression in ovarian cancer: A meta-analysis. *Arch. Gynecol. Obstet.* **2016**, *294*, 1019–1029. [CrossRef] [PubMed]

64. Elzarkaa, A.A.; Sabaa, B.E.; Abdelkhalik, D.; Mansour, H.; Melis, M.; Shaalan, W.; Farouk, M.; Malik, E.; Soliman, A.A. Clinical relevance of CD44 surface expression in advanced stage serous epithelial ovarian cancer: A prospective study. *J. Cancer Res. Clin. Oncol.* **2016**, *142*, 949–958. [CrossRef] [PubMed]

65. Bonneau, C.; Rouzier, R.; Geyl, C.; Cortez, A.; Castela, M.; Lis, R.; Darai, E.; Touboul, C. Predictive markers of chemoresistance in advanced stages epithelial ovarian carcinoma. *Gynecol. Oncol.* **2015**, *136*, 112–120. [CrossRef] [PubMed]

66. Bourguignon, L.Y.; Peyrollier, K.; Xia, W.; Gilad, E. Hyaluronan-CD44 interaction activates stem cell marker nanog, stat-3-mediated mdr1 gene expression, and ankyrin-regulated multidrug efflux in breast and ovarian tumor cells. *J. Biol. Chem.* **2008**, *283*, 17635–17651. [CrossRef] [PubMed]

67. Klemba, A.; Purzycka-Olewiecka, J.K.; Wcislo, G.; Czarnecka, A.M.; Lewicki, S.; Lesyng, B.; Szczylik, C.; Kieda, C. Surface markers of cancer stem-like cells of ovarian cancer and their clinical relevance. *Contemp. Oncol.* **2018**, *22*, 48–55. [CrossRef] [PubMed]

68. Luo, L.; Zeng, J.; Liang, B.; Zhao, Z.; Sun, L.; Cao, D.; Yang, J.; Shen, K. Ovarian cancer cells with the CD117 phenotype are highly tumorigenic and are related to chemotherapy outcome. *Exp. Mol. Pathol.* **2011**, *91*, 596–602. [CrossRef] [PubMed]

69. Shaw, T.J.; Vanderhyden, B.C. AKT mediates the pro-survival effects of kit in ovarian cancer cells and is a determinant of sensitivity to imatinib mesylate. *Gynecol. Oncol.* **2007**, *105*, 122–131. [CrossRef] [PubMed]

70. Ruscito, I.; Cacsire Castillo-Tong, D.; Vergote, I.; Ignat, I.; Stanske, M.; Vanderstichele, A.; Ganapathi, R.N.; Glajzer, J.; Kulbe, H.; Trillsch, F.; et al. Exploring the clonal evolution of CD133/aldehyde-dehydrogenase-1 (ALDH1)-positive cancer stem-like cells from primary to recurrent high-grade serous ovarian cancer (HGSOC). A study of the ovarian cancer therapy-innovative models prolong survival (OCTIPS) consortium. *Eur. J. Cancer* **2017**, *79*, 214–225. [PubMed]

71. Liang, J.; Yang, B.; Cao, Q.; Wu, X. Association of vasculogenic mimicry formation and CD133 expression with poor prognosis in ovarian cancer. *Gynecol. Obstet. Investig.* **2016**, *81*, 529–536. [CrossRef] [PubMed]

72. Zhou, Q.; Chen, A.; Song, H.; Tao, J.; Yang, H.; Zuo, M. Prognostic value of cancer stem cell marker CD133 in ovarian cancer: A meta-analysis. *Int. J. Clin. Exp. Med.* **2015**, *8*, 3080–3088. [PubMed]

73. Baba, T.; Convery, P.A.; Matsumura, N.; Whitaker, R.S.; Kondoh, E.; Perry, T.; Huang, Z.; Bentley, R.C.;

Mori, S.; Fujii, S.; et al. Epigenetic regulation of CD133 and tumorigenicity of CD133+ ovarian cancer cells. *Oncogene* **2009**, *28*, 209–218. [CrossRef] [PubMed]

74. Curley, M.D.; Therrien, V.A.; Cummings, C.L.; Sergent, P.A.; Koulouris, C.R.; Friel, A.M.; Roberts, D.J.; Seiden, M.V.; Scadden, D.T.; Rueda, B.R.; et al. CD133 expression defines a tumor initiating cell population in primary human ovarian cancer. *Stem Cells* **2009**, *27*, 2875–2883. [CrossRef] [PubMed]

75. Silva, I.A.; Bai, S.; McLean, K.; Yang, K.; Griffith, K.; Thomas, D.; Ginestier, C.; Johnston, C.; Kueck, A.; Reynolds, R.K.; et al. Aldehyde dehydrogenase in combination with CD133 defines angiogenic ovarian cancer stem cells that portend poor patient survival. *Cancer Res.* **2011**, *71*, 3991–4001. [CrossRef] [PubMed]

76. Roy, L.; Bobbs, A.; Sattler, R.; Kurkewich, J.L.; Dausinas, P.B.; Nallathamby, P.; Cowden Dahl, K.D. CD133 promotes adhesion to the ovarian cancer metastatic niche. *Cancer Growth Metastasis* **2018**, *11*. [CrossRef] [PubMed]

77. Landen, C.N., Jr.; Goodman, B.; Katre, A.A.; Steg, A.D.; Nick, A.M.; Stone, R.L.; Miller, L.D.; Mejia, P.V.; Jennings, N.B.; Gershenson, D.M.; et al. Targeting aldehyde dehydrogenase cancer stem cells in ovarian cancer. *Mol. Cancer Ther.* **2010**, *9*, 3186–3199. [CrossRef] [PubMed]

78. Wang, Y.C.; Yo, Y.T.; Lee, H.Y.; Liao, Y.P.; Chao, T.K.; Su, P.H.; Lai, H.C. Aldh1-bright epithelial ovarian cancer cells are associated with CD44 expression, drug resistance, and poor clinical outcome. *Am. J. Pathol.* **2012**, *180*, 1159–1169. [CrossRef] [PubMed]

79. Zhang, H.; Qiu, J.; Ye, C.; Yang, D.; Gao, L.; Su, Y.; Tang, X.; Xu, N.; Zhang, D.; Xiong, L.; et al. Ror1 expression correlated with poor clinical outcome in human ovarian cancer. *Sci. Rep.* **2014**, *4*, 5811. [CrossRef] [PubMed]

80. Zhang, S.; Cui, B.; Lai, H.; Liu, G.; Ghia, E.M.; Widhopf, G.F., 2nd; Zhang, Z.; Wu, C.C.; Chen, L.; Wu, R.; et al. Ovarian cancer stem cells express ror1, which can be targeted for anti-cancer-stem-cell therapy. *Proc. Natl. Acad. Sci. USA* **2014**, *111*, 17266–17271. [CrossRef] [PubMed]

81. Zhao, W.; Ji, X.; Zhang, F.; Li, L.; Ma, L. Embryonic stem cell markers. *Molecules* **2012**, *17*, 6196–6236. [CrossRef] [PubMed]

82. Yu, Z.; Pestell, T.G.; Lisanti, M.P.; Pestell, R.G. Cancer stem cells. *Int. J. Biochem. Cell Biol.* **2012**, *44*, 2144–2151. [CrossRef] [PubMed]

83. Wang, J.; Rao, S.; Chu, J.; Shen, X.; Levasseur, D.N.; Theunissen, T.W.; Orkin, S.H. A protein interaction network for pluripotency of embryonic stem cells. *Nature* **2006**, *444*, 364–368. [CrossRef] [PubMed]

84. Wen, Y.; Hou, Y.; Huang, Z.; Cai, J.; Wang, Z. Sox2 is required to maintain cancer stem cells in ovarian cancer. *Cancer Sci.* **2017**, *108*, 719–731. [CrossRef] [PubMed]

85. Di, J.; Duiveman-de Boer, T.; Zusterzeel, P.L.; Figdor, C.G.; Massuger, L.F.; Torensma, R. The stem cell markers OCT4A, nanog and C-MYC are expressed in ascites cells and tumor tissue of ovarian cancer patients. *Cell. Oncol.* **2013**, *36*, 363–374. [CrossRef] [PubMed]

86. Ning, Y.X.; Luo, X.; Xu, M.; Feng, X.; Wang, J. Let-7d increases ovarian cancer cell sensitivity to a genistein analog by targeting c-MYC. *Oncotarget* **2017**, *8*, 74836–74845. [CrossRef] [PubMed]

87. Zhou, S.; Schuetz, J.D.; Bunting, K.D.; Colapietro, A.M.; Sampath, J.; Morris, J.J.; Lagutina, I.; Grosveld, G.C.; Osawa, M.; Nakauchi, H.; et al. The ABC transporter BCRP1/ABCG2 is expressed in a wide variety of stem cells and is a molecular determinant of the side-population phenotype. *Nat. Med.* **2001**, *7*, 1028–1034. [CrossRef] [PubMed]

88. Garson, K.; Vanderhyden, B.C. Epithelial ovarian cancer stem cells: Underlying complexity of a simple paradigm. *Reproduction* **2015**, *149*, R59–R70. [CrossRef] [PubMed]

89. Hu, L.; McArthur, C.; Jaffe, R.B. Ovarian cancer stem-like side-population cells are tumourigenic and chemoresistant. *Br. J. Cancer* **2010**, *102*, 1276–1283. [CrossRef] [PubMed]

90. Kobayashi, Y.; Seino, K.; Hosonuma, S.; Ohara, T.; Itamochi, H.; Isonishi, S.; Kita, T.; Wada, H.; Kojo, S.; Kiguchi, K. Side population is increased in paclitaxel-resistant ovarian cancer cell lines regardless of resistance to cisplatin. *Gynecol. Oncol.* **2011**, *121*, 390–394. [CrossRef] [PubMed]

91. Szotek, P.P.; Pieretti-Vanmarcke, R.; Masiakos, P.T.; Dinulescu, D.M.; Connolly, D.; Foster, R.; Dombkowski, D.; Preffer, F.; Maclaughlin, D.T.; Donahoe, P.K. Ovarian cancer side population defines cells with stem cell-like characteristics and mullerian inhibiting substance responsiveness. *Proc. Natl. Acad. Sci. USA* **2006**, *103*, 11154–11159. [CrossRef] [PubMed]

92. Karmakar, S.; Seshacharyulu, P.; Lakshmanan, I.; Vaz, A.P.; Chugh, S.; Sheinin, Y.M.; Mahapatra, S.; Batra, S.K.; Ponnusamy, M.P. HPAF1/PD2 interacts with OCT3/4 to promote self-renewal of ovarian cancer stem cells. *Oncotarget* **2017**, *8*, 14806–14820. [CrossRef] [PubMed]

93.   Peng, S.; Maihle, N.J.; Huang, Y. Pluripotency factors LIN28 and OCT4 identify a sub-population of stem cell-like cells in ovarian cancer. *Oncogene* **2010**, *29*, 2153–2159. [CrossRef] [PubMed]

94.   Varas-Godoy, M.; Rice, G.; Illanes, S.E. The crosstalk between ovarian cancer stem cell niche and the tumor microenvironment. *Stem Cells Int.* **2017**, *2017*. [CrossRef] [PubMed]

95.   Vathipadiekal, V.; Saxena, D.; Mok, S.C.; Hauschka, P.V.; Ozbun, L.; Birrer, M.J. Identification of a potential ovarian cancer stem cell gene expression profile from advanced stage papillary serous ovarian cancer. *PLoS ONE* **2012**, *7*, e29079. [CrossRef] [PubMed]

96.   Ponnusamy, M.P.; Batra, S.K. Ovarian cancer: Emerging concept on cancer stem cells. *J. Ovarian Res.* **2008**, *1*, 4. [CrossRef] [PubMed]

97.   Cowden Dahl, K.D.; Dahl, R.; Kruichak, J.N.; Hudson, L.G. The epidermal growth factor receptor responsive MIR-125a represses mesenchymal morphology in ovarian cancer cells. *Neoplasia* **2009**, *11*, 1208–1215. [CrossRef] [PubMed]

98.   Roy, L.; Bobbs, A.; Cowden Dahl, K. Indiana University School of Medicine-South Bend, University of Notre Dame. Unpublished data, 2016.

99.   Visvader, J.E.; Lindeman, G.J. Cancer stem cells: Current status and evolving complexities. *Cell Stem Cell* **2012**, *10*, 717–728. [CrossRef] [PubMed]

100.   Li, H.; Zeng, J.; Shen, K. PI3K/AKT/mTOR signaling pathway as a therapeutic target for ovarian cancer. *Arch. Gynecol. Obstet.* **2014**, *290*, 1067–1078. [CrossRef] [PubMed]

101.   Altomare, D.A.; Wang, H.Q.; Skele, K.L.; De Rienzo, A.; Klein-Szanto, A.J.; Godwin, A.K.; Testa, J.R. AKT and mTOR phosphorylation is frequently detected in ovarian cancer and can be targeted to disrupt ovarian tumor cell growth. *Oncogene* **2004**, *23*, 5853–5857. [CrossRef] [PubMed]

102.   Cai, J.; Xu, L.; Tang, H.; Yang, Q.; Yi, X.; Fang, Y.; Zhu, Y.; Wang, Z. The role of the PTEN/PI3K/AKT pathway on prognosis in epithelial ovarian cancer: A meta-analysis. *Oncologist* **2014**, *19*, 528–535. [CrossRef] [PubMed]

103.   Luo, X.; Dong, Z.; Chen, Y.; Yang, L.; Lai, D. Enrichment of ovarian cancer stem-like cells is associated with epithelial to mesenchymal transition through an miRNA-activated AKT pathway. *Cell Prolif.* **2013**, *46*, 436–446. [CrossRef] [PubMed]

104.   Seo, E.J.; Kwon, Y.W.; Jang, I.H.; Kim, D.K.; Lee, S.I.; Choi, E.J.; Kim, K.H.; Suh, D.S.; Lee, J.H.; Choi, K.U.; et al. Autotaxin regulates maintenance of ovarian cancer stem cells through lysophosphatidic acid-mediated autocrine mechanism. *Stem Cells* **2016**, *34*, 551–564. [CrossRef] [PubMed]

105.   Ali, A.Y.; Kim, J.Y.; Pelletier, J.F.; Vanderhyden, B.C.; Bachvarov, D.R.; Tsang, B.K. AKT confers cisplatin chemoresistance in human gynecological carcinoma cells by modulating ppm1d stability. *Mol. Carcinog.* **2015**, *54*, 1301–1314. [CrossRef] [PubMed]

106.   Chau, W.K.; Ip, C.K.; Mak, A.S.; Lai, H.C.; Wong, A.S. C-kit mediates chemoresistance and tumor-initiating capacity of ovarian cancer cells through activation of Wnt/BETA-catenin-ATP-binding cassette G2 signaling. *Oncogene* **2013**, *32*, 2767–2781. [CrossRef] [PubMed]

107.   Yoshikawa, T.; Miyamoto, M.; Aoyama, T.; Soyama, H.; Goto, T.; Hirata, J.; Suzuki, A.; Nagaoka, I.; Tsuda, H.; Furuya, K.; et al. JAK2/STAT3 pathway as a therapeutic target in ovarian cancers. *Oncol. Lett.* **2018**, *15*, 5772–5780. [CrossRef] [PubMed]

108.   Abubaker, K.; Luwor, R.B.; Zhu, H.; McNally, O.; Quinn, M.A.; Burns, C.J.; Thompson, E.W.; Findlay, J.K.; Ahmed, N. Inhibition of the JAK2/STAT3 pathway in ovarian cancer results in the loss of cancer stem cell-like characteristics and a reduced tumor burden. *BMC Cancer* **2014**, *14*, 317. [CrossRef] [PubMed]

109.   Saini, U.; Suarez, A.A.; Naidu, S.; Wallbillich, J.J.; Bixel, K.; Wanner, R.A.; Bice, J.; Kladney, R.D.; Lester, J.; Karlan, B.Y.; et al. STAT3/PIAS3 levels serve as "early signature" genes in the development of high-grade serous carcinoma from the fallopian tube. *Cancer Res.* **2018**, *78*, 1739–1750. [CrossRef] [PubMed]

110.   Rosen, D.G.; Mercado-Uribe, I.; Yang, G.; Bast, R.C., Jr.; Amin, H.M.; Lai, R.; Liu, J. The role of constitutively active signal transducer and activator of transcription 3 in ovarian tumorigenesis and prognosis. *Cancer* **2006**, *107*, 2730–2740. [CrossRef] [PubMed]

111.   Burgos-Ojeda, D.; Wu, R.; McLean, K.; Chen, Y.C.; Talpaz, M.; Yoon, E.; Cho, K.R.; Buckanovich, R.J. CD24$^+$ ovarian cancer cells are enriched for cancer-initiating cells and dependent on JAK2 signaling for growth and metastasis. *Mol. Cancer Ther.* **2015**, *14*, 1717–1727. [CrossRef] [PubMed]

112.   Rinkenbaugh, A.L.; Baldwin, A.S. The NF-κB pathway and cancer stem cells. *Cells* **2016**, *5*, 16. [CrossRef] [PubMed]

113. Gonzalez-Torres, C.; Gaytan-Cervantes, J.; Vazquez-Santillan, K.; Mandujano-Tinoco, E.A.; Ceballos-Cancino, G.; Garcia-Venzor, A.; Zampedri, C.; Sanchez-Maldonado, P.; Mojica-Espinosa, R.; Jimenez-Hernandez, L.E.; et al. NF-κB participates in the stem cell phenotype of ovarian cancer cells. *Arch. Med. Res.* **2017**, *48*, 343–351. [CrossRef] [PubMed]

114. Leizer, A.L.; Alvero, A.B.; Fu, H.H.; Holmberg, J.C.; Cheng, Y.C.; Silasi, D.A.; Rutherford, T.; Mor, G. Regulation of inflammation by the NF-κB pathway in ovarian cancer stem cells. *Am. J. Reprod. Immunol.* **2011**, *65*, 438–447. [CrossRef] [PubMed]

115. House, C.D.; Jordan, E.; Hernandez, L.; Ozaki, M.; James, J.M.; Kim, M.; Kruhlak, M.J.; Batchelor, E.; Elloumi, F.; Cam, M.C.; et al. NF-κB promotes ovarian tumorigenesis via classical pathways that support proliferative cancer cells and alternative pathways that support ALDH(+) cancer stem-like cells. *Cancer Res.* **2017**, *77*, 6927–6940. [CrossRef] [PubMed]

116. Takebe, N.; Harris, P.J.; Warren, R.Q.; Ivy, S.P. Targeting cancer stem cells by inhibiting Wnt, notch, and hedgehog pathways. *Nat. Rev. Clin. Oncol.* **2011**, *8*, 97–106. [CrossRef] [PubMed]

117. Chen, X.; Thiaville, M.M.; Chen, L.; Stoeck, A.; Xuan, J.; Gao, M.; Shih, I.M.; Wang, T.L. Defining notch3 target genes in ovarian cancer. *Cancer Res.* **2012**, *72*, 2294–2303. [CrossRef] [PubMed]

118. Park, J.T.; Li, M.; Nakayama, K.; Mao, T.L.; Davidson, B.; Zhang, Z.; Kurman, R.J.; Eberhart, C.G.; Shih, I.M.; Wang, T.L. Notch3 gene amplification in ovarian cancer. *Cancer Res.* **2006**, *66*, 6312–6318. [CrossRef] [PubMed]

119. Choi, J.H.; Park, J.T.; Davidson, B.; Morin, P.J.; Shih, I.M.; Wang, T.L. Jagged-1 and notch3 juxtacrine loop regulates ovarian tumor growth and adhesion. *Cancer Res.* **2008**, *68*, 5716–5723. [CrossRef] [PubMed]

120. Park, J.T.; Chen, X.; Trope, C.G.; Davidson, B.; Shih, I.M.; Wang, T.L. Notch3 overexpression is related to the recurrence of ovarian cancer and confers resistance to carboplatin. *Am. J. Pathol.* **2010**, *177*, 1087–1094. [CrossRef] [PubMed]

121. Qin, S.; Li, Y.; Cao, X.; Du, J.; Huang, X. Nanog regulates epithelial-mesenchymal transition and chemoresistance in ovarian cancer. *Biosci. Rep.* **2017**, *37*. [CrossRef] [PubMed]

122. Steg, A.D.; Katre, A.A.; Goodman, B.; Han, H.D.; Nick, A.M.; Stone, R.L.; Coleman, R.L.; Alvarez, R.D.; Lopez-Berestein, G.; Sood, A.K.; et al. Targeting the notch ligand jagged1 in both tumor cells and stroma in ovarian cancer. *Clin. Cancer Res.* **2011**, *17*, 5674–5685. [CrossRef] [PubMed]

123. Grigoryan, T.; Wend, P.; Klaus, A.; Birchmeier, W. Deciphering the function of canonical Wnt signals in development and disease: Conditional loss- and gain-of-function mutations of beta-catenin in mice. *Genes Dev.* **2008**, *22*, 2308–2341. [CrossRef] [PubMed]

124. Gavert, N.; Ben-Ze'ev, A. Beta-catenin signaling in biological control and cancer. *J. Cell. Biochem.* **2007**, *102*, 820–828. [CrossRef] [PubMed]

125. Clevers, H. Wnt/beta-catenin signaling in development and disease. *Cell* **2006**, *127*, 469–480. [CrossRef] [PubMed]

126. Asem, M.S.; Buechler, S.; Wates, R.B.; Miller, D.L.; Stack, M.S. Wnt5a signaling in cancer. *Cancers* **2016**, *8*, 79. [CrossRef] [PubMed]

127. Schindler, A.J.; Watanabe, A.; Howell, S.B. LGR5 and LGR6 in stem cell biology and ovarian cancer. *Oncotarget* **2018**, *9*, 1346–1355. [CrossRef] [PubMed]

128. Flesken-Nikitin, A.; Hwang, C.I.; Cheng, C.Y.; Michurina, T.V.; Enikolopov, G.; Nikitin, A.Y. Ovarian surface epithelium at the junction area contains a cancer-prone stem cell niche. *Nature* **2013**, *495*, 241–245. [CrossRef] [PubMed]

129. Kessler, M.; Hoffmann, K.; Brinkmann, V.; Thieck, O.; Jackisch, S.; Toelle, B.; Berger, H.; Mollenkopf, H.J.; Mangler, M.; Sehouli, J.; et al. The notch and Wnt pathways regulate stemness and differentiation in human fallopian tube organoids. *Nat. Commun.* **2015**, *6*, 8989. [CrossRef] [PubMed]

130. Ng, A.; Tan, S.; Singh, G.; Rizk, P.; Swathi, Y.; Tan, T.Z.; Huang, R.Y.; Leushacke, M.; Barker, N. LGR5 marks stem/progenitor cells in ovary and tubal epithelia. *Nat. Cell Biol.* **2014**, *16*, 745–757. [CrossRef] [PubMed]

131. Anastas, J.N.; Moon, R.T. Wnt signalling pathways as therapeutic targets in cancer. *Nat. Rev. Cancer* **2013**, *13*, 11–26. [CrossRef] [PubMed]

132. Barbolina, M.V.; Burkhalter, R.J.; Stack, M.S. Diverse mechanisms for activation of Wnt signalling in the ovarian tumour microenvironment. *Biochem. J.* **2011**, *437*, 1–12. [CrossRef] [PubMed]

133. Liao, X.; Siu, M.K.; Au, C.W.; Wong, E.S.; Chan, H.Y.; Ip, P.P.; Ngan, H.Y.; Cheung, A.N. Aberrant activation

of hedgehog signaling pathway in ovarian cancers: Effect on prognosis, cell invasion and differentiation. *Carcinogenesis* **2009**, *30*, 131–140. [CrossRef] [PubMed]

134. Ray, A.; Meng, E.; Reed, E.; Shevde, L.A.; Rocconi, R.P. Hedgehog signaling pathway regulates the growth of ovarian cancer spheroid forming cells. *Int. J. Oncol.* **2011**, *39*, 797–804. [PubMed]

135. Bhattacharya, R.; Kwon, J.; Ali, B.; Wang, E.; Patra, S.; Shridhar, V.; Mukherjee, P. Role of hedgehog signaling in ovarian cancer. *Clin. Cancer Res.* **2008**, *14*, 7659–7666. [CrossRef] [PubMed]

136. Kudo, K.; Gavin, E.; Das, S.; Amable, L.; Shevde, L.A.; Reed, E. Inhibition of gli1 results in altered c-JUN activation, inhibition of cisplatin-induced upregulation of ERCC1, XPD and XRCC1, and inhibition of platinum-DNA adduct repair. *Oncogene* **2012**, *31*, 4718–4724. [CrossRef] [PubMed]

137. Song, X.; Yan, L.; Lu, C.; Zhang, C.; Zhu, F.; Yang, J.; Jing, H.; Zhang, Y.; Qiao, J.; Guo, H. Activation of hedgehog signaling and its association with cisplatin resistance in ovarian epithelial tumors. *Oncol. Lett.* **2018**, *15*, 5569–5576. [CrossRef] [PubMed]

138. Merchant, A.A.; Matsui, W. Targeting hedgehog—A cancer stem cell pathway. *Clin. Cancer Res.* **2010**, *16*, 3130–3140. [CrossRef] [PubMed]

9

Cancer Associated Fibroblasts: Naughty Neighbors that Drive Ovarian Cancer Progression

Subramanyam Dasari [1,†], **Yiming Fang** [1,†] **and Anirban K. Mitra** [1,2,3,*]

1   Medical Sciences Program, Indiana University School of Medicine, Bloomington, IN 47401, USA; sudasari@iu.edu (S.D.); yimfang@iu.edu (Y.F.)
2   Indiana University Melvin and Bren Simon Cancer Center, Indianapolis, IN 46202, USA
3   Department of Medical and Molecular Genetics, Indiana University School of Medicine, Indianapolis, IN 46202, USA
*   Correspondence: anmitra@indiana.edu
†   These authors contributed equally to this work.

Abstract: Ovarian cancer is the most lethal gynecologic malignancy, and patient prognosis has not improved significantly over the last several decades. In order to improve therapeutic approaches and patient outcomes, there is a critical need for focused research towards better understanding of the disease. Recent findings have revealed that the tumor microenvironment plays an essential role in promoting cancer progression and metastasis. The tumor microenvironment consists of cancer cells and several different types of normal cells recruited and reprogrammed by the cancer cells to produce factors beneficial to tumor growth and spread. These normal cells present within the tumor, along with the various extracellular matrix proteins and secreted factors, constitute the tumor stroma and can compose 10–60% of the tumor volume. Cancer associated fibroblasts (CAFs) are a major constituent of the tumor microenvironment, and play a critical role in promoting many aspects of tumor function. This review will describe the various hypotheses about the origin of CAFs, their major functions in the tumor microenvironment in ovarian cancer, and will discuss the potential of targeting CAFs as a possible therapeutic approach.

Keywords: ovarian cancer; tumor microenvironment; cancer associated fibroblasts; fibroblast; cross-talk; invasion; angiogenesis; ECM; chemoresistance; therapy

1. Introduction

Ovarian cancer is the deadliest of all the gynecologic malignancies, and is the fifth leading cause of cancer related deaths among women in the United States. There has been only a modest improvement in ovarian cancer patient prognosis over the last several decades [1,2]. Therefore, there is a critical need for focused research to improve our understanding of the disease and develop novel therapies that are more effective. In the past, most of the research efforts were focused on the cancer cells in isolation. However, recent research has identified the tumor microenvironment as a key factor in promoting cancer progression [3–7]. The cancer cells recruit various normal cells and reprogram them to produce factors beneficial to tumor growth and spread. These normal cells present within the tumor constitute the tumor stroma and can compose 10–60% of the tumor volume [3].

In order to survive and proliferate, the cancer cells productively interact with their microenvironment. The tumor microenvironment is complex and contains a variety of cells constituting the tumor stroma. Tumors however, can only grow if their complex tissue environment provides them with a milieu of factors and conditions that can sustain their growth and spread [8]. A complicated bidirectional interaction is therefore happening at the interface between the genetically unstable malignant cells and the genetically stable stroma, a process that will determine the degree of tumor promotion and proliferation, invasiveness, potential for spread, and even patient prognosis [9].

The tumor stroma consists of cellular components like the cancer associated fibroblasts (CAFs), immune cells, endothelial cells, pericytes, adipocytes, and so forth, as well as acellular components like the extra cellular matrix proteins (ECMs) [3–7]. Each of these tumor microenvironmental elements has been shown to play important roles in tumor growth and progression in various cancers, including ovarian cancer. CAFs are an important constituent of the tumor stroma, and this review will focus on providing an overview of the origin, function, and potential targeting of CAFs in ovarian cancer therapy.

2. Origin of CAFs

There are several hypotheses about the origin of CAFs, which include the reprogramming of the resident normal fibroblasts by the cancer cells, and differentiation of mesenchymal stem cells (Figure 1). A less widely accepted theory is that they are already present as a small subpopulation of normal fibroblasts, which are selected for by the cancer cells [10]. These subpopulations may have acquired a mutation, or epigenetic alterations, independent of the tumor cells, which transform them into activated fibroblasts. A proinflammatory microenvironment resulting in the generation of reactive oxygen species may promote acquisition of genetic lesions [11]. As the tumor develops in their vicinity, these subpopulations might be selected for by the cancer cells for their ability to support tumor growth [10]. Since mutations are not commonly found in the tumor stroma, and CAFs are not believed to have clonal populations with distinct genetic changes, this hypothesis has not gained much traction [12]. Fibroblasts are mesenchymal cells that are generally present in the basement membrane and serve as a scaffold, secreting ECMs, and growth and trophic factors [13,14]. They are generally in a quiescent "inactive" state, but retain some plasticity, and are capable of getting "activated" by various physiological stimuli. During development, dermal fibroblasts play a role in tissue patterning, and can differentiate into multiple kind of cells, including hair follicle cells, papillary cells, reticular cells, and pre-adipocytes [15]. The fibroblasts get activated at the site of wound healing by factors such as insulin-like growth factors (IGFs), transforming growth factor beta 1,2,3 (TGF-β 1,2,3), and platelet-derived growth factor (PDGF), among others. These activated fibroblasts express α-smooth muscle actin (α-SMA), which makes them contractile, and helps in wound closure. These α-SMA expressing fibroblasts are called myofibroblasts. They secrete various ECMs and extracellular proteases, which help in the initial wound healing and development of the scar. They also secrete factors like TGF-β to stimulate epithelial to mesenchymal transition in the epithelial cells around the wound. This enables the epithelial cells to move and close the wound. Thereafter, as the wound heals, epithelialization is promoted by epidermal growth factors (EGFs) and the keratinocyte growth factor (KGF) produced by the fibroblasts [16].

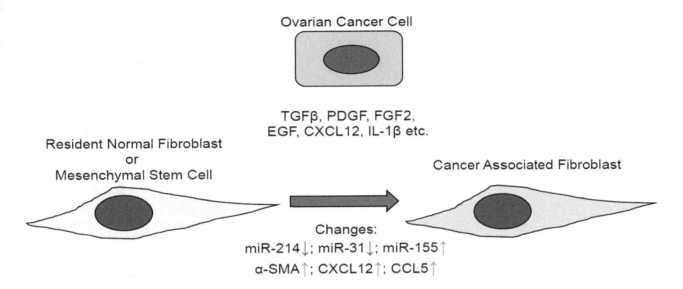

Figure 1. Formation of cancer associated fibroblasts (CAFs) through the reprogramming of resident normal fibroblasts or mesenchymal stem cells by ovarian cancer cells. TGF-β: transforming growth factor beta; PDGF: platelet-derived growth factor; FGF: fibroblast growth factor; EGF: epidermal growth factors; CXCL12: C-X-C Motif Chemokine Ligand 12; CCL5: C-C Motif Chemokine Ligand 5; ↑: upregulated;↓: downregulated.

CAFs display several traits of the activated fibroblasts found in healing wounds, including upregulation of TGF-β, increased secretion of ECMs, extra cellular proteases, and expression of α-SMA. It is believed that cancer cells can recruit the resident normal fibroblasts and reprogram them into CAFs. Several reports have demonstrated evidence in support of this hypothesis in ovarian cancer [7]. Ovarian cancer cells produce factors including TGF-β and PDGF, that can change normal fibroblasts into "activated" CAFs. We have previously shown that ovarian cancer cells can induce a change in expression of a set of 3 microRNAs in the resident normal omental fibroblasts, which reprograms them into CAFs [7]. miR-214 and miR-31 were found to decrease, while miR-155 expression increased, in the normal fibroblasts because of their interaction with the metastasizing ovarian cancer cells. This resulted in their reprogramming into CAFs (Figure 1). It was the first report of a set of microRNAs reprogramming normal fibroblasts into CAFs. Simultaneous inhibition of miR-214 and miR-31, along with overexpression of miR-155, could convert normal fibroblasts into CAFs. These results supported previous findings in other cancers, which demonstrated the absence of mutations in CAFs. Moreover, CAFs can be isolated from tumors and cultured in vitro for several passages, and yet retain their phenotype and their ability to support cancer cell functions. This suggested a potential role of epigenetic regulation [17]. The role of microRNAs in reprogramming of normal fibroblasts into CAFs further revealed a potential mechanism. Interestingly, overexpressing miR-214 and miR-31 and inhibiting miR-155 simultaneously in CAFs could revert them back into normal fibroblasts. This offers a potential opportunity to normalize a key component of the tumor microenvironment. Research on targeting the tumor microenvironment has revealed that the normalization of the tumor microenvironment is a more effective approach as compared to attempts at obliterating it altogether. The latter typically leads to the cancer cells becoming more aggressive. Depleting α-SMA positive CAFs in a transgenic mouse model of pancreatic ductal adenocarcinoma through induction of thymidine kinase by ganciclovir administration, either early in the tumor precursor stage or late carcinoma stage, led to the development of undifferentiated tumors, which were highly invasive and resulted in decreased survival [18]. Since this was observed when the CAFs were ablated in the precursor lesions or in the late carcinomas, it indicated that irrespective of tumor stage, in the absence of the microenvironmental support, the more aggressive cancer cell clones are selected. These findings are similar to the increased metastasis observed upon pericyte depletion [19].

Other hypotheses about the origin of CAFs include the recruitment of mesenchymal stem cells by the cancer cells to the tumor [10,20]. Human pancreatic cancer cells were shown to recruit bone marrow derived progenitors when injected in mice [21]. The resulting tumors had about 40% myofibroblasts derived from bone marrow cells. Similarly, CAFs were shown to be derived from mesenchymal stem cells in ovarian cancer and supported tumor growth through the secretion of the paracrine factor IL-6 [22]. Ovarian cancer cells have been reported to secrete IL-1β that leads to the decreased expression of p53 protein in the ovarian fibroblasts, converting them into CAFs [23]. The decreased p53 resulted in increased secretion of IL-8, growth regulated oncogene-alpha (GRO-α), IL-6, IL-1β, and vascular endothelial growth factor (VEGF) by the CAFs. Mesenchymal stem cell derived CAFs were also shown to regulate ovarian cancer stem cells through bone morphogenetic protein secretion, which resulted in resistance to chemotherapy [24,25]. The mesothelial cells lining the peritoneum and the omentum have also been reported as a source of CAFs in ovarian cancer peritoneal and omental metastasis [26]. The mesothelial cells have been shown to undergo mesothelial to mesenchymal transition under the influence of ovarian cancer cell secreted TGF-β, which can form a subpopulation of the CAFs in ovarian cancer metastatic tumors [27]. Others have demonstrated that ovarian cancer cells interact with the mesothelial cells in a β1-integrin-dependent manner to induce mesothelial to mesenchymal transition and convert them into CAFs [28].

3. CAF Markers

Since CAFs in the tumor microenvironment are functionally very similar to the activated fibroblasts in healing wounds, they both share several markers. CAFs express α-SMA, which is also a marker of myofibroblasts in wound healing [10]. Ovarian cancer CAFs also express α-SMA, while normal fibroblasts do not [29]. However, the expression of α-SMA is only one of many changes that occur in activated fibroblasts [30]. The levels of expression of α-SMA may also vary between CAFs. As evidenced by the findings of Mhawech-Fauceglia et al., the CAFs in ovarian tumors are predominantly α-SMA positive, but not all of them stain for the protein [29]. This indicates the existence of a certain level heterogeneity within the CAF population.

In addition to α-SMA, many other markers have been reported to distinguish CAFs from normal fibroblasts. They include fibroblast activated protein (FAP), S100A4, and platelet derived growth factor receptor, among others [7,29,31]. FAP, a cell surface serine protease, has emerged as a specific marker of CAFs in ovarian cancer [32]. While each of them has been shown to be an effective marker by different groups, there is no clear consensus about a universal marker for CAFs. The probable reason for this is that CAFs are a heterogeneous population, with some expressing one marker and others expressing other markers. α-SMA and PDGF positive CAFs do not overlap with S100A4 positive CAFs in pancreatic cancer [33]. The mutual exclusivity and heterogeneity in CAF marker expression may impart unique functions; for example, FAP and podoplanin positive CAFs were found to be immunosuppressive through a nitric oxide-dependent mechanism, while FAP positive and podoplanin negative CAFs were not immunosuppressive in lung adenocarcinoma [34]. For prostate cancer, CAFs expressing high CD90 had greater tumor promoting capacity than CAFs expressing low CD90 [35]. Pancreatic ductal adenocarcinomas have a subpopulation of CAFs that are distinct from those expressing α-SMA. These CAFs express proinflammatory mediators like IL-6, and mediate a paracrine interaction with the carcinoma cells [36]. In ovarian cancer, the expression levels of different CAF markers, CD10, podoplanin, FAP, Platelet-derived growth factor receptor alpha (PDGFRα), Platelet-derived growth factor receptor beta (PDGFRβ), S100 calcium binding protein A4 (S100A4), α-SMA, snail family transcriptional repressor 2 (SNAI2, commonly known as Slug), Zinc finger E-box-binding homeobox 1 (ZEB1), and twist family bHLH transcription factor 1 (TWIST1), clustered the CAFs into different subgroups showing different protein expression patterns [31].

Due to the continuous reciprocal interactions of CAFs with cancer cells, it is quite possible that the CAFs can undergo dynamic changes in their marker expression and functions depending on the heterogeneity of the cancer cells within the tumors. A recent study identified a unique subset of CAFs expressing the metallo-endopeptidase CD10 and the complement anaphylatoxin receptor GPR77 [37]. These CAFs were enriched following neoadjuvant chemotherapy, and were shown to promote cancer stem cell self-renewal through the secretion of IL-6 and IL-8. Therefore, their abundance in the tumors of breast cancer patients predicted a poor prognosis. Similarly, the evolving ovarian cancer metastatic tumors are metabolically reprogrammed by CAFs through the secretion of C-C Motif Chemokine Ligand 5 (CCL5), C-X-C motif chemokine ligand 10 (CXCL10), and IL-6 to utilize glycogen [38]. The CAFs with activated p38 MAP kinase signaling were capable of inducing such reprogramming. Therefore, considering the heterogeneity of CAFs, it is important to take into account their functional effects in promoting tumor progression as well as the potential of dynamic changes in them.

4. CAF Functions

CAFs have multiple functions in the tumor microenvironment, which directly or indirectly promote tumor progression. Most of these functions are mediated through the secretion of paracrine factors, ECMs, and proteases, as well as through cell surface receptors and direct contact with cancer cells. These functions and their underlying mechanisms are detailed below, outlined in Figure 2, and listed in Table 1.

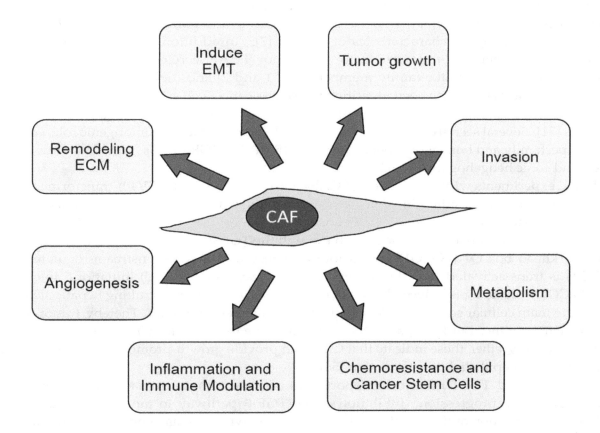

Figure 2. Functions of CAFs contributing towards tumor progression. ECM: extra cellular matrix; EMT: epithelial–mesenchymal transition.

Table 1. Functional roles of cancer associated fibroblasts (CAFs) in tumor progression.

No.	Functional Role of CAF	References
1	Promoting of tumor growth	[39]
2	Promoting tumor invasion	[3,40]
3	Inducing EMT in cancer cells	[41,42]
4	Remodeling the ECM	[43,44]
5	Inducing angiogenesis	[45,46]
6	Inflammation and immune modulation	[7,47]
7	Promoting chemoresistance and cancer stem cells	[48,49]
8	Reprogramming cancer metabolism	[3,4,38]

ECM: extra cellular matrix; EMT: epithelial–mesenchymal transition.

4.1. Promoting Tumor Growth

CAFs have predominantly been demonstrated to have tumor-promoting functions. They stimulate cancer cell survival, growth, and invasion, enhance the stiffness of the extracellular matrix, contribute to angiogenesis by releasing pro-angiogenic factors, contribute to a pro-inflammatory milieu, and impact on the activation state of various immune cells [50]. CAFs are crucial in tumor-stroma communication through modulation of the extracellular matrix, fibrogenesis, and chemoattraction of other stromal cells. Several studies have demonstrated that tumor–CAF crosstalk promotes growth and invasion of the particular cancer cells [39]. CAFs produce autocrine and paracrine cytokines that promote the growth and biological characteristics of tumors [7]. In addition to classical growth factors, including EGF and hepatocyte growth factor (HGF), novel CAF secreted proteins (secreted frizzled related protein 1, and IGF like family member (IGF) 1 and 2) and membrane molecules (integrin α11 and syndecan 1) have also been identified to possess cancer cell supporting roles. These factors directly or indirectly stimulate tumor growth and survival, or enhance their migratory and invasive properties [51]. Several secreted molecular regulators of CAFs have a pro-tumorigenic role, such as the TGF-β superfamily and bone morphogenic proteins (BMPs), PDGFs, EGFs, fibroblast growth factors (FGFs), and sonic hedgehog (SHH) [52].

Initial experiments with co-injection of CAFs with simian virus 40 (SV40)-transformed prostate epithelial cells in mice resulted in tumors resembling prostatic intraepithelial neoplasia, whereas normal fibroblasts did not. Similarly, co-transplantation of myofibroblasts with Ras-transformed hepatocytes strongly enhances tumor growth through the TGF-β/PDGF axis [39]. In addition, CAFs induce forkhead box Q1 (FOXQ1) expression; as a result, N-myc downstream-regulated gene 1 (NDRG1) is trans-activated to enhance hepatocellular carcinoma (HCC) initiation. Interestingly, pSTAT6/CCL26 signaling is induced by the FOXQ1/NDRG1 axis, thus recruiting hepatic stellate cells (HSCs), the main cellular source of CAFs, to the tumor microenvironment. Thereby, tumor-initiating properties are enhanced at least partly through a positive feedback loop between CAFs and HCC cells [53]. Taken together, these indicate that CAFs can provide growth-promoting signals to epithelial cells, and support epithelial transformation [54].

Tumor-derived TGF-β1 has been reported to activate tumor stroma, and thereby facilitate tumor growth and progression. Inhibition of the TGF-β pathway in mouse fibroblasts through conditional inactivation of the *TGFBR2* gene is associated with increased oncogenic potential of the adjacent epithelia [55]. An invasive breast cancer cohort study, using a randomized tamoxifen trial, demonstrated that TGF-β receptor type-2 expression in cancer-associated fibroblasts regulates breast cancer cell growth and survival, and is a prognostic marker in pre-menopausal breast cancer [56]. Mesenchymal stem cell derived CAFs recruited to the stroma of the dysplastic stomach express IL-6, Wnt5a, and bone morphogenetic protein 4, which promote tumor growth through DNA hypomethylation [57]. In oral squamous cell carcinoma (OCC), CAFs promote the production of endogenous reactive oxygen species (ROS) through CCL2 expression, which induces the cell cycle regulatory proteins, and promotes OCC proliferation, migration, and invasion [58]. CAFs have also been reported to promote Th2 polarization of the tumor microenvironment, and stimulate tumor growth and metastasis by recruiting tumor-associated macrophages (TAMs), myeloid derived suppressor cells (MDSCs), and T regulatory cells (T_{regs}) [8,59].

In ovarian cancer, CAFs promote tumor invasion and growth through the secretion of a number of chemokines, cytokines, and growth factors like CCL5, IL-6, IL-8, HB-EGF, and TGF-α, among others [7]. These secreted factors were regulated by the decreased expression of miR-214 and miR-31, and an increased expression of miR-155, in CAFs induced by ovarian cancer cells. CCL5 was a target of miR-214 and miR-31, and was responsible for homing of the ovarian cancer cells onto plugs of CAFs in vitro [7]. Inhibiting CCL5 with a neutralizing antibody was sufficient to reduce tumor growth of co-injected CAFs and ovarian cancer cells in mice [7].

4.2. Promoting Tumor Invasion

Tumor invasion is a key hallmark of cancer and is essential for successful dissemination of the cancer cells. Myofibroblasts have the inherent ability to invade through the ECM in the basement membrane during wound healing. Similarly, CAFs have the ability to invade through matrix, and have been widely reported to promote invasiveness of cancer cells [3]. There are several potential mechanisms by which CAFs can directly or indirectly promote cancer cell invasiveness. These include secretion of factors and proteases that help in the invasion. Zhu et al. (2016) [40] reported that Gal-1-regulated CAF activation promotes breast cancer cell metastasis by upregulating MMP-9 expression in breast cancer. Recent studies have shown that breast CAFs overexpress the chemokine CXCL1, a key regulator of tumor invasion and chemo-resistance. TGF-β negatively regulates CXCL1 expression in CAFs through Smad2/3 binding to the promoter, and through suppression of HGF/c-Met autocrine signaling [60]. CAFs can also induce changes in the cancer cells, which helps in their invasiveness. They have been reported to promote the metastatic activity of breast cancer cells by activating the transcription of HOTAIR via TGF-β1 secretion [61].

CAFs can serve as engines for collective invasion of directly interacting cancer cells through heterotypic interactions between the N-cadherin expressed on CAFs with the E-cadherin on cancer cells [62]. Interestingly, a dual mechanism is involved. CAFs favor invasion of cancer cells by pulling them away from the tumor, while cancer cells further enhance their spread by polarizing CAF migration away from the tumor. Along similar lines, vimentin is reported to be necessary for lung adenocarcinoma metastasis by maintaining heterotypic tumor cell–CAF interactions during collective invasion [63]. Cdc42EP3—a member of the BORG family of Cdc42 effectors—is highly expressed in CAFs, and regulates the actin and septin fibrillar networks. Coordination between the actin and the septin networks in CAFs is required for force-mediated matrix remodeling, promoting cancer cell invasion, angiogenesis, and tumor growth [64].

In ovarian cancer we have previously shown that CAFs can promote coordinated invasion of the cancer cells, which promotes metastasis [7]. Using a novel 3D live confocal imaging-based co-invasion assay, we observed that the CAFs derived from ovarian cancer omental metastasis are able to closely interact with ovarian cancer cells and invade through matrigel by forming distinct networks of CAFs and cancer cells, which invaded together. Cancer cells alone invaded at a slower rate and failed to form the network consisting of cellular associations. The mechanism of CAF–cancer cell interactions reported by Labernadie et al. [62] involving heterophilic E-cadherin/N-cadherin junctions could potentially be playing a role in these interactions between the CAFs and ovarian cancer cells. A comparison of gene expression profiles of CAFs from omental metastasis with normal omental fibroblasts revealed that the CAFs secrete multiple chemokines and cytokines that can potentially regulate invasion and motility of cancer cells [7]. Among them, CCL5 was identified as a key CAF derived mediator of metastasis, which was itself regulated by miR-214 and miR-31. Both these microRNAs are downregulated in CAFs during the reprogramming of normal fibroblasts by metastasizing ovarian cancer cells [7]. Zhao et al.

(2017) identified STAT4 as a key regulator of ovarian cancer metastasis via Wnt7a-induced activation of CAFs [65]. The concomitant increased production of CXCL12, IL6, and VEGFA by CAFs within the tumor microenvironment could enable peritoneal metastasis of ovarian cancer via induction of the EMT program. They also established a model of promotion of ovarian cancer metastasis by STAT4 via tumor-derived Wnt7a-induced activation of CAFs [65]. CAFs promote ovarian cancer cell proliferation, migration, and invasion through the paracrine FGF-1 factor. The FGF-1/FGFR-4 signaling axis regulates the stromal microenvironment in ovarian carcinomas. CAFs also activate the expression of Snail1 and MMP3, as well as reduce the expression of E-cadherin [66].

4.3. Inducing EMT in Cancer Cells

An epithelial-mesenchymal transition (EMT) is a biological process that allows a polarized epithelial cell, which normally interacts with the basement membrane via its basal surface, to undergo multiple biochemical changes that enable it to assume a mesenchymal cell phenotype, which includes enhanced migratory capacity, invasiveness, elevated resistance to apoptosis, and greatly increased production of ECM components. The completion of an EMT is signaled by the degradation of the underlying basement membrane and the formation of a mesenchymal cell that can migrate away from the epithelial layer in which it originated [67]. The idea that epithelial cells can downregulate epithelial characteristics and acquire mesenchymal characteristics arose in the early 1980s from observations made by Elizabeth Hay [68]. Over the subsequent years, the importance of EMT in cancer progression has been well established. The heterotypic interactions of cancer cells with the microenvironment, including CAFs, has been shown to be a key inducer of EMT.

Coculturing CAFs with lung cancer cells can induce miR-33b downregulation and promote epithelial cells EMT. miR-33b overexpression in lung cancer cells can counteract CAF-induced EMT. Interestingly, Snail1 expression in fibroblasts activates the inductive effects of CAFs on lung cancer cells. Snail1-expressing cancer-associated fibroblasts induce lung cancer cell epithelial-mesenchymal transition through miR-33b [41]. CAF conditioned medium induced epithelial-mesenchymal transition (EMT) by regulating the expression of EMT-associated markers E-cadherin and vimentin, and modulated metastasis-related genes MMP-2 and VEGF, both in vitro and in vivo. Further studies demonstrated that CAFs enhanced the metastatic potential of lung cancer cells by secreting IL-6 and subsequently activating the JAK2/STAT3 signaling pathway [42]. TGF-β1 secreted by CAFs can induce EMT in the interacting cancer cells and promote metastasis [69,70]. In ovarian tumors, CAF derived exosomes contain higher levels of TGF-β1 compared to those derived from normal omental fibroblasts [71]. Theses exosomes, upon uptake by ovarian cancer cells, induce EMT through the activation of SMADs. Activation of STAT3 by microenvironmental IL-6 can also induce EMT in ovarian cancer cells [72]. CAFs were reported to be the major source of IL-6 in the tumor microenvironment of ovarian tumors [72]. Therefore, CAFs can make cancer cells more aggressive by inducing EMT in them through various paracrine mechanisms.

4.4. Remodeling the ECM

Every organ has an ECM with unique composition, providing physical support for tissue integrity and elasticity. It is a dynamic structure that is constantly remodeled to control tissue homeostasis [73]. Dysregulation of ECM composition, structure, stiffness, and abundance contributes to several pathological conditions, such as fibrosis and invasive cancer. Typically, tumors have much stiffer ECMs, causing altered dynamics of the biophysical and biochemical interactions of the cancer cells with their microenvironment [74]. The increased stiffness of the matrix promotes invasiveness and motility of the cancer cells through improved invadosome and lamella formation [75]. Matrix stiffness drives EMT and metastasis through the TWIST1–G3BP2 mechanotransduction pathway in breast cancer [76]. A 9-gene matrisome gene signature has been identified through the analysis of available databases, and is associated with tumor progression through promotion of EMT, angiogenesis, hypoxia, inflammation, and altered metabolism in several cancers, including ovarian cancer [43]. Altered ECMs and ECM remodeling enzymes, like matrix metalloproteinases (MMPs), tissue inhibitors of metalloproteinases (TIMPs), and lysyl oxidases (LOXs), work to create a stiffer microenvironment permissive for tumor cell growth, migration, and invasion [44]. The increased secretion of fibronectin and LOXs by breast cancer CAFs contribute towards the remodeling of the ECMs in these tumors, promoting invasion and metastasis [77]. TGF-β activates the secretion of versican by CAFs in high-grade serous ovarian tumors, which induces the expression of MMP9 and CD44 by the cancer cells, resulting in ECM remodeling and invasion [78]. A recent study has demonstrated the role of ovarian cancer cell derived inhibin βA in effectively inducing CAFs, which then secrete increased amounts of collagens and other ECMs [79]. Therefore, CAFs serve the important function of remodeling the ECMs through altered secretion of the matrisome components, and provide the ideal microenvironmental stiffness for tumor progression.

4.5. Inducing Angiogenesis

As the tumor grows, the cancer cells are further removed from the existing blood vessels, and as a result, experience depleted levels of oxygen and nutrients. This typically places a limit to the tumor size, as cell proliferation in the regions well supplied by the blood vessels is balanced by cell death in the regions deprived of oxygen and nutrients. Therefore, in order to progress, the tumors must induce angiogenesis. It is the formation of a new vascular network to supply nutrients and oxygen, and remove waste products. Multiple factors, like VEGF, basic fibroblast growth factor (bFGF), interleukin-8 (IL-8), placenta-like growth factor (PLGF), TGF-β, platelet-derived endothelial growth factor (PD-EGF), pleiotrophin, activated hypoxia-inducible factor-1α (HIF-1α), and so forth, have been shown to trigger angiogenesis [80,81]. Many of these pro-angiogenic factors are contributed by the tumor microenvironment [82]. CAFs induce angiogenesis directly, as well as indirectly, through VEGFA, PDGFC, FGF2, CXCL12, osteopontin, and CSF3 secretion, ECM production, and recruitment of myeloid cells [82]. SDF-1 secreted by breast cancer CAFs has been involved in mobilization of endothelial precursor cells from bone marrow, thereby inducing de novo angiogenesis, as well as in tumor growth through a paracrine effect on CXCR4 expressing cancer cells [45]. Similarly, fibroblast-derived SDF-1 synergized with IL-8 in the promotion of a complete angiogenic response in recruited endothelial cells in pancreatic cancer [46]. SDF-1 is induced in breast cancer CAFs by oxidative stress-mediated activation of HIF-1 [83]. Chloride intracellular channel protein 3 (CLIC3) secreted by breast cancer CAFs induces angiogenesis through an active transglutaminase-2 (TGM2) mediated mechanism [84]. MMP-13 secreted by CAFs promotes tumor angiogenesis by releasing VEGF entrapped in the ECM, thereby leading to increased invasion of endothelial cells in squamous cell carcinoma and melanoma [85]. Ovarian cancer CAFs can indirectly induce angiogenesis through increased secretion of pro-inflammatory factors IL-6, COX-2, and CXCL1 [86]. Ovarian cancer cell expression HOXA9 induces CAFs to secrete CXCL12, IL-6, and VEGF-A expression, which promotes angiogenesis [87]. Ovarian cancer CAFs have also been shown to induce angiogenesis by secreting VEGF-C as a result of induction by Sonic Hedgehog (SHH) from ovarian cancer cells [88]. While angiogenesis can be induced by cancer cells as well as the tumor microenvironment, CAFs are important direct or indirect contributors to the process, and hence towards cancer progression.

4.6. Inflammation and Immune Modulation

Inflammation is a normal physiological response that is initiated in injured tissue and helps in its healing. In clinical settings, chronic inflammation and cancer are closely related, and cancer is referred to as "wounds that never heal". During tissue injury associated with wounding, cell proliferation is enhanced while the tissue regenerates; proliferation and inflammation subside after the assaulting agent is removed or the repair completed. In contrast, proliferating neoplastic cells continue to proliferate in microenvironments rich in inflammatory cells, and growth and survival factors, that support their growth [89]. Pro-inflammatory cytokines are secreted by cancer cells and CAFs to attract immune cells to the tumor. Macrophages actively attracted into tumor regions along defined chemotactic gradients start to differentiate into tumor-associated macrophages (TAMs), which further enhance the growth and metastasis of cancer cells [52]. CAFs are functionally required for mediating inflammation during squamous cell carcinogenesis, starting at the earliest pre-neoplastic stages [90]. A recent paper demonstrated that CAFs associated to incipient neoplasia exhibit a pro-inflammatory signature, leading them to mainly overexpress SDF-1, IL-6, and IL-1β, as well as to recruit proangiogenic macrophages. This gene set is under the transcriptional control of nuclear factor-κB (NF-κB) and cyclooxygenase 2 (COX-2), thereby strengthening the link between CAFs and inflammatory mediators in tumor progression [47]. We have demonstrated that ovarian cancer CAFs produce an array of chemokines and cytokines, which can potentially induce a proinflammatory response [7]. These chemokines and cytokines were directly or indirectly regulated by miR-214, miR-31, and miR-155 in CAFs [7]. Several other groups have also shown many chemokines and cytokines, including IL-6, COX-2, and CXCL1, to be involved in tumor-related inflammation in epithelial ovarian cancer [50,91].

CAFs in the tumor microenvironment exert immunomodulatory effects through secretion of immunomodulatory factors that polarize responsive immune populations, such as macrophages [92]. In order for the tumor to survive, any immune response directed toward the tumor cells needs to be suppressed [52]. CAFs play important roles in shaping the tumor immunosuppressive microenvironment in oral squamous cell carcinoma by inducing the protumor M2 macrophages [93]. Immunosuppressive activity of CAFs has been reported in head and neck squamous cell carcinoma through increased expression levels of IL-6, CXCL8, and TGF1 [94]. Genetic ablation of Chitinase 3-like 1 (Chi3L1) in fibroblasts in vivo attenuated tumor growth, macrophage recruitment, and reprogramming to an M2-like phenotype, enhanced tumor infiltration by CD8+ and CD4+ T cells, and promoted a Th1 phenotype. These results indicate that CAF-derived Chi3L1 promotes tumor growth and shifts the balance of the immune milieu towards type 2 immunity [95]. Activation of the PD1/PDL1 signaling pathway in T-cells leads to T-cell exhaustion and immune suppression. IL6 secreted by CAFs in hepatocellular carcinoma activates neutrophils in the tumor microenvironment, and induces PDL1 expression in them through the JAK-STAT3 pathway. The PDL1 expressing neutrophils inhibit T-cell mediated immunity and create a protumor microenvironment [96]. Being the most abundant cellular component of the stroma, CAFs can exert their effects indirectly on tumor progression through secreted factors that help evolve a proinflammatory and immunosuppressive microenvironment for the cancer cells to thrive in.

4.7. Promoting Chemoresistance and Cancer Stem Cells

The eventual development of chemoresistance is the cause of most ovarian cancer related mortalities. The role of the tumor microenvironment in this process has generated great interest in recent years. Glutathione and cysteine released by fibroblasts in ovarian tumors contribute towards the depletion of platinum in the nuclei of the adjacent ovarian cancer cells, and thus impart resistance to platinum based chemotherapies [97]. CAFs can also induce therapy resistance by reducing the bioavailability of the drugs, by causing tumor microvessel leakiness. CAFs induce the *lipoma-preferred partner* (LPP) gene in microvascular endothelial cells through a calcium-dependent FAK/ERK/MLC2/CREB signaling pathway [48]. In one study, the increased *LPP* enhanced the endothelial cell motility and permeability through increased focal adhesions and stress fiber formation [48]. CAFs can also induce chemoresistance in cancer cells by inducing apoptosis resistance. CAFs activate STAT3 signaling in ovarian cancer cells resulting in the development of chemoresistance through the increased expression of the antiapoptotic survivin and Bcl-2 [49]. CAFs in pancreatic ductal adenocarcinoma can similarly decrease apoptosis and increase the chemoresistance of the cancer cells by the induction of transcriptional downregulation of caspases by promoter hypermethylation [98]. Ovarian cancer apoptosis was also inhibited by CAF derived exosomes that transfer miR-21 to the cancer cells. The miR-21 then downregulated its direct target apoptotic protease activating factor 1 (APAF1), conferring chemoresistance [99].

Cancer stem cells are known to be resistant to cytotoxic chemotherapy and can give rise to tumor relapse. CD10 and GPR77 expressing CAFs induce cancer stem cells in breast and lung cancer through the consistent secretion of IL-6 and IL-8 [37]. These CAFs also increase the take rate of patient derived xenograft tumors, and inhibition of GPR77 abolishes this effect [37]. In one study, autophagic CAFs in luminal breast cancer induced stemness in the cancer cells through the secretion of high-mobility group box 1 (HMGB1), resulting in the activation of toll-like receptor 4 in the cancer cells [100]. In endocrine resistant metastatic breast cancer, the transfer of CAF derived exosomes containing miR-221 activated an ER^{lo}/$Notch^{hi}$ feed-forward loop that generated $CD133^{hi}$ cancer stem cells [101]. In ovarian cancer, the evidence of induction of cancer stem cells is limited, with a few reports indicating the role of CAF derived fibroblast growth factor 4 and IL-6 in inducing cancer stem cells [102,103]. Targeting the FHF4/FGFR2 axis that mediates the CAF-cancer stem cell signaling prevented the CAFs from inducing cancer stem cells [102]. Insulin growth factor receptor activation in ovarian cancer cells by CAFs, and the resulting increased Nanog expression, is also reported to promote cancer stem cells in ovarian cancer [104]. Overall, the potential role of CAFs in providing a stem cell niche for cancer stem cells is an idea that needs to be systematically researched.

4.8. Reprogramming Cancer Cell Metabolism

Cancer cells have an altered metabolism to cope with their different growth rate, nutrient availability, and the hypoxia they experience as compared to normal cells. This altered metabolism is considered one of the hallmarks of cancer, and the tumor microenvironment is a major contributor towards this phenomenon [3,4,38,105]. CAFs have been reported to secrete vesicles, which created hypoxia mimicking conditions in the cancer cells, causing reductive carboxylation of glutamine in them, and decreased oxidative phosphorylation [106]. The CAF derived vesicles are also carriers of metabolites feeding into the tricarboxylic acid cycle in the cancer cells. This brings forth a novel mechanism by which CAFs can influence the cancer cells through the transfer of metabolites and pushing away from an oxygen based energy metabolism. Using stable isotope labeling of amino acids in cell culture (SILAC) in cocultures of CAFs with ovarian cancer cells, a recent study demonstrated how the CAFs can help ovarian cancer cells switch from utilizing lipids to using glycogen reserves for energy [38]. As the metastatic tumor grows and depletes the adipocytes in the omentum, the IL-6, CXCL10, and CCL5 secreted by the CAFs induce the ovarian cancer cells to start utilizing glycogen. The activation of p38 MAP kinase in the CAFs drives the cytokine secretion, which in turn activates glycogen phosphorylase in the ovarian cancer cells [38]. This demonstrates that the dynamic changes happening in the tumor microenvironment as the tumor progresses, forces the cancer cells to reset their energy sources. CAFs can orchestrate this switch by turning off glycogen synthesis and activating glycogen utilization for glycolysis. Therefore, targeting the key enzyme in this process, glycogen phosphorylase, would be a potential therapeutic option to treat ovarian cancer metastasis.

5. Targeting CAFs Clinically

Since CAFs contribute towards so many critical aspects essential for tumor progression, strategies targeting CAFs to treat ovarian cancer can be potentially effective. Moreover, since CAFs themselves are genetically stable and do not have the propensity to mutate, acquiring resistance against these therapies would be less likely. Since CAFs overexpress FAP, a humanized antibody (sibrotuzumab) directed against human FAP has been tested in phase 1 clinical trials to demonstrate that it is safe to administer to patients with high levels of FAP expression in their tumors [107]. However, it did not have any beneficial effect in a phase II trial for metastatic colorectal cancer [108]. A fusion protein consisting of an anti-FAP antibody fused with IL-2 (RO6874281) is presently under clinical trials as a combination therapy with atezolizumab—an anti-PDL-1 antibody—for advanced or metastatic solid tumors (ClinicalTrials.gov: NCT03386721). In addition, a phase I clinical trial is ongoing to test RO6874281 as a single agent, or in combination with trastuzumab or cetuximab, for solid tumor, and breast, head, and neck tumors (ClinicalTrials.gov: NCT02627274). As TGF-β plays an essential role in stromal-epithelial interaction and CAF induction, targeting TGF-β is a potentially promising approach to target CAFs as well as cancer cells. Transgenic mice expressing a TGF-β antagonist were resistant to metastasis to multiple organs while not exhibiting the adverse pathological outcomes observed in TGF-β-null mice [109]. Transcription profiling of CAFs microdissected from ovarian cancer patient tumors identified a subpopulation that had activation of SMAD signaling [110]. These CAFs were markers of poor patient progression, and targeting SMAD signaling with calcitriol inhibited tumor progression in mice. At present there are as many as 60 active clinical trials on TGF-β in cancers (clinicaltrials.gov). However, it is very difficult to differentiate the role of CAF derived TGF-β from other stromal sources and cancer cell autocrine TGF-β signaling. The HGF-cMet pathway, involving the cross-talk between CAFs and cancer cells, plays a role in cancer metastasis, and is another potential target for blocking CAF–cancer cell interaction. Targeting c-Met or HGF has shown promising tumor growth inhibition and gemcitabine sensitization in vivo [111,112]. There are 69 active studies on cMet listed in clinicaltrials.gov. Targeting CAF can decrease the immunosuppressive microenvironment of the tumor, as well as lead to CD8+ T-cell activation, and enhance anti-tumor immunity [18,113].

While several strategies to target CAFs in tumors have been attempted, much remains to be studied before it can be effectively translated to the clinic. Strategies like targeting TGF-β may benefit from attacking both the cancer and stromal compartments. Importantly, the potential of combining such therapies with existing platinum and taxane based chemotherapies should be tested for ovarian cancer. However, previous experiences with targeting the tumor microenvironment have taught us that an approach towards normalization is preferable to an eradication of the tumor stroma. This is because the latter approach tends to give rise to more aggressive cancer cells. Therefore, targeting CAFs should aim for reverting them back to normal fibroblasts, rather than depleting them altogether.

6. Conclusions

CAFs are an important constituent of the ovarian cancer tumor microenvironment, and have been demonstrated to play an important role in tumor progression, metastasis, and chemoresistance. While a universal CAF marker has not been identified, several markers have been demonstrated in unique subpopulations, indicating that CAFs are heterogenous in this context, and this may also dictate their function. Continuous reciprocal interactions of CAFs with cancer cells and other components of the microenvironment shape their fate, marker expression, and function in the tumor. Continuing research towards a better understanding of their plasticity, regulation, function, and heterogeneity would greatly enhance the way we perceive tumors, and will determine how we treat them. Strategies to "normalize" CAFs and deprive the cancer cells of the gamut of factors provided by them may be an effective approach to complement existing therapies targeting the cancer cells.

Author Contributions: Conceptualization, manuscript preparation, figures, and funding acquisition, A.K.M.; Literature review and draft preparation, S.D., Y.F., and A.K.M.; Editing, S.D. and A.K.M.

References

1.   Torre, L.A.; Trabert, B.; DeSantis, C.E.; Miller, K.D.; Samimi, G.; Runowicz, C.D.; Gaudet, M.M.; Jemal, A.; Siegel, R.L. Ovarian cancer statistics. *CA Cancer J. Clin.* **2018**, *68*, 284–296. [CrossRef] [PubMed]
2.   Siegel, R.L.; Miller, K.D.; Jemal, A. Cancer statistics, 2016. *CA Cancer J. Clin.* **2016**, *66*, 7–30. [CrossRef] [PubMed]
3.   Hanahan, D.; Coussens, L.M. Accessories to the crime: Functions of cells recruited to the tumor microenvironment. *Cancer Cell* **2012**, *21*, 309–322. [CrossRef] [PubMed]
4.   Ladanyi, A.; Mukherjee, A.; Kenny, H.A.; Johnson, A.; Mitra, A.K.; Sundaresan, S.; Nieman, K.M.; Pascual, G.; Benitah, S.A.; Montag, A.; et al. Adipocyte-induced CD36 expression drives ovarian cancer progression and metastasis. *Oncogene* **2018**, *37*, 2285–2301. [CrossRef] [PubMed]

5.   Tomar, S.; Plotnik, J.P.; Haley, J.; Scantland, J.; Dasari, S.; Sheikh, Z.; Emerson, R.; Lenz, D.; Hollenhorst, P.C.; Mitra, A.K. ETS1 induction by the microenvironment promotes ovarian cancer metastasis through focal adhesion kinase. *Cancer Lett.* **2018**, *414*, 190–204. [CrossRef] [PubMed]

6.   Mitra, A.K.; Chiang, C.Y.; Tiwari, P.; Tomar, S.; Watters, K.M.; Peter, M.E.; Lengyel, E. Microenvironment-induced downregulation of miR-193b drives ovarian cancer metastasis. *Oncogene* **2015**, *34*, 5923–5932. [CrossRef] [PubMed]

7.   Mitra, A.K.; Zillhardt, M.; Hua, Y.; Tiwari, P.; Murmann, A.E.; Peter, M.E.; Lengyel, E. MicroRNAs reprogram normal fibroblasts into cancer-associated fibroblasts in ovarian cancer. *Cancer Discov.* **2012**, *2*, 1100–1108. [CrossRef] [PubMed]

8.   Goubran, H.A.; Kotb, R.R.; Stakiw, J.; Emara, M.E.; Burnouf, T. Regulation of Tumor Growth and Metastasis: The Role of Tumor Microenvironment. *Cancer Growth Metastasis* **2014**, *7*, 9–18. [CrossRef] [PubMed]

9.   Joyce, J.A.; Pollard, J.W. Microenvironmental regulation of metastasis. *Nat. Rev. Cancer* **2009**, *9*, 239–252. [CrossRef] [PubMed]

10. Orimo, A.; Weinberg, R.A. Stromal fibroblasts in cancer: A novel tumor-promoting cell type. *Cell Cycle* **2006**, *5*, 1597–1601. [CrossRef] [PubMed]

11. Legrand, A.J.; Poletto, M.; Pankova, D.; Clementi, E.; Moore, J.; Castro-Giner, F.; Ryan, A.J.; O'Neill, E.; Markkanen, E.; Dianov, G.L. Persistent DNA strand breaks induce a CAF-like phenotype in normal fibroblasts. *Oncotarget* **2018**, *9*, 13666–13681. [CrossRef] [PubMed]

12. Qiu, W.; Hu, M.; Sridhar, A.; Opeskin, K.; Fox, S.; Shipitsin, M.; Trivett, M.; Thompson, E.R.; Ramakrishna, M.; Gorringe, K.L.; et al. No evidence of clonal somatic genetic alterations in cancer-associated fibroblasts from human breast and ovarian carcinomas. *Nat. Genet.* **2008**, *40*, 650–655. [CrossRef] [PubMed]

13. Li, H.; Fan, X.; Houghton, J. Tumor microenvironment: The role of the tumor stroma in cancer. *J. Cell Biochem.* **2007**, *101*, 805–815. [CrossRef] [PubMed]

14. Kalluri, R.; Zeisberg, M. Fibroblasts in cancer. *Nat. Rev. Cancer* **2006**, *6*, 392–401. [CrossRef] [PubMed]

15. Thulabandu, V.; Chen, D.; Atit, R.P. Dermal fibroblast in cutaneous development and healing. *Wiley Interdiscip. Rev. Dev. Biol.* **2018**, *7*, e307. [CrossRef] [PubMed]

16. Tomasek, J.J.; Gabbiani, G.; Hinz, B.; Chaponnier, C.; Brown, R.A. Myofibroblasts and mechano-regulation of connective tissue remodelling. *Nat. Rev. Mol. Cell Biol.* **2002**, *3*, 349–363. [CrossRef] [PubMed]

17. Hu, M.; Yao, J.; Cai, L.; Bachman, K.E.; van den Brule, F.; Velculescu, V.; Polyak, K. Distinct epigenetic changes in the stromal cells of breast cancers. *Nat. Genet.* **2005**, *37*, 899–905. [CrossRef] [PubMed]

18. Ozdemir, B.C.; Pentcheva-Hoang, T.; Carstens, J.L.; Zheng, X.; Wu, C.C.; Simpson, T.R.; Laklai, H.; Sugimoto, H.; Kahlert, C.; Novitskiy, S.V.; et al. Depletion of carcinoma-associated fibroblasts and fibrosis induces immunosuppression and accelerates pancreas cancer with reduced survival. *Cancer Cell* **2014**, *25*, 719–734. [CrossRef] [PubMed]

19. Cooke, V.G.; LeBleu, V.S.; Keskin, D.; Khan, Z.; O'Connell, J.T.; Teng, Y.; Duncan, M.B.; Xie, L.; Maeda, G.; Vong, S.; et al. Pericyte depletion results in hypoxia-associated epithelial-to-mesenchymal transition and metastasis mediated by met signaling pathway. *Cancer Cell* **2012**, *21*, 66–81. [CrossRef] [PubMed]

20. Direkze, N.C.; Hodivala-Dilke, K.; Jeffery, R.; Hunt, T.; Poulsom, R.; Oukrif, D.; Alison, M.R.; Wright, N.A. Bone marrow contribution to tumor-associated myofibroblasts and fibroblasts. *Cancer Res.* **2004**, *64*, 8492–8495. [CrossRef] [PubMed]

21. Ishii, G.; Sangai, T.; Oda, T.; Aoyagi, Y.; Hasebe, T.; Kanomata, N.; Endoh, Y.; Okumura, C.; Okuhara, Y.; Magae, J.; et al. Bone-marrow-derived myofibroblasts contribute to the cancer-induced stromal reaction. *Biochem. Biophys. Res. Commun.* **2003**, *309*, 232–240. [CrossRef]

22. Spaeth, E.L.; Dembinski, J.L.; Sasser, A.K.; Watson, K.; Klopp, A.; Hall, B.; Andreeff, M.; Marini, F. Mesenchymal Stem Cell Transition to Tumor-Associated Fibroblasts Contributes to Fibrovascular Network Expansion and Tumor Progression. *PLoS ONE* **2009**, *4*, e4992. [CrossRef] [PubMed]

23. Schauer, I.G.; Zhang, J.; Xing, Z.; Guo, X.; Mercado-Uribe, I.; Sood, A.K.; Huang, P.; Liu, J. Interleukin-1β promotes ovarian tumorigenesis through a p53/NF-κB-mediated inflammatory response in stromal fibroblasts. *Neoplasia* **2013**, *15*, 409–420. [CrossRef] [PubMed]

24. McLean, K.; Gong, Y.; Choi, Y.; Deng, N.; Yang, K.; Bai, S.; Cabrera, L.; Keller, E.; McCauley, L.; Cho, K.R.; et al. Human ovarian carcinoma-associated mesenchymal stem cells regulate cancer stem cells and tumorigenesis via altered BMP production. *J. Clin. Investig.* **2011**, *121*, 3206–3219. [CrossRef] [PubMed]

25. Coffman, L.G.; Choi, Y.J.; McLean, K.; Allen, B.L.; di Magliano, M.P.; Buckanovich, R.J. Human carcinoma-associated mesenchymal stem cells promote ovarian cancer chemotherapy resistance via a BMP4/HH signaling loop. *Oncotarget* **2016**, *7*, 6916–6932. [CrossRef] [PubMed]
26. Rynne-Vidal, A.; Jimenez-Heffernan, J.A.; Fernandez-Chacon, C.; Lopez-Cabrera, M.; Sandoval, P. The Mesothelial Origin of Carcinoma Associated-Fibroblasts in Peritoneal Metastasis. *Cancers* **2015**, *7*, 1994–2011. [CrossRef] [PubMed]
27. Kenny, H.A.; Chiang, C.Y.; White, E.A.; Schryver, E.M.; Habis, M.; Romero, I.L.; Ladanyi, A.; Penicka, C.V.; George, J.; Matlin, K.; et al. Mesothelial cells promote early ovarian cancer metastasis through fibronectin secretion. *J. Clin. Investig.* **2014**, *124*, 4614–4628. [CrossRef] [PubMed]
28. Sandoval, P.; Jimenez-Heffernan, J.A.; Rynne-Vidal, A.; Perez-Lozano, M.L.; Gilsanz, A.; Ruiz-Carpio, V.; Reyes, R.; Garcia-Bordas, J.; Stamatakis, K.; Dotor, J.; et al. Carcinoma-associated fibroblasts derive from mesothelial cells via mesothelial-to-mesenchymal transition in peritoneal metastasis. *J. Pathol.* **2013**, *231*, 517–531. [CrossRef] [PubMed]
29. Mhawech-Fauceglia, P.; Wang, D.; Samrao, D.; Kim, G.; Lawrenson, K.; Meneses, T.; Liu, S.; Yessaian, A.; Pejovic, T. Clinical Implications of Marker Expression of Carcinoma-Associated Fibroblasts (CAFs) in Patients with Epithelial Ovarian Carcinoma After Treatment with Neoadjuvant Chemotherapy. *Cancer Microenviron.* **2014**, *7*, 33–39. [CrossRef] [PubMed]
30. Strutz, F.; Zeisberg, M. Renal fibroblasts and myofibroblasts in chronic kidney disease. *J. Am. Soc. Nephrol.* **2006**, *17*, 2992–2998. [CrossRef] [PubMed]
31. Fukagawa, D.; Sugai, T.; Osakabe, M.; Suga, Y.; Nagasawa, T.; Itamochi, H.; Sugiyama, T. Protein expression patterns in cancer-associated fibroblasts and cells undergoing the epithelial-mesenchymal transition in ovarian cancers. *Oncotarget* **2018**, *9*, 27514–27524. [CrossRef] [PubMed]
32. Lai, D.; Ma, L.; Wang, F. Fibroblast activation protein regulates tumor-associated fibroblasts and epithelial ovarian cancer cells. *Int. J. Oncol.* **2012**, *41*, 541–550. [CrossRef] [PubMed]
33. Sugimoto, H.; Mundel, T.M.; Kieran, M.W.; Kalluri, R. Identification of fibroblast heterogeneity in the tumor microenvironment. *Cancer Biol. Ther.* **2006**, *5*, 1640–1646. [CrossRef] [PubMed]
34. Cremasco, V.; Astarita, J.L.; Grauel, A.L.; Keerthivasan, S.; MacIsaac, K.D.; Woodruff, M.C.; Wu, M.; Spel, L.; Santoro, S.; Amoozgar, Z.; et al. FAP delineates heterogeneous and functionally divergent stromal cells in immune-excluded breast tumors. *Cancer Immunol. Res.* **2018**, *18*, e0098. [CrossRef] [PubMed]
35. Zhao, H.; Peehl, D.M. Tumor-promoting phenotype of CD90hi prostate cancer-associated fibroblasts. *Prostate* **2009**, *69*, 991–1000. [CrossRef] [PubMed]
36. Ohlund, D.; Handly-Santana, A.; Biffi, G.; Elyada, E.; Almeida, A.S. Distinct populations of inflammatory fibroblasts and myofibroblasts in pancreatic cancer. *J. Exp. Med.* **2017**, *214*, 579–596. [PubMed]
37. Su, S.; Chen, J.; Yao, H.; Liu, J.; Yu, S.; Lao, L.; Wang, M.; Luo, M.; Xing, Y.; Chen, F.; et al. CD10(+) GPR77(+) Cancer-Associated Fibroblasts Promote Cancer Formation and Chemoresistance by Sustaining Cancer Stemness. *Cell* **2018**, *172*, 841–856. [CrossRef] [PubMed]
38. Curtis, M.; Kenny, H.A.; Ashcroft, B.; Mukherjee, A.; Johnson, A.; Zhang, Y.; Helou, Y.; Batlle, R.; Liu, X.; Gutierrez, N.; et al. Fibroblasts Mobilize Tumor Cell Glycogen to Promote Proliferation and Metastasis. *Cell Metab.* **2018**, in press. [CrossRef] [PubMed]
39. Van Zijl, F.; Mair, M.; Csiszar, A.; Schneller, D.; Zulehner, G.; Huber, H.; Eferl, R.; Beug, H.; Dolznig, H.; Mikulits, W. Hepatic tumor–stroma crosstalk guides epithelial to mesenchymal transition at the tumor edge. *Oncogene* **2009**, *28*, 4022–4033. [CrossRef] [PubMed]
40. Zhu, X.; Wang, K.; Zhang, K.; Xu, F.; Yin, Y.; Zhu, L.; Zhou, F. Galectin-1 knockdown in carcinoma-associated fibroblasts inhibits migration and invasion of human MDA-MB-231 breast cancer cells by modulating MMP-9 expression. *Acta Biochim. Biophys. Sin. (Shanghai)* **2016**, *48*, 462–467. [CrossRef] [PubMed]
41. You, J.; Li, M.; Tan, Y.; Cao, L.; Gu, Q.; Yang, H.; Hu, C. Snail1-expressing cancer-associated fibroblasts induce lung cancer cell epithelial-mesenchymal transition through miR-33b. *Oncotarget* **2017**, *8*, 114769–114786. [CrossRef] [PubMed]
42. Wang, L.; Cao, L.; Wang, H.; Liu, B.; Zhang, Q.; Meng, Z.; Wu, X.; Zhou, Q.; Xu, K. Cancer-associated fibroblasts enhance metastatic potential of lung cancer cells through IL-6/STAT3 signaling pathway. *Oncotarget* **2017**, *8*, 76116–76128. [CrossRef] [PubMed]
43. Yuzhalin, A.E.; Urbonas, T.; Silva, M.A.; Muschel, R.J.; Gordon-Weeks, A.N. A core matrisome gene signature predicts cancer outcome. *Br. J. Cancer* **2018**, *118*, 435–440. [CrossRef] [PubMed]

44. Choe, C.; Shin, Y.S.; Kim, C.; Choi, S.J.; Lee, J.; Kim, S.Y.; Cho, Y.B.; Kim, J. Crosstalk with cancer-associated fibroblasts induces resistance of non-small cell lung cancer cells to epidermal growth factor receptor tyrosine kinase inhibition. *OncoTargets Ther.* **2015**, *8*, 3665–3678. [CrossRef] [PubMed]

45. Orimo, A.; Gupta, P.B.; Sgroi, D.C.; Arenzana-Seisdedos, F.; Delaunay, T.; Naeem, R.; Carey, V.J.; Richardson, A.L.; Weinberg, R.A. Stromal fibroblasts present in invasive human breast carcinomas promote tumor growth and angiogenesis through elevated SDF-1/CXCL12 secretion. *Cell* **2005**, *121*, 335–348. [CrossRef] [PubMed]

46. Matsuo, Y.; Ochi, N.; Sawai, H.; Yasuda, A.; Takahashi, H.; Funahashi, H.; Takeyama, H.; Tong, Z.; Guha, S. CXCL8/IL-8 and CXCL12/SDF-1alpha co-operatively promote invasiveness and angiogenesis in pancreatic cancer. *Int. J. Cancer* **2009**, *124*, 853–861. [CrossRef] [PubMed]

47. Kojima, Y.; Acar, A.; Eaton, E.N.; Mellody, K.T.; Scheel, C.; Ben-Porath, I.; Onder, T.T.; Wang, Z.C.; Richardson, A.L.; Weinberg, R.A.; et al. Autocrine TGF-β and stromal cell-derived factor-1 (SDF-1) signaling drives the evolution of tumor-promoting mammary stromal myofibroblasts. *Proc. Nat. Acad. Sci. USA* **2010**, *107*, 20009–20014. [CrossRef] [PubMed]

48. Leung, C.S.; Yeung, T.L.; Yip, K.P.; Wong, K.K.; Ho, S.Y.; Mangala, L.S.; Sood, A.K.; Lopez-Berestein, G.; Sheng, J.; Wong, S.T.; et al. Cancer-associated fibroblasts regulate endothelial adhesion protein LPP to promote ovarian cancer chemoresistance. *J. Clin. Investig.* **2018**, *128*, 589–606. [CrossRef] [PubMed]

49. Yan, H.; Guo, B.Y.; Zhang, S. Cancer-associated fibroblasts attenuate Cisplatin-induced apoptosis in ovarian cancer cells by promoting STAT3 signaling. *Biochem. Biophys. Res. Commun.* **2016**, *470*, 947–954. [CrossRef] [PubMed]

50. Schauer, I.G.; Sood, A.K.; Mok, S.; Liu, J. Cancer-Associated Fibroblasts and Their Putative Role in Potentiating the Initiation and Development of Epithelial Ovarian Cancer. *Neoplasia* **2011**, *13*, 393–405. [CrossRef] [PubMed]

51. Chen, J.S.; Liang, L.L.; Xu, H.X.; Chen, F.; Shen, S.L.; Chen, W.; Chen, L.Z.; Su, Q.; Zhang, L.J.; Bi, J.; et al. miR-338-3p inhibits epithelial-mesenchymal transition and metastasis in hepatocellular carcinoma cells. *Oncotarget* **2017**, *8*, 71418–71429. [CrossRef] [PubMed]

52. Xing, F.; Saidou, J.; Watabe, K. Cancer associated fibroblasts (CAFs) in tumor microenvironment. *Front. Biosci.* **2010**, *15*, 166–179. [CrossRef]

53. Luo, Q.; Wang, C.Q.; Yang, L.Y.; Gao, X.M.; Sun, H.T.; Zhang, Y.; Zhang, K.L.; Zhu, Y.; Zheng, Y.; Sheng, Y.Y.; et al. FOXQ1/NDRG1 axis exacerbates hepatocellular carcinoma initiation via enhancing crosstalk between fibroblasts and tumor cells. *Cancer Lett.* **2018**, *417*, 21–34. [CrossRef] [PubMed]

54. Olumi, A.F.; Grossfeld, G.D.; Hayward, S.W.; Carroll, P.R.; Tlsty, T.D.; Cunha, G.R. Carcinoma-associated fibroblasts direct tumor progression of initiated human prostatic epithelium. *Cancer Res.* **1999**, *59*, 5002–5011. [PubMed]

55. Bhowmick, N.A.; Chytil, A.; Plieth, D.; Gorska, A.E.; Dumont, N.; Shappell, S.; Washington, M.K.; Neilson, E.G.; Moses, H.L. TGF-β signaling in fibroblasts modulates the oncogenic potential of adjacent epithelia. *Science* **2004**, *303*, 848–851. [CrossRef] [PubMed]

56. Busch, S.; Acar, A.; Magnusson, Y.; Gregersson, P.; Ryden, L.; Landberg, G. TGF-β receptor type-2 expression in cancer-associated fibroblasts regulates breast cancer cell growth and survival and is a prognostic marker in pre-menopausal breast cancer. *Oncogene* **2015**, *34*, 27–38. [CrossRef] [PubMed]

57. Quante, M.; Tu, S.P.; Tomita, H.; Gonda, T.; Wang, S.S.; Takashi, S.; Baik, G.H.; Shibata, W.; Diprete, B.; Betz, K.S.; et al. Bone marrow-derived myofibroblasts contribute to the mesenchymal stem cell niche and promote tumor growth. *Cancer Cell* **2011**, *19*, 257–272. [CrossRef] [PubMed]

58. Li, X.; Xu, Q.; Wu, Y.; Li, J.; Tang, D.; Han, L.; Fan, Q. A CCL2/ROS autoregulation loop is critical for cancer-associated fibroblasts-enhanced tumor growth of oral squamous cell carcinoma. *Carcinogenesis* **2014**, *35*, 1362–1370. [CrossRef] [PubMed]

59. Liao, D.; Luo, Y.; Markowitz, D.; Xiang, R.; Reisfeld, R.A. Cancer associated fibroblasts promote tumor growth and metastasis by modulating the tumor immune microenvironment in a 4T1 murine breast cancer model. *PLoS ONE* **2009**, *4*, e7965. [CrossRef] [PubMed]

60. Fang, W.B.; Mafuvadze, B.; Yao, M.; Zou, A.; Portsche, M.; Cheng, N. TGF-β Negatively Regulates CXCL1 Chemokine Expression in Mammary Fibroblasts through Enhancement of Smad2/3 and Suppression of HGF/c-Met Signaling Mechanisms. *PLoS ONE* **2015**, *10*, e0135063. [CrossRef] [PubMed]

61. Ren, Y.; Jia, H.H.; Xu, Y.Q.; Zhou, X.; Zhao, X.H.; Wang, Y.F.; Song, X.; Zhu, Z.Y.; Sun, T.; Dou, Y.; et al. Paracrine and epigenetic control of CAF-induced metastasis: The role of HOTAIR stimulated by TGF-ss1 secretion. *Mol. Cancer* **2018**, *17*, 5. [CrossRef] [PubMed]

62. Labernadie, A.; Kato, T.; Brugués, A.; Serra-Picamal, X.; Derzsi, S.; Arwert, E.; Weston, A.; González-Tarragó, V.; Elosegui-Artola, A.; Albertazzi, L.; et al. A mechanically active heterotypic E-cadherin/N-cadherin adhesion enables fibroblasts to drive cancer cell invasion. *Nat. Cell Biol.* **2017**, *19*, 224. [CrossRef] [PubMed]

63. Richardson, A.M.; Havel, L.S.; Koyen, A.E.; Konen, J.M.; Shupe, J.; Wiles, W.G.T.; Martin, W.D.; Grossniklaus, H.E.; Sica, G.; Gilbert-Ross, M.; et al. Vimentin Is Required for Lung Adenocarcinoma Metastasis via Heterotypic Tumor Cell-Cancer-Associated Fibroblast Interactions during Collective Invasion. *Clin. Cancer Res.* **2018**, *24*, 420–432. [CrossRef] [PubMed]

64. Calvo, F.; Ranftl, R.; Hooper, S.; Farrugia, A.J.; Moeendarbary, E.; Bruckbauer, A.; Batista, F.; Charras, G.; Sahai, E. Cdc42EP3/BORG2 and Septin Network Enables Mechano-transduction and the Emergence of Cancer-Associated Fibroblasts. *Cell Rep.* **2015**, *13*, 2699–2714. [CrossRef] [PubMed]

65. Zhao, L.; Ji, G.; Le, X.; Luo, Z.; Wang, C.; Feng, M.; Xu, L.; Zhang, Y.; Lau, W.B.; Lau, B.; et al. An integrated analysis identifies STAT4 as a key regulator of ovarian cancer metastasis. *Oncogene* **2017**, *36*, 3384–3396. [CrossRef] [PubMed]

66. Sun, Y.; Fan, X.; Zhang, Q.; Shi, X.; Xu, G.; Zou, C. Cancer-associated fibroblasts secrete FGF-1 to promote ovarian proliferation, migration, and invasion through the activation of FGF-1/FGFR4 signaling. *Tumour Biol.* **2017**, *39*, e1010428317712592. [CrossRef] [PubMed]

67. Kalluri, R.; Weinberg, R.A. The basics of epithelial-mesenchymal transition. *J. Clin. Investig.* **2009**, *119*, 1420–1428. [CrossRef] [PubMed]

68. Lamouille, S.; Xu, J.; Derynck, R. Molecular mechanisms of epithelial–mesenchymal transition. *Nat. Rev. Mol. Cell Biol.* **2014**, *15*, 178–196. [CrossRef] [PubMed]

69. Zhuang, J.; Lu, Q.; Shen, B.; Huang, X.; Shen, L.; Zheng, X.; Huang, R.; Yan, J.; Guo, H. TGFβ1 secreted by cancer-associated fibroblasts induces epithelial-mesenchymal transition of bladder cancer cells through lncRNA-ZEB2NAT. *Sci. Rep.* **2015**, *5*, e11924. [CrossRef] [PubMed]

70. Yu, Y.; Xiao, C.H.; Tan, L.D.; Wang, Q.S.; Li, X.Q.; Feng, Y.M. Cancer-associated fibroblasts induce epithelial-mesenchymal transition of breast cancer cells through paracrine TGF-β signalling. *Br. J. Cancer* **2014**, *110*, 724–732. [CrossRef] [PubMed]

71. Li, W.; Zhang, X.; Wang, J.; Li, M.; Cao, C.; Tan, J.; Ma, D.; Gao, Q. TGFβ1 in fibroblasts-derived exosomes promotes epithelial-mesenchymal transition of ovarian cancer cells. *Oncotarget* **2017**, *8*, 96035–96047. [PubMed]

72. Wang, L.; Zhang, F.; Cui, J.Y.; Chen, L.; Chen, Y.T.; Liu, B.W. CAFs enhance paclitaxel resistance by inducing EMT through the IL6/JAK2/STAT3 pathway. *Oncol. Rep.* **2018**, *39*, 2081–2090. [PubMed]

73. Bonnans, C.; Chou, J.; Werb, Z. Remodelling the extracellular matrix in development and disease. *Nat. Rev. Mol. Cell Biol.* **2014**, *15*, 786–801. [CrossRef] [PubMed]

74. DuFort, C.C.; Paszek, M.J.; Weaver, V.M. Balancing forces: Architectural control of mechanotransduction. *Nat. Rev. Mol. Cell Biol.* **2011**, *12*, 308–319. [CrossRef] [PubMed]

75. Kai, F.; Laklai, H.; Weaver, V.M. Force Matters: Biomechanical Regulation of Cell Invasion and Migration in Disease. *Trends Cell Biol.* **2016**, *26*, 486–497. [CrossRef] [PubMed]

76. Wei, S.C.; Fattet, L.; Tsai, J.H.; Guo, Y.; Pai, V.H.; Majeski, H.E.; Chen, A.C.; Sah, R.L.; Taylor, S.S.; Engler, A.J.; et al. Matrix stiffness drives epithelial-mesenchymal transition and tumour metastasis through a TWIST1-G3BP2 mechanotransduction pathway. *Nat. Cell Biol.* **2015**, *17*, 678–688. [CrossRef] [PubMed]

77. Tang, X.; Hou, Y.; Yang, G.; Wang, X.; Tang, S.; Du, Y.E.; Yang, L.; Yu, T.; Zhang, H.; Zhou, M.; et al. Stromal miR-200s contribute to breast cancer cell invasion through CAF activation and ECM remodeling. *Cell Death Differ.* **2016**, *23*, 132–145. [CrossRef] [PubMed]

78. Yeung, T.L.; Leung, C.S.; Wong, K.K.; Samimi, G.; Thompson, M.S.; Liu, J.; Zaid, T.M.; Ghosh, S.; Birrer, M.J.; Mok, S.C. TGF-β modulates ovarian cancer invasion by upregulating CAF-derived versican in the tumor microenvironment. *Cancer Res.* **2013**, *73*, 5016–5028. [CrossRef] [PubMed]

79. Nagaraja, A.S.; Dood, R.L.; Armaiz-Pena, G.; Kang, Y.; Wu, S.Y.; Allen, J.K.; Jennings, N.B.; Mangala, L.S.; Pradeep, S.; Lyons, Y.; et al. Adrenergic-mediated increases in INHBA drive CAF phenotype and collagens. *JCI Insight* **2017**, *2*, e93076. [CrossRef] [PubMed]

80. Kerbel, R.; Folkman, J. Clinical translation of angiogenesis inhibitors. *Nat. Rev. Cancer* **2002**, *2*, 727–739. [CrossRef] [PubMed]

81. Nishida, N.; Yano, H.; Nishida, T.; Kamura, T.; Kojiro, M. Angiogenesis in Cancer. *Vasc. Health Risk Manag.* **2006**, *2*, 213–219. [CrossRef] [PubMed]

82. De Palma, M.; Biziato, D.; Petrova, T.V. Microenvironmental regulation of tumour angiogenesis. *Nat. Rev. Cancer* **2017**, *17*, 457–474. [CrossRef] [PubMed]

83. Toullec, A.; Gerald, D.; Despouy, G.; Bourachot, B.; Cardon, M.; Lefort, S.; Richardson, M.; Rigaill, G.; Parrini, M.C.; Lucchesi, C.; et al. Oxidative stress promotes myofibroblast differentiation and tumour spreading. *EMBO Mol. Med.* **2010**, *2*, 211–230. [CrossRef] [PubMed]

84. Hernandez-Fernaud, J.R.; Ruengeler, E.; Casazza, A.; Neilson, L.J.; Pulleine, E.; Santi, A.; Ismail, S.; Lilla, S.; Dhayade, S.; MacPherson, I.R.; et al. Secreted CLIC3 drives cancer progression through its glutathione-dependent oxidoreductase activity. *Nat. Commun.* **2017**, *8*, e14206.

85. Lederle, W.; Hartenstein, B.; Meides, A.; Kunzelmann, H.; Werb, Z.; Angel, P.; Mueller, M.M. MMP13 as a stromal mediator in controlling persistent angiogenesis in skin carcinoma. *Carcinogenesis* **2010**, *31*, 1175–1184. [CrossRef] [PubMed]

86. Erez, N.; Glanz, S.; Raz, Y.; Avivi, C.; Barshack, I. Cancer associated fibroblasts express pro-inflammatory factors in human breast and ovarian tumors. *Biochem. Biophys. Res. Commun.* **2013**, *437*, 397–402. [CrossRef] [PubMed]

87. Ko, S.Y.; Barengo, N.; Ladanyi, A.; Lee, J.S.; Marini, F.; Lengyel, E.; Naora, H. HOXA9 promotes ovarian cancer growth by stimulating cancer-associated fibroblasts. *J. Clin. Investig.* **2012**, *122*, 3603–3617. [CrossRef] [PubMed]

88. Wei, R.; Lv, M.; Li, F.; Cheng, T.; Zhang, Z.; Jiang, G.; Zhou, Y.; Gao, R.; Wei, X.; Lou, J.; et al. Human CAFs promote lymphangiogenesis in ovarian cancer via the Hh-VEGF-C signaling axis. *Oncotarget* **2017**, *8*, 67315–67328. [CrossRef] [PubMed]

89. Arnold, K.M.; Opdenaker, L.M.; Flynn, D.; Sims-Mourtada, J. Wound Healing and Cancer Stem Cells: Inflammation as a Driver of Treatment Resistance in Breast Cancer. *Cancer Growth Metastasis* **2015**, *8*, 1–13. [CrossRef] [PubMed]

90. Erez, N.; Truitt, M.; Olson, P.; Arron, S.T.; Hanahan, D. Cancer-Associated Fibroblasts Are Activated in Incipient Neoplasia to Orchestrate Tumor-Promoting Inflammation in an NF-κB-Dependent Manner. *Cancer Cell* **2010**, *17*, 135–147. [CrossRef] [PubMed]

91. Yang, G.; Rosen, D.G.; Liu, G.; Yang, F.; Guo, X.; Xiao, X.; Xue, F.; Mercado-Uribe, I.; Huang, J.; Lin, S.H.; et al. CXCR2 promotes ovarian cancer growth through dysregulated cell cycle, diminished apoptosis, and enhanced angiogenesis. *Clin. Cancer Res.* **2010**, *16*, 3875–3886. [CrossRef] [PubMed]

92. Lakins, M.A.; Ghorani, E.; Munir, H.; Martins, C.P.; Shields, J.D. Cancer-associated fibroblasts induce antigen-specific deletion of CD8 + T Cells to protect tumour cells. *Nat. Commun.* **2018**, *9*, e948. [CrossRef] [PubMed]

93. Takahashi, H.; Sakakura, K.; Kudo, T.; Toyoda, M.; Kaira, K.; Oyama, T.; Chikamatsu, K. Cancer-associated fibroblasts promote an immunosuppressive microenvironment through the induction and accumulation of protumoral macrophages. *Oncotarget* **2017**, *8*, 8633–8647. [CrossRef] [PubMed]

94. Takahashi, H.; Sakakura, K.; Kawabata-Iwakawa, R.; Rokudai, S.; Toyoda, M.; Nishiyama, M.; Chikamatsu, K. Immunosuppressive activity of cancer-associated fibroblasts in head and neck squamous cell carcinoma. *Cancer Immunol. Immunother.* **2015**, *64*, 1407–1417. [CrossRef] [PubMed]

95. Cohen, N.; Shani, O.; Raz, Y.; Sharon, Y.; Hoffman, D.; Abramovitz, L.; Erez, N. Fibroblasts drive an immunosuppressive and growth-promoting microenvironment in breast cancer via secretion of Chitinase 3-like 1. *Oncogene* **2017**, *36*, 4457–4468. [CrossRef] [PubMed]

96. Cheng, Y.; Li, H.; Deng, Y.; Tai, Y.; Zeng, K.; Zhang, Y.; Liu, W.; Zhang, Q.; Yang, Y. Cancer-associated fibroblasts induce PDL1+ neutrophils through the IL6-STAT3 pathway that foster immune suppression in hepatocellular carcinoma. *Cell Death Dis.* **2018**, *9*, e422. [CrossRef] [PubMed]

97. Wang, W.; Kryczek, I.; Dostal, L.; Lin, H.; Tan, L.; Zhao, L.; Lu, F.; Wei, S.; Maj, T.; Peng, D.; et al. Effector T Cells Abrogate Stroma-Mediated Chemoresistance in Ovarian Cancer. *Cell* **2016**, *165*, 1092–1105. [CrossRef] [PubMed]

98. Muerkoster, S.S.; Werbing, V.; Koch, D.; Sipos, B.; Ammerpohl, O.; Kalthoff, H.; Tsao, M.S.; Folsch, U.R.; Schafer, H. Role of myofibroblasts in innate chemoresistance of pancreatic carcinoma—Epigenetic downregulation of caspases. *Int. J. Cancer* **2008**, *123*, 1751–1760. [CrossRef] [PubMed]

99. Au Yeung, C.L.; Co, N.N.; Tsuruga, T.; Yeung, T.L.; Kwan, S.Y.; Leung, C.S.; Li, Y.; Lu, E.S.; Kwan, K.; Wong, K.K. Exosomal transfer of stroma-derived miR21 confers paclitaxel resistance in ovarian cancer cells through targeting. *APAF1* **2016**, *7*, e11150. [CrossRef] [PubMed]

100. Zhao, X.L.; Lin, Y.; Jiang, J.; Tang, Z.; Yang, S.; Lu, L.; Liang, Y.; Liu, X.; Tan, J.; Hu, X.G.; et al. High-mobility group box 1 released by autophagic cancer-associated fibroblasts maintains the stemness of luminal breast cancer cells. *J. Pathol.* **2017**, *243*, 376–389. [CrossRef] [PubMed]

101. Sansone, P.; Berishaj, M.; Rajasekhar, V.K.; Ceccarelli, C.; Chang, Q.; Strillacci, A.; Savini, C.; Shapiro, L.; Bowman, R.L.; Mastroleo, C.; et al. Evolution of Cancer Stem-like Cells in Endocrine-Resistant Metastatic Breast Cancers Is Mediated by Stromal Microvesicles. *Cancer Res.* **2017**, *77*, 1927–1941. [CrossRef] [PubMed]

102. Yasuda, K.; Torigoe, T.; Mariya, T.; Asano, T.; Kuroda, T.; Matsuzaki, J.; Ikeda, K.; Yamauchi, M.; Emori, M.; Asanuma, H.; et al. Fibroblasts induce expression of FGF4 in ovarian cancer stem-like cells/cancer-initiating cells and upregulate their tumor initiation capacity. *Lab Investig.* **2014**, *94*, 1355–1369. [CrossRef] [PubMed]

103. Pasquier, J.; Rafii, A. Role of the microenvironment in ovarian cancer stem cell maintenance. *Biomed. Res. Int.* **2013**, *2013*, e630782. [CrossRef] [PubMed]

104. Kalluri, R. The biology and function of fibroblasts in cancer. *Nat. Rev. Cancer* **2016**, *16*, 582–598. [CrossRef] [PubMed]

105. Nieman, K.M.; Kenny, H.A.; Penicka, C.V.; Ladanyi, A.; Buell-Gutbrod, R.; Zillhardt, M.R.; Romero, I.L.; Carey, M.S.; Mills, G.B.; Hotamisligil, G.S.; et al. Adipocytes promote ovarian cancer metastasis and provide energy for rapid tumor growth. *Nat. Med.* **2011**, *17*, 1498–1503. [CrossRef] [PubMed]

106. Zhao, H.; Yang, L.; Baddour, J.; Achreja, A.; Bernard, V.; Moss, T.; Marini, J.C.; Tudawe, T.; Seviour, E.G.; San Lucas, F.A.; et al. Tumor microenvironment derived exosomes pleiotropically modulate cancer cell metabolism. *Elife* **2016**, *5*, e10250. [CrossRef] [PubMed]

107. Scott, A.M.; Wiseman, G.; Welt, S.; Adjei, A.; Lee, F.T.; Hopkins, W.; Divgi, C.R.; Hanson, L.H.; Mitchell, P.; Gansen, D.N.; et al. A Phase I dose-escalation study of sibrotuzumab in patients with advanced or metastatic fibroblast activation protein-positive cancer. *Clin. Cancer Res.* **2003**, *9*, 1639–1647. [PubMed]

108. Hofheinz, R.D.; Al-Batran, S.E.; Hartmann, F.; Hartung, G.; Jager, D.; Renner, C.; Tanswell, P.; Kunz, U.; Amelsberg, A.; Kuthan, H.; et al. Stromal antigen targeting by a humanised monoclonal antibody: An early phase II trial of sibrotuzumab in patients with metastatic colorectal cancer. *Onkologie* **2003**, *26*, 44–48. [CrossRef] [PubMed]

109. Yang, Y.A.; Dukhanina, O.; Tang, B.; Mamura, M.; Letterio, J.J.; MacGregor, J.; Patel, S.C.; Khozin, S.; Liu, Z.Y.; Green, J.; et al. Lifetime exposure to a soluble TGF-β antagonist protects mice against metastasis without adverse side effects. *J. Clin. Investig.* **2002**, *109*, 1607–1615. [CrossRef] [PubMed]

110. Yeung, T.-L.; Sheng, J.; Leung, C.S.; Li, F.; Kim, J.; Ho, S.Y.; Matzuk, M.M.; Lu, K.H.; Wong, S.T.C.; Mok, S.C. Systematic Identification of Druggable Epithelial–Stromal Crosstalk Signaling Networks in Ovarian Cancer. *J. Natl. Cancer Inst.* **2018**, *10*, e097. [CrossRef] [PubMed]

111. Brandes, F.; Schmidt, K.; Wagner, C.; Redekopf, J.; Schlitt, H.J.; Geissler, E.K.; Lang, S.A. Targeting cMET with INC280 impairs tumour growth and improves efficacy of gemcitabine in a pancreatic cancer model. *BMC Cancer* **2015**, *15*, e71. [CrossRef] [PubMed]

112. Chen, L.; Li, C.; Zhu, Y. The HGF inhibitory peptide HGP-1 displays promising in vitro and in vivo efficacy for targeted cancer therapy. *Oncotarget* **2015**, *6*, 30088–30101. [CrossRef] [PubMed]

113. Ohshio, Y.; Teramoto, K.; Hanaoka, J.; Tezuka, N.; Itoh, Y.; Asai, T.; Daigo, Y.; Ogasawara, K. Cancer-associated fibroblast-targeted strategy enhances antitumor immune responses in dendritic cell-based vaccine. *Cancer Sci.* **2015**, *106*, 134–142. [CrossRef] [PubMed]

10

Targeting the Microenvironment in High Grade Serous Ovarian Cancer

Nkechiyere G. Nwani [1], Livia E. Sima [1], Wilberto Nieves-Neira [1,2] and Daniela Matei [1,2,*]

[1]   Department of Obstetrics and Gynecology, Northwestern University, Chicago, IL 60611, USA; Nnwani@northwestern.edu (N.G.N.); Livia.sima@northwestern.edu (L.E.S.); wilberto.nieves-neira@nm.org (W.N.-N.)

[2]   Robert H. Lurie Comprehensive Cancer Center, Chicago, IL 60611, USA

[*]   Correspondence: daniela.matei@northwestern.edu

Abstract: Cancer–stroma interactions play a key role in cancer progression and response to standard chemotherapy. Here, we provide a summary of the mechanisms by which the major cellular components of the ovarian cancer (OC) tumor microenvironment (TME) including cancer-associated fibroblasts (CAFs), myeloid, immune, endothelial, and mesothelial cells potentiate cancer progression. High-grade serous ovarian cancer (HGSOC) is characterized by a pro-inflammatory and angiogenic signature. This profile is correlated with clinical outcomes and can be a target for therapy. Accumulation of malignant ascites in the peritoneal cavity allows for secreted factors to fuel paracrine and autocrine circuits that augment cancer cell proliferation and invasiveness. Adhesion of cancer cells to the mesothelial matrix promotes peritoneal tumor dissemination and represents another attractive target to prevent metastasis. The immunosuppressed tumor milieu of HGSOC is permissive for tumor growth and can be modulated therapeutically. Results of emerging preclinical and clinical trials testing TME-modulating therapeutics for the treatment of OC are highlighted.

Keywords: high-grade serous ovarian cancer; tumor microenvironment; angiogenesis; immune response; metastasis; therapeutic targeting strategies

1. Introduction

High-grade serous ovarian cancer (HGSOC) comprises the majority of epithelial ovarian tumors, is associated with a p53-mutated signature and is characterized by initial sensitivity to platinum and a unique pattern of dissemination in the peritoneal space. The peritoneum consists of mesothelial cells that cover and protect the viscera. The sub-peritoneal stroma contains a collagen-based matrix, activated fibroblasts, blood vessels, and lymphatics. This unique milieu permits accumulation of factors secreted by both cancer and stromal cells and enables metastatic seeding and tumor proliferation. The immune component of the peritoneal milieu consists of monocytes/macrophages and cytotoxic T cells. Several studies have demonstrated an "activated" phenotype of the peritoneal environment associated with ovarian cancer (OC), as opposed to its quiescent state in benign conditions [1]. The pro-inflammatory signature associated with cancer favors angiogenesis and exerts chemotactic and protective effects on cancer cells. Chemokines, cytokines, and growth factors commonly secreted in the tumor microenvironment (TME) include the stromal cell-derived factor (SDF1), interleukin-6 (IL-6), interleukin (IL-8), monocyte chemoattractant protein 1 (MCP1), Chemokine (C-C motif) ligand 5 and 7 (CCL5 and CCL7), transforming growth factor-β1 TGF β1, tumor necrosis factor-α (TNFα), fibroblast growth factor (FGF), and others [1–4]. While tumor cells play a role in the secretion of factors that modulate angiogenesis, non-transformed tumor infiltrating cells such as fibroblasts, myeloid cells, immune cells, and endothelial precursors also play a crucial role modulating neo-vascularization [5]. OC metastasis commonly involves the omentum, an adipocyte-rich organ. Lipid transfer between adipocytes and cancer cells mediated by fatty acid binding protein 4 (FABP4), through a "symbiotic" process between cancer cells and the fatty microenvironment was described as a key regulator of peritoneal metastasis [6]. As the rich TME protects cancer cells from noxious stimuli promoting tumor growth (Figure 1), its disruption through targeted therapy could arrest cancer progression. Indeed, over the past decade, several classes of novel agents targeting the ovarian TME have been developed and tested clinically. The most active agents are antiangiogenic therapies, which have been recently approved by the Food and Drug Administraton FDA for OC. Other emerging strategies, particularly immunotherapy, are in various stages of development. Here, several targeted therapies directed against the main components of the TME will be reviewed.

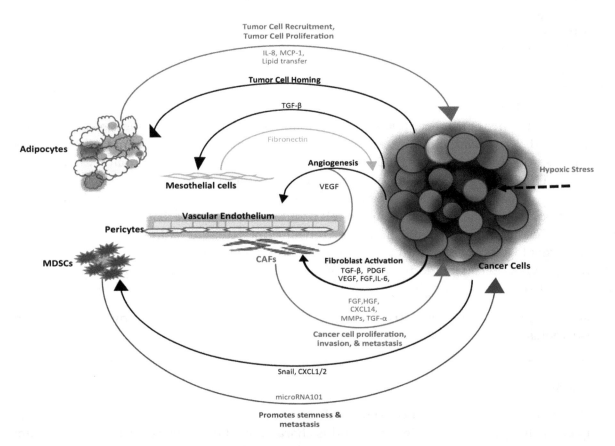

Figure 1. The interplay between cancer and stromal cells in the tumor microenvironent TME regulates tumor growth and metastasis: as tumors grow, hypoxic stress and low nutrient availability drives the release of tumor-secreted growth factors and cytokines that exert paracrine effects on the surrounding stroma. Sustained exposure to tumor-derived transforming growth factor-β (TGF-β), platelet-derived growth factor (PDGF), fibroblast growth factor (FGF) and vascular endothelial growth factor (VEGF) drives fibroblasts trans-differentiation into (cancer associated fibroblasts) CAFs. These factors also act upon endothelial cells, pericytes and immune cells to stimulate angiogenesis. CAF-derived FGF and hepatocyte growth factor (HGF) promote tumor cell proliferation, CAF-derived matrix metalloproteinases (MMPs) promote invasion while chemokine ligand 14 (CXCL14) and transforming growth factor-α (TGF-α) enhance metastasis. Ovarian cancer (OC) cell-derived TGF-β1 upregulates fibronectin secretion in mesothelial cells, which in turn enhances spheroid adhesion to the peritoneal wall. Adipocytes facilitate cells proliferation by providing energy dense lipids to the metastasized cancer cells. Cancer cells expressing Snail and chemokine (C-X-C motif) ligand 1/2 (CXCL1/2) recruit myeloid-derived suppressor cells (MDSCs) to the tumor site; conversely MDSC-secreted microRNA101 reprograms tumor cells to a stemness phenotype.

2. Fibroblasts

Fibroblasts represent the preeminent cellular component of connective tissues, the structural scaffold of many organs in the body. They are a heterogeneous population of mesenchymal-derived cells that maintain the composition of the extracellular matrix (ECM) [7,8]. As such, fibroblasts produce and deposit most of the proteins that comprise the ECM, including collagens, proteoglycans, tenascin, fibronectin, and laminin. Tissue homeostasis involves a tightly orchestrated balance of ECM synthesis and metabolism; in addition to ECM production, fibroblasts are also responsible for matrix metabolism. They produce several ECM-degrading matrix metalloproteinases (MMPs) and their inhibitors, tissue inhibitors of metalloproteinases (TIMPs) [9]. It has been observed that fibroblasts within the tumor milieu are phenotypically similar to activated fibroblasts associated with granulating tissue (wound healing) [10]. These cancer-associated fibroblasts (CAFs) function as tumor-promoting cells; playing important roles in tumor initiation and progression [11–13]. Although resident fibroblasts are a major source of CAFs, they can also arise from the trans-differentiation of other cell populations including epithelial cells, endothelial cells, pericytes, adipocytes and bone marrow-derived mesenchymal stem cells [14]. During tumorigenesis the trans-differentiation of the aforementioned cells into CAFs is driven by sustained exposure to tumor-derived factors including TGF-β, PDGF-BB, basic fibroblast growth factor (bFGF), vascular endothelial growth factor (VEGF), as well as microRNAs, reactive oxygen species (ROS), matrix metalloproteases (MMPs) and extracellular vesicles [15–19].

Current evidence suggests the mechanisms/downstream effectors that coordinate CAF activation vary and are contingent on CAF origin. For example, it was shown that SKOV3 cells stimulate normal fibroblasts conversion through TGF-β mediated induction of ROS and CLIC4, which led to the subsequent increase in the expression CAF markers αSMA and FAP. On the other hand, Jeon et al., demonstrated that cancer cell-derived lysophosphatidic acid induced TGF-β in adipose tissue-derived mesenchymal stem cells which then promoted their trans-differentiation into CAFs [18,20]. Likewise, expression of HOXA9, a differentiation related gene, was linked to paracrine secretion of TGF-β2 by OC cells, inducing adipose and mesenchymal stem cells to become CAFs [21]. It is unknown whether other stromal cells such as pericytes and endothelial could also contribute to the reactive stroma associated with HGSOC.

The role of fibroblasts in cancer progression is complex. Early studies provided evidence that fibroblasts possess anti-tumorigenic function by forming a restrictive stroma. However, the atypical cancer-stroma interactions promote fibroblasts to develop tumor-permissive properties [22–24]. Recent reports illustrate how the reciprocal cancer cell–fibroblast communication potentiates tumor growth and progression in OC models. For example, CAFs have been shown to suppress the immune response through miR141/200a-mediated expression of CAF-derived CXCL12. This chemokine promotes infiltration of immunosuppressive CD25+ FOXP3+ T lymphocytes in the HGSOC milieu, which in turn allows tumor growth [25]. CAFs have also been shown to drive tumor cell proliferation, migration and invasion by producing high amounts of mitogenic factors, hepatocyte growth factor (HGF) and FGF [26–28]. Additionally, CAF-secreted IL-8 and SDF-1 drive angiogenesis to facilitate oxygen and nutrients delivery to the tumor tissue [29,30]. Fibroblasts treated with SKOV3-derived extracellular vesicles acquired an activated phenotype; in turn these fibroblast enhanced tumor and endothelial cells proliferation [17]. In another study, OC cell-derived TNF-α induced TGF-α transcription in stromal fibroblasts. In turn, TGF-α secreted by these fibroblasts promoted metastasis via induction of EGFR signaling in cancer cells [31]. CAFs also produce metabolites that are essential to cancer cells' survival, such as lactate that is absorbed and utilized by oxidative phosphorylation in adjacent cancer cells [32]. The chemokine ligand 14 (CXCL14) is a CAFs secreted protein that is associated with a poor prognosis in OC. It was discovered that CXCL14 induced LINC00092 expression in OC cells, which resulted enhanced metastasis. LINC0009 interacted with 6-phosphofructo-2-kinase/fructose-2,6-biphosphatase 2 (PFKFB2) to induce a glycolytic phenotype in ovarian cancer cells. These interactions are necessary for maintaining the CAF-phenotype, thereby unearthing a positive feedback loop between CAF-cancer cells interactions that sustain a tumor-permissive microenvironment [33].

Cancer invasion and metastasis is also closely associated with MMPs secreted by CAFs and tumor cells and increased MMP expression has been associated with poor prognosis for various cancers [34]. In addition to modifying the ECM, MMPs can facilitate tumor growth and invasion by increasing the bioavailability of ECM tethered growth factors. For instance, CAF-secreted matrix metalloproteinase-13 (MMP-13) enhanced tumor cells invasion through proteolytic cleavage of matrix-bound VEGF and angiogenesis [35].

An additional factor involved in CAF-tumor cell cross-talk is the fibroblast activation protein (FAP). FAP is exclusively expressed on activated fibroblasts, and increased expression is associated with poor prognosis in many tumors [36]. In OC, FAP promoted HO-8910PM tumor cell proliferation, invasion and migration via interactions with integrin $\alpha3\beta1$ and urokinase-type plasminogen activator receptor (uPAR) signaling complex [37]. Moreover, elevated stromal FAP expression was a strong predictive marker of platinum resistance and relapse [38]. Due to the adverse effects of CAFs on cancer recurrence and patient survival, there has been extensive investment in developing strategies to effectively target CAFs.

3. Therapies Targeting Fibroblasts

FAP is overexpressed in many epithelial cancers including OC, and its expression is often associated with poor prognosis [36,38], cancer cell migration, invasion and immunosuppression [39–41]. As such, FAP has emerged as a potential therapeutic target to abate the tumor promoting effects of CAFs. The catalytic activity of FAP was shown to be necessary for tumor proliferation. However, inhibition of FAP enzymatic activity by small molecules has had little success in clinical trials [42,43]. In a transgenic mouse model, targeted depletion of FAP-expressing CAFs resulted in increased cancer cell death. Mechanistically, this effect was dependent on TNF-α and IFN-γ, which are known to be involved in CD8$^+$ T cell mediated cancer cell death [41]. Furthermore, pre-clinical studies using vaccines against FAP showed promising results for colon and lung cancer. Vaccines targeting FAP-expressing cells significantly suppressed tumor growth by eliciting CD8$^+$ or a combined CD8$^+$ and CD4$^+$-T cell response respectively [40,44].

TGF-β, a cytokine abundantly secreted by fibroblasts and detectable in ascites fluid, contributes to the development of a tumor-promoting microenvironment. Several TGF-β targeting agents have been evaluated in clinical trials. These include small molecule kinase, antisense oligonucleotides, and TGF-β-ligand traps [45,46]. In a mouse model of peritoneal metastasis, the TGF-β inhibitor A-83-01 improved overall survival [47,48]. Likewise, the transforming growth factor-β receptor 1 (TβRI) kinase inhibitor galunisertib inhibited tumor growth in a partly TME-dependent manner in various PDX tumors [49]. TGF-β inhibitors have also been shown to enhance the efficacy of conventional therapeutics. For example, combination treatment with TGF-β receptor inhibitor LY2109761 and cisplatin significantly blocked the growth of cisplatin-resistant ovarian xenografts [50]. Despite promising initial preclinical results, advancement of TGF-β signaling inhibitors to the clinical arena has been slow, marred by initial concerns over systemic (cardiac) toxicity, which fortunately appears to be limited in humans [51].

Several other tyrosine kinase inhibitors (TKI) have been employed to mitigate the pro-tumorigenic effects of growth factors secreted by fibroblasts in the tumor milieu, such as the platelet derived growth factor (PDGF) and fibroblast growth factor (FGF). PDGF-D over-expression was associated with lymph node metastasis and platinum resistance in ovarian cancer [52] and imatinib, a PDGFR inhibitor, was shown to inhibit OC cell growth [53]. While the precise effects of imatinib on ovarian stroma are not well defined, previous research demonstrated that this TKI suppressed angiogenesis in cervical tumors [54]. Dasatinib, another FDA approved TKI, which also targets the PDGF receptor has been shown to partially revert lung cancer-derived CAFs to a normal phenotype [55]. Clinical trials tested the PDGFR inhibitors imatinib and sorafenib in patients with recurrent platinum resistant OC and demonstrated modest clinical activity [56,57].

4. Angiogenesis

Angiogenesis is the process whereby new blood vessels sprout from the pre-existing vasculature. Angiogenesis is a tightly regulated and transient process observed in biological processes such as development, wound healing and reproduction [58]. However, pathological angiogenesis is a rate-limiting event in metastasis. As tumors increase in size (>1–2 mm^2), nutrient and oxygen availability are reduced and an angiogenic switch is activated; the newly formed blood vessels are able to deliver nutrients and oxygen necessary for cancer cell proliferation, facilitate waste expulsion, and also provide the primary route by which cancer cells migrate to secondary sites (metastasis) [59]. In fact, tumor vascularity serves as an indicator of metastatic potential for many cancers with highly vascularized tumors having greater incidence of metastasis and reduced survival [60,61]. In cancers, angiogenesis is driven by reduced levels of anti-angiogenic factors, and sustained overproduction of pro-angiogenic molecules by tumor and host cells [58]. Angiogenesis is triggered by growth factors such as VEGF, PDGF, (FGF), angiopoietin (Ang), as well as the chemokines IL-8 and interleukin-6 (IL-6) [59,62,63]. The association between HGSOC and an angiogenic signature was recognized more than two decades ago and has remained a staple in the study of this tumor's biology. VEGF is the most extensively studied angiogenic factor in pathological angiogenesis; it is overexpressed in HGSOC and secreted into malignant ascites [64–67]. Increased VEGF expression is associated with reduced survival rates in patients with OC [68–70]. In a cohort of 222 HGSOC specimens, high levels of VEGF-A were correlated with increased microvessel density and with infiltration by immune cells [71]. Interestingly, high levels of VEGF-A were associated with BRCA-mutated ovarian tumors [71]. Although cancer cells are a major source of angiogenic factors, non-neoplastic cells (immune cells, adipocytes, and CAFs) in the TME also produce the angiogenic factors required to sustain tumor growth and progression [72]. As such, there has been considerable focus on developing therapeutics to inhibit the angiogenic signaling as a means of mitigating cancer progression.

5. Anti-Angiogenic Therapy (AAT)

VEGF is the most extensively studied pro-angiogenic factor and therapies targeting this pathway use either inhibition of the ligand or of its receptor, vascular endothelial growth factor receptor (VEGFR). VEGF-A is a secreted glycoprotein that belongs a family of related growth factors that includes VEGF-B, VEGF-C, VEGF-D and VEGF-E and placental growth factor (PLGF), which have varying functions in angiogenesis [73]. The VEGF system functions as a mitogenic factor for endothelial cells, induces endothelial cell migration and differentiation, and protects immature endothelial cell against apoptosis [74,75]. VEGF exerts these functions by binding to the tyrosine kinase receptors VEGFR-1 (Flt-1) and VEGFR-2 (KDR/Flk-1) on the cell surface, causing them to dimerize and become activated [76]. Bevacizumab (Avastin, Roche, Basel, Switzerland), is a humanized monoclonal antibody against VEGF that binds and inactivates VEGF, thus inhibiting endothelial cell activation and proliferation. Bevacizumab was shown to reduce tumor growth and prolong survival in murine ovarian cancer models [77,78]. Clinical trials using bevacizumab as a single agent and in combination with other therapeutics have been successful and bevacizumab is currently FDA approved for use in the front-line setting, as well as in recurrent disease [79,80].

The first clinical trial to test the efficacy of bevacizumab in OC was performed by the Gynecologic Oncology Group (protocol GOG 170D) and tested the drug in 62 patients with recurrent, platinum-resistant disease. In this trial, 21% of patients exhibited objective clinical responses and 40.3% survived progression-free for at least 6 months. Median progression-free survival (PFS) and overall survival (OS) were 4.7 and 17 months respectively [81]. This initial success led to the development of combination therapies using bevacizumab with chemotherapy. In the ICON7 phase III trial, the efficacy of bevacizumab in combination with platinum and paclitaxel was tested in patients with advanced or metastatic epithelial ovarian cancer after cytoreductive surgery. Bevacizumab was continued for 12 additional cycles or until progression of disease. Progression-free survival at 42 months was increased from 22.4 months with chemotherapy alone to 24.1 months with combination treatment ($p = 0.04$). Interestingly, PFS and OS were most significantly increased in patients at high risk for progression. In this group, survival at 42 months was 28.8 months for patients receiving standard therapy vs. 36.6 months for patients receiving carboplatin/platinum and bevacizumab [82]. Similar results were observed in GOG protocol 218, where chemotherapy plus bevacizumab followed by bevacizumab maintenance improved PFS (but not OS) compared to platinum and paclitaxel alone after cytoreductive surgery [79]. In another randomized phase III clinical trial (AURELIA Trial), bevacizumab in combination with physician's choice chemotherapy was tested in women with recurrent platinum-resistant OC. The median PFS was 3.4 months for patients who received chemotherapy alone versus 6.7 months for patients treated with bevacizumab and chemotherapy [83]. These results summarized in Table 1 led to the approval and widespread clinical use of the first therapy targeting the ovarian cancer TME.

Table 1. Pivotal trials demonstrating Bevacizumab (Bev) clinical activity in OC.

Study	Course of Treatment	Target	TME Component	Patient Population	Phase Trial Size	Trial Endpoint	Clinical Outcome
ICON7	Chemo ± Bevac	VEGF-A	Endothelium	High risk ovarian cancer, stage IIIC or IV	Phase III N = 1528	PFS	At 42 months 22.4 vs. 24.1 months $p = 0.04$
GOG218	Chemo vs. Chemo + Bevac initiation vs. Chemo + Bevac Throughout	VEGF-A	Endothelium	New Diagnosed Stage III or IV OC	Phase III N = 1873	PFS, OS	Median PFS; 10.3 vs. 11.2 vs. 14.1 months; OS; *ns*
AURELIA	Chemo ± Bevac	VEGF-A	Endothelium	Recurrent OC PL-R	Phase III N = 361	PFS, OS	Median PFS; 3.4 vs. 6.7 months. OS; 13.3 vs. 16.6 months
OCEANS	Chemo ± Bevac	VEGF-A	Endothelium	Recurrent OC PL-S	Phase III N = 484	PFS	Median PFS 8.4 vs. 12.4 months
GOG213	Chemo ± Bevac	VEGF-A	Endothelium	Recurrent OC PL-S	Phase III N = 674	ORR	Median overall survival 37.3 vs. 42.2 months

Other modalities to block this pathway are in development. For example, aflibercept is a recombinant fusion protein of VEGFR1 and VEGFR 2 extracellular domain, which functions as a decoy receptor and inhibits VEGF-mediated signaling by trapping VEGF-A, VEGF-B, placental growth factor-1 (PlGF-1) and (PlGF-2). Aflibercept was shown to reduce ascites and decrease the peritoneal dissemination of OC xenograft models [53,84–86]. A phase II trial tested the efficacy of aflibercept in patients with advanced platinum-resistant OC and malignant ascites. Patients who required three or more previous paracenteses per month were given intravenous aflibercept 4 mg/kg every two weeks. The primary study endpoint was repeat paracentesis response rate (RPRR), and a response was defined as a minimum two-fold increase in time to repeat paracentesis compared with the baseline interval. Ten out of 16 patients treated achieved a response; RPRR was 62.5% (95% CI 35.4–84.8%). Median time to repeat paracentesis was 76.0 days (95% CI 64.0–178.0), 4.5 times longer than the baseline (16.8 days) and the median PFS was 59.5 days (95% CI 41.0–83.0) [87], demonstrating that targeting this growth factor in the TME leads to appreciable clinical benefits.

However, angiogenesis is a complex phenomenon tightly regulated by complementary and cross-talking pathways, which allows for the development of resistance [88]. Thus, inhibitors that concurrently block multiple receptors were tested in an effort to improve the efficacy of AAT. Cediranib (AZD2171, AstraZeneca) is a receptor tyrosine kinase inhibitor that inhibits vascular endothelial receptor 1–3 (VEGFR 1–3), platelet-derived growth factor-α and β (PDGFR-α and -β), and c-kit. A phase II clinical trial assessed the efficacy of cediranib in patients with recurrent gynecologic cancers who had received less than two lines of platinum-based chemotherapy. Of 46 patients treated, eight patients (17%) had partial responses (PR), six patients (13%) stable disease (SD), and there were no complete responses (CRs) [89]. In another phase II trial, the efficacy of single-agent cediranib was assessed in 74 patients with persistent/recurrent OC following one round of platinum-based chemotherapy. The patients were stratified into two groups; 39 platinum-sensitive (PL-S) and 35 platinum-resistant (PL-R), and the primary endpoint was objective response rate at 16 weeks. In the platinum sensitive (PL-S) group, 10 patients (26%) demonstrated partial responses (PR) and 20 (51%) had stable disease (SD). There were no confirmed PR in the platinum resistant (PL-R) group and 23 patients (66%) had SD. The median PFS was 7.2 months for PL-S and 3.7 months for PL-R groups, and the median OS was 27.7 and 11.9 months respectively [90]. Currently cediranib is being evaluated in combination with olaparib, a poly (ADP-ribose) polymerase PARP inhibitor in women with recurrent OC.

Nintedanib is another tyrosine kinase inhibitor for VEGFR-1-3, FGFR 1-3, PDGFR α and β. Nintedanib was tested as maintenance treatment after chemotherapy in a randomized trial. PFS at 36-weeks was 5.0% vs. 16.3% in placebo and nintedanib treated patients [91]. However, in a subsequent phase III trial (AGO-OVAR 12) nintedanib combined with platinum-based therapy did not induce a significant survival advantage after debulking surgery. The median PFS was 17.2 vs. 16.6 months for patients treated with nintedanib and placebo, respectively. A post-hoc analysis showed that nintedanib and platinum-based therapy combination improved PFS in non-high-risk patients [92]. Pazopanib (GW786034) is tyrosine kinase inhibitor for VEGFR-1, -2 and -3 PDGFR-α and -β and c-kit. An ongoing clinical phase II trial (MITO-11) is evaluating the safety and activity of pazopanib in combination with paclitaxel in patients with platinum-resistant or refractory OC. The median progression-free survival was 3.5 months in patients treated with weekly paclitaxel vs. 6.3 months in patients treated with weekly paclitaxel and pazopanib. The median overall survival was 14.8 months in paclitaxel treated vs. 18.7 months in patients treated with paclitaxel and pazopanib [93]. In all, these and other trials have convincingly demonstrated the activity of AAT in HGSOC, leading to the approval of bevacizumab for treatment in both the adjuvant and recurrent settings. New trials are evaluating the efficacy of anti-angiogenic drugs in combination with immune modulators or PARP inhibitors for treatment of gynecologic malignancies.

6. Interactions with the Mesothelial Matrix

In order to form secondary tumors, disseminated OC cell spheroids floating in the peritoneal cavity rely on their capacity to adhere to the mesothelial lining covering the peritoneal cavity and abdominal organs. During dissemination from the primary site, OC cells lose E-cadherin expression (Figure 2, upper left) and upregulate $\alpha 5$ integrin, which was proposed as a therapeutic target [94]. Secondary site invasion occurs upon displacement of the mesothelial monolayer cells (Figure 2, lower right), with cancer cells invading and submerging into the subjacent environment. The clearance of mesothelial cells is enabled by traction forces mediated by myosin and generated by the adhesion complex molecules, $\alpha 5$ integrin and talin-1, and is more efficiently accomplished by reprogrammed mesenchymal-like OC cells [95,96]. Other receptors that play a role in OC cell adhesion to mesothelium include CD44 and $\beta 1$ integrin (Iβ1) [97]. OC cell-derived TGF-β1 upregulates fibronectin (FN) expression in mesotheial cells [98]. The adhesion of OC cells to the FN matrix secreted by mesothelial cells [98] is dependent upon $\alpha 5 \beta 1$ integrin clustering and talin recruitment to stabilize the adhesions (Figure 2) [95]. Integrin clustering is induced by secreted tissue transglutaminase (TG2), which forms a bridge connecting Iβ1 and FN together at the cell surface [99]. This event induces downstream RhoA activation and suppression of Src–p190RhoGAP signaling. A focus of our laboratory's work was to understand the role played by the TG2-Iβ1-FN ternary complex in the process of OC metastasis and to test it as a new therapeutic target. By using OC orthotopic and ip xenografts, we showed that TG2 knock-down blocked peritoneal dissemination of ovarian tumors through a mechanism dependent on β1-integrin mediated cell adhesion and signaling [100,101]. Our recent results also demonstrate that engagement of integrin β1 facilitated by TG2 activates β-catenin signaling and stemness associated pathways in in vivo and organoid models of HGSOC [102,103].

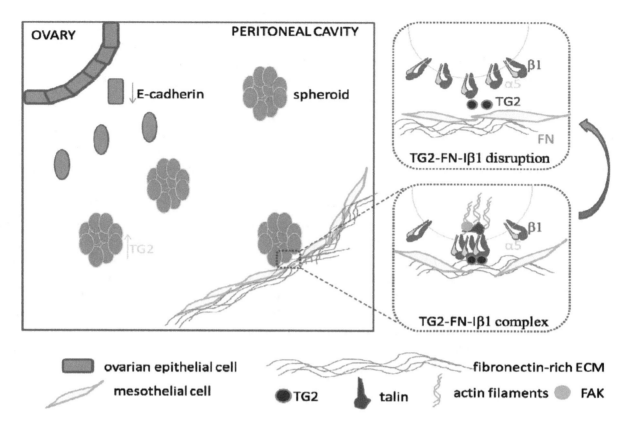

Figure 2. Ovarian cancer cells adhere to the mesothelial lining during tumor dissemination in the peritoneal cavity. Upon activation of EMT (epithelial-to-mesenchymal transition), cells progressively shed from the primary tumor into the peritoneal cavity (blue square). During the EMT process, there is a decrease in E-cadherin expression and increase in proteins associated to a mesenchymal phenotype, such as vimentin, tissue transglutaminase (TG2) and integrins. Cells that survive in the environment of the peritoneal cavity form spheroids. Spheroids attach to the fibronectin (FN) rich matrix secreted by the mesothelial cells, clear the subjacent monolayer and invade the underling tissue. These adhesion and invasion processes are mediated by interactions of integrin-β1 receptors with the FN fibrils in the ECM. Upon FN binding, α5β1 integrin receptors undergo clustering, which is enhanced by molecular bridges with TG2. Next, talin is recruited to the adhesion complex and provides the necessary traction force for the mesothelial monolayer displacement (red dotted bottom square). Also, "outside-in" signaling downstream of β1 integrin is activated, inducing focal adhesion kinase (FAK) phosphorylation. Therapeutic strategies targeting the TG2-FN-Iβ1 complex aim at interfering with the cell adhesion process and consequently preventing OC metastasis (red dotted top square).

7. Targeting Ovarian Cancer Cell Adhesion to the Peritoneal Matrix

Several strategies have been tested in an effort to block OC peritoneal dissemination. Treatment with blocking antibodies against integrins and the CD44 receptor were shown to inhibit OC cells adhesion to the mesothelial layer for short time intervals [104–106]. As α5β1 integrin is expressed on both OC cells as well as on the endothelial cells forming microvessels [107], it was expected that targeting this heterodimer (Figure 2, top square) will interfere with tumor growth and metastasis in many types of solid cancers, including OC [108]. Currently several drugs targeting integrins are under development (reviewed in [109]).

Volociximab, a chimeric antibody that binds α5β1 integrin with high affinity, was shown to block growth and dissemination of OC xenograft models [94]. However, the phase II clinical trial testing volociximab in patients with recurrent, platinum-resistant OC failed to demonstrate benefit although the drug was well tolerated [110]. Intetumumab (CNTO-95), a human αv-integrin specific monoclonal antibody that targets both αvβ3- and αvβ5-integrins showed anti-tumor and anti-angiogenic effects in xenografts models of breast cancer [111,112]. In a phase I clinical trial including patients with advanced solid tumors, one patient with ovarian carcinosarcoma had stable disease for six months [113]. Other integrin-blocking antibodies, such as etaracizumab, the humanized version of anti-αvβ3-integrin LM609 had minimal therapeutic benefit in other cancers [114]. Cilengitide is a stable cyclic pentapeptide containing an Arg-Gly-Asp (RGD) motif which allows selective binding to αvβ3 and αvβ5 integrins [115]. Cilengitide was tested in brain tumors and was found to not increase OS in glioblastoma patients during a phase III trial [116]. Given that αvβ3 integrin expression by tumor cells correlates with a favorable prognosis in OC patients [117], targeting this integrin might be a less appropriate strategy for OC. The initial disappointment with integrin targeting strategies may be related to their prior testing in the recurrent, advanced setting as single agents. Development of combination regimens and testing of these blocking antibodies in patients with low volume metastatic disease might overcome the lack of clinical success with this intervention.

FN is one of the most abundant ECM proteins in the omentum and peritoneum [118]. Adhesion of OC cells to FN via α5β1 integrin impacts "outside-in signaling" by inducing phosphorylation of focal adhesion kinase (FAK) either directly [119] or through c-Met [108]. This can further lead to activation of mitogenic pathways [120] which support tumor growth [121]. The β1 integrin–FN interaction is further enhanced by the bridging activity of TG2, a protein we discovered to be overexpressed in OC [122]. Previous work in our group has emphasized the importance of TG2 in the OC metastatic process, by providing evidence of its involvement in promoting OC cells' epithelial-to-mesenchymal transition through activation of non-canonical NF-κB [123], increasing cell proliferation by regulating β-catenin signaling [102], enhancing peritoneal dissemination [100], and increasing invasion by regulating MMP-2 [124]. As proof of principle that the TG2-FN-Iβ1 complex represents an interesting target in OC, we used a function-blocking antibody which targeted the FN binding domain of TG2, and showed that this antibody blocked OC spheroid proliferation and tumor initiating capacity by disrupting the interaction between OC stem cells and their niche [103].

To discover potent and selective TG2-FN inhibitors we used both virtual docking and high throughput screening strategies. Through an initial in silico docking approach, we identified a small molecule inhibitor capable of disrupting this complex and of blocking cancer cell adhesion to the FN matrix [125]. Subsequent efforts used an AlphaLISA-based assay adapted to high-throughput screening and applied to the ChemDiv library leading to the discovery and validation of several small molecules [126]. One hit selected from this screen (TG53) was validated in vitro to be an efficient inhibitor of OC cell adhesion to FN, migration and invasion. Future efforts focus on optimizing this compound through structure–activity relationship-based strategies to generate more selective, potent and drug-like compounds which block the TG2-FN protein–protein interaction and ultimately prevent OC metastasis.

8. Tumor Immune Response in Ovarian Cancer

Preclinical models and retrospective cohort analyses of human tumor specimens have demonstrated that the interaction between cancer cells and the host immune defense plays an important role harnessing tumor progression. There are several immune cell subsets relevant for tumor progression and response to immunotherapy [127]. These are classified in two categories: immune reactive and immune suppressive cells. The immune reactive cells include primarily cytotoxic T lymphocytes and activated CD4+ T cells. The immune suppressive cells are myeloid lineage subpopulations known as myeloid-derived suppressor cells (MDSCs), tumor-associated macrophages (TAMs, especially M2 subtype), dendritic cells (DCs) and the lymphocyte subsets of T helper cells (Th2 subtype) and T regulatory cells (Tregs). A seminal study showed that the presence of CD3+ tumor infiltrating lymphocytes (TILs) in OC is associated with increased survival [128]. The 5-year overall survival (OS) was 38% for patients whose tumors contained T cells compared to 4.5% for those whose tumors were devoid of T cells. Subsequently, a strong association between the presence of CD8+ TILs and favorable clinical outcomes of HGSOC was recognized [129–131]. The CD8+ to T regulatory (Tregs) cells ratio was also shown to correlate with increased survival of OC patients [130]. More recently, the presence of CD8[+] cells expressing the TNFR-family receptor CD137 (4-1BB) was reported as a prognostic marker associated with improved survival of OC patients [132]. A recent study evaluated the immune TME landscape in differentially growing metastases after several therapy cycles in an OC patient and reported heterogeneity in immune infiltrates that explained the evolution of tumor masses over nine years period [133]. This unique report revealed a correlation between the regressing or stable metastases and the presence of oligoclonal expanding T cells. Conversely, progressing tumors showed a lack of infiltration with anti-cancer lymphocytes. This study reinforces the importance of the tumor immune microenvironment to the outcome of OC disease. In all, these and other studies [134] strongly support the role of anti-tumor immunity as a key regulator in the evolution of the disease.

Enhancing the naturally occurring immune defense could therefore play an important role harnessing disease progression. Immunotherapy has demonstrated efficacy in various malignancies [135,136]. Several immune modulatory approaches (vaccines, IL2, CTLA-4 directed antibodies, adoptive transfer of activated T cells) have been tested in OC, with promising results in early interventions [137,138]. However, the impact of immunotherapy on the survival of OC patients remains unproven and predictive markers of positive outcomes remain undefined, highlighting the need to further optimize such strategies.

9. Immune Checkpoint Inhibitors

Recent advances have brought attention to the programmed cell death protein-1 (PD-1) mechanism used by cancer cells to evade immune surveillance, which can be effectively targeted by inhibitory antibodies [139]. This strategy demonstrated impressive clinical activity in several solid tumors (melanoma, lymphoma, renal, lung, and bladder cancer) leading to new FDA-approved interventions [140–142]. PD-1 signaling blocks T-cell activation keeping nascent T-cells in check and preventing immune responses against normal tissues. During cancer progression, this inhibitory pathway is activated by upregulating the expression of PD ligands (PD-L1 and PD-L2) on tumor and immune cells and permits evasion from immune surveillance [139]. The significance of the PD1 pathway to OC progression has been investigated; however, the emerging evidence is conflicting. On one hand, initial studies showed that the increased PD-L1 expression in ovarian tumors correlates with decreased intra-tumoral CD8[+] lymphocytes and worse patient survival [143]. Presence of dendritic cells expressing PD1 in the OC microenvironment was also found to be associated with decreased numbers of TILs and suppressed T cell activity [144], consistent with the concept that PD-L1 represents an escape mechanism. On the other hand, more recent studies using specific PD1 and PD-L1 detection antibodies provide evidence to the contrary. Two reports showed that expression of PD-L1 on immune cells in the tumor milieu, including on tumor associated macrophages (TAMs), is associated with increased total numbers of TILs and better survival in HGSOC [145,146]. It remains unresolved how expression of the PD1 pathway elements can be causally linked to a favorable prognosis in OC. It is possible that expression of PD-L1 reflects an active immune TME (defined by increased TILs density) able to attack and eliminate the tumor, or that PD-L1[+] TILs have a yet to be defined regulatory role in the immune response mechanism. Additional support for clinical interventions targeting this pathway includes that PD-1/PD-L1 blockade restored anti-tumor immunity in an OC xenograft model [147]. Two recent clinical trials tested PD-1 (pembrolizumab) and PD-L1 (avelumab) inhibitory antibodies in women with recurrent OC, reporting response rates of 11% (pembrolizumab) and 10% (avelumab), with 23% and 40% additional patients experiencing stable disease, respectively [148,149]. These early data suggest that immune checkpoint blockade in OC has defined, albeit modest activity.

Another emerging concept refers to the tumor neoantigen load as an important regulator of anti-tumor immune response and a marker for response to treatment [150,151]. Along these lines, a recent study showed that BRCA 1 and 2 mutated ovarian tumors are characterized by increased neoantigen load and that this correlates with increased number of TILs, increased expression of PD1 and PDL1, and is linked to improved clinical outcome [152]. These data support exploring

PD1 blockade in OC and continued investigation of the complex immune milieu associated with ovarian tumors. Therefore, identifying rational combinations to enhance the activity of PD1 blocking antibodies in OC and further analysis of the immune tumor milieu to identify predictive markers is necessary. Our group is exploring the combination of the PD1 inhibitor pembrolizumab and the DNA hypomethylating agent guadecitabine in women with recurrent platinum-resistant ovarian cancer (NCT02901899), testing the hypothesis that epigenomic priming will enhance the activity of immune checkpoint inhibitors.

10. Targeting Tumor Associated Macrophages (TAMs) and Myeloid-Derived Suppressor Cells (MDSCs)

Myeloid cells are frequently observed in the stroma of growing tumors [153]. The role of myeloid suppressor cells has been recognized first in late 1970s. In 2007, the term myeloid-derived suppressor cells (MDSCs) was coined for "bone marrow-derived cells of myeloid lineage comprising myeloid precursors and immature macrophages, granulocytes, and DCs, characterized by their high potential to suppress T cells" [154]. Immature myeloid suppressor cells were shown even earlier to accumulate in a variety of immune-related diseases, including cancer [155,156]. MDSC subsets were found to be responsible for immune suppression in 10 pre-clinical models of tumorigenesis [157]. In OC, macrophages are mainly found in ascites or infiltrate of the omentum. TAMs in the omentum were shown to harbor predominantly the M2 phenotype and to facilitate tumor progression [158,159]. Peritoneal TAMs support this process by secreting cytokines such as IL-6 and IL-8 [160]. In the ascites, M2 macrophage-like TAMs were found in the center of spheroids, where they participated in mechanisms supporting tumor cell proliferation and migration during OC metastasis [161]. The main signaling pathway involved in TAMs cross-talk to floating spheroid cancer cells was EGF–EGFR. TAMs promoted cancer cell invasiveness by activating the NF-κB and JNK signaling pathways [162]. Reversely, peritoneal macrophages were shown to adopt the M2 phenotype under the influence of OC cells expressing homeobox gene HOXA9 [163]. PD-L1 was primarily expressed by CD68+ TAMs rather than tumor cells in HGSOC, and often colocalized with both cytotoxic T cells as well as T regulatory cells and was a positive prognostic marker [146].

The contribution of MDSCs defined as harboring Lin−CD45+CD33+ markers combination was studied in a cohort of patients with HGSOC [164]. MDSCs comprised 37% of non-neoplastic cells in the TME and were responsible for inhibiting T-cell immunity, by blocking both T cell proliferation and effector function. Increased tumor MDSCs inversely correlated with CD8+ TILs and overall survival in advanced OC [165]. Interestingly, the corresponding Lin−CD45+CD33+ fraction in patients' blood did not have the same properties. MDSCs were shown to support metastasis and a cancer stem cell phenotype. Mechanistically, it was shown that tumor-resident MDSCs enhance stemness via microRNA101, which targets co-repressor gene C-terminal binding protein-2 (CtBP2) 3'-UTR region and interferes with its binding at NANOG, OCT4/3, and SOX2 promoters in primary OC cells [164]. Primary ovarian tumors expressing high levels of Snail were shown to recruit increased number of CD33+ MDSCs through secretion of the CXCR2 ligands CXCL1/2 [166,167]. Therefore, blocking CXCR2 would represent a therapeutic approach for Snail-high OC tumors.

Targeting immature myeloid cells and their cross-talk with other immune cells and cancer cells is a potential strategy of combating tumor progression. Several classes of therapeutics targeting MDSCs or TAMs have been described and were recently reviewed [167]. They include agents which promote MDSCs apoptosis, antibodies that induce MDSCs and/or TAMs depletion, compounds that induce immature myeloid cells differentiation (such as retinoic acid, vitamin D3 or HDACi), inhibitors of immune suppression function (sildenafil, triterpenoids, inhibitors of COX-2, inducible nitric oxide), compounds which block recruitment (by targeting chemokines and chemokine receptors) or MDSCs proliferation, and lastly TAM reprogramming factors. Given that TAMs and MDSCs mediate resistance to immunotherapy targeting, this immune suppressive cell population could increase the success rate of checkpoint blockade inhibitors [168].

Several strategies have been tested in preclinical models, but progress towards clinical is still ongoing. For example, almetuzumab, which targets CD52 expressed by vascular leukocytes and Tie2$^+$ monocytes, was shown to have anti-myeloid and anti-angiogenic properties in OC models [169]. Anti-CD52 therapy decreased tumor growth in an OC murine model. Additionally, ovarian TAMs express high levels of folate receptor-2, which can be targeted by using methotrexate loaded G5-dendrimers (G5-MTX) [170]. Noteworthy, these G5-MTX nanoparticles were shown to overcome resistance to anti-VEGF-A therapy in OC preclinical models. Epigenetic modulators have also been shown to alter the myeloid population, triggering anti-tumor immune responses. For example, the bromodomain inhibitor JQ1 significantly reduced PD-L1 expression on TAMs and dendritic cells, induced increased T cell cytotoxic activity and suppressed OC tumor growth in preclinical models [171]. A combination of histone deacetylase inhibitors (HDACi) and DNA methyltransferase inhibitor (DNMTi) was shown to reduce TAMs and increase T and NK cell activation, delaying tumor progression in preclinical models [172]. The combination of DNMTi/HDACi also synergized with the immune checkpoint inhibitors. Clinical trials testing HDACi and DNMTi with anti-PD1 therapy in patients with recurrent OC are ongoing. Lastly, catumaxomab is a humanized antibody that targets three different cell types: tumor cells (via epithelial cell adhesion molecule (EpCAM) binding); T-cells (via CD3 binding); and accessory cells (macrophages, dendritic cells, and natural killer cells) via type I, IIa, and III Fcγ receptors (FcγR). Subsequently, catumaxomab induces several effects, including T-cell-mediated tumor lysis, antibody-dependent cell-mediated cytotoxicity, and phagocytosis via activation of NK cells and TAMs. Catumaxomab is administered intra-peritoneally and was shown to be clinically active in patients with malignant ascites, leading to its approval in Europe for the treatment of EpCAM$^+$ tumors associated with ascites, including HGSOC [173].

11. Conclusions

New targets at the interface between HGSOC cells and the TME have been characterized. Targeted treatments, alone or in combination with chemotherapy, are emerging and, in some situations, are already impacting clinical outcomes in women with HGSOC. Anti-angiogenic therapy in combination with chemotherapy has significantly improved the survival of women with advanced OC and has become part of the standard approach. In contrast, CAFs-directed strategies or therapeutics targeting cell adhesion to the matrix remain less impressive. Future development of combination and sequencing strategies based on a refined understanding of tumor biology and cross-talking pathways is critically needed. While immune interventions are still being optimized, early results suggest that combination strategies are needed to overcome the immune tolerant milieu of HGSOC. This could be due to silencing of tumor antigen and low tumor mutational burden, which render the ovarian tumors to be "cold", or to an infiltration of immunosuppressive cells. Therefore, current approaches investigate dual immune targeting or combinations with interventions that de-repress tumor antigens through epigenetic reprogramming or which increase the tumor mutational burden by inducing DNA damage. It is clear that in order to improve clinical outcomes in this fatal malignancy, interventions affecting both cancer cells and the stroma need to be implemented. Thus, we anticipate that clinical trials will continue to explore rationally designed combinations and/or sequences of therapies targeting vulnerabilities of both tumor cells and the TME.

References

1.   Freedman, R.S.; Deavers, M.; Liu, J.; Wang, E. Peritoneal inflammation—A microenvironment for epithelial ovarian cancer (eoc). *J. Transl. Med.* **2004**, *2*, 23. [CrossRef] [PubMed]
2.   Said, N.; Socha, M.J.; Olearczyk, J.J.; Elmarakby, A.A.; Imig, J.D.; Motamed, K. Normalization of the ovarian cancer microenvironment by sparc. *Mol. Cancer Res.* **2007**, *5*, 1015–1030. [CrossRef] [PubMed]
3.   Hurteau, J.; Rodriguez, G.C.; Whitaker, R.S.; Shah, S.; Mills, G.; Bast, R.C.; Berchuck, A. Transforming growth factor-beta inhibits proliferation of human ovarian cancer cells obtained from ascites. *Cancer* **1994**, *74*, 93–99. [CrossRef]

4.   Gopinathan, G.; Milagre, C.; Pearce, O.M.; Reynolds, L.E.; Hodivala-Dilke, K.; Leinster, D.A.; Zhong, H.; Hollingsworth, R.E.; Thompson, R.; Whiteford, J.R.; et al. Interleukin-6 stimulates defective angiogenesis. *Cancer Res.* **2015**, *75*, 3098–3107. [CrossRef] [PubMed]

5.   Nozawa, H.; Chiu, C.; Hanahan, D. Infiltrating neutrophils mediate the initial angiogenic switch in a mouse model of multistage carcinogenesis. *Proc. Natl. Acad. Sci. USA* **2006**, *103*, 12493–12498. [CrossRef] [PubMed]

6.   Nieman, K.M.; Kenny, H.A.; Penicka, C.V.; Ladanyi, A.; Buell-Gutbrod, R.; Zillhardt, M.R.; Romero, I.L.; Carey, M.S.; Mills, G.B.; Hotamisligil, G.S.; et al. Adipocytes promote ovarian cancer metastasis and provide energy for rapid tumor growth. *Nat. Med.* **2011**, *17*, 1498–1503. [CrossRef] [PubMed]

7.   Tarin, D.; Croft, C.B. Ultrastructural features of wound healing in mouse skin. *J. Anat.* **1969**, *105*, 189–190. [PubMed]

8.   Chang, H.Y.; Chi, J.T.; Dudoit, S.; Bondre, C.; van de Rijn, M.; Botstein, D.; Brown, P.O. Diversity, topographic differentiation, and positional memory in human fibroblasts. *Proc. Natl. Acad. Sci. USA* **2002**, *99*, 12877–12882. [CrossRef] [PubMed]

9.   McAnulty, R.J. Fibroblasts and myofibroblasts: Their source, function and role in disease. *Int. J. Biochem. Cell Biol.* **2007**, *39*, 666–671. [CrossRef] [PubMed]

10.   Ryan, G.B.; Cliff, W.J.; Gabbiani, G.; Irle, C.; Montandon, D.; Statkov, P.R.; Majno, G. Myofibroblasts in human granulation tissue. *Hum. Pathol.* **1974**, *5*, 55–67. [CrossRef]

11.   Kalluri, R.; Zeisberg, M. Fibroblasts in cancer. *Nat. Rev. Cancer* **2006**, *6*, 392–401. [CrossRef] [PubMed]

12.   Bhowmick, N.A.; Chytil, A.; Plieth, D.; Gorska, A.E.; Dumont, N.; Shappell, S.; Washington, M.K.; Neilson, E.G.; Moses, H.L. Tgf-beta signaling in fibroblasts modulates the oncogenic potential of adjacent epithelia. *Science* **2004**, *303*, 848–851. [CrossRef] [PubMed]

13.   Liao, D.; Luo, Y.; Markowitz, D.; Xiang, R.; Reisfeld, R.A. Cancer associated fibroblasts promote tumor growth and metastasis by modulating the tumor immune microenvironment in a 4t1 murine breast cancer model. *PLoS ONE* **2009**, *4*, e7965. [CrossRef] [PubMed]

14.   Kendall, R.T.; Feghali-Bostwick, C.A. Fibroblasts in fibrosis: Novel roles and mediators. *Front. Pharmacol.* **2014**, *5*, 123. [CrossRef] [PubMed]

15.   Hanahan, D.; Coussens, L.M. Accessories to the crime: Functions of cells recruited to the tumor microenvironment. *Cancer Cell* **2012**, *21*, 309–322. [CrossRef] [PubMed]

16.   Madar, S.; Goldstein, I.; Rotter, V. 'Cancer associated fibroblasts'—More than meets the eye. *Trends Mol. Med.* **2013**, *19*, 447–453. [CrossRef] [PubMed]

17.   Giusti, I.; Francesco, M.D.; Ascenzo, S.; Palmerini, M.G.; Macchiarelli, G.; Carta, G.; Dolo, V. Ovarian cancer-derived extracellular vesicles affect normal human fibroblast behavior. *Cancer Biol. Ther.* **2018**, *19*, 722–734. [CrossRef] [PubMed]

18.   Yao, Q.; Qu, X.; Yang, Q.; Wei, M.; Kong, B. Clic4 mediates tgf-beta1-induced fibroblast-to-myofibroblast transdifferentiation in ovarian cancer. *Oncol. Rep.* **2009**, *22*, 541–548. [PubMed]

19.   Fang, T.; Lv, H.; Lv, G.; Li, T.; Wang, C.; Han, Q.; Yu, L.; Su, B.; Guo, L.; Huang, S.; et al. Tumor-derived exosomal mir-1247-3p induces cancer-associated fibroblast activation to foster lung metastasis of liver cancer. *Nat. Commun.* **2018**, *9*, 191. [CrossRef] [PubMed]

20.   Jeon, E.S.; Moon, H.J.; Lee, M.J.; Song, H.Y.; Kim, Y.M.; Cho, M.; Suh, D.S.; Yoon, M.S.; Chang, C.L.; Jung, J.S.; et al. Cancer-derived lysophosphatidic acid stimulates differentiation of human mesenchymal stem cells to myofibroblast-like cells. *Stem Cells* **2008**, *26*, 789–797. [CrossRef] [PubMed]

21.   Ko, S.Y.; Barengo, N.; Ladanyi, A.; Lee, J.S.; Marini, F.; Lengyel, E.; Naora, H. Hoxa9 promotes ovarian cancer growth by stimulating cancer-associated fibroblasts. *J. Clin. Investig.* **2012**, *122*, 3603–3617. [CrossRef] [PubMed]

22.   Dotto, G.P.; Weinberg, R.A.; Ariza, A. Malignant transformation of mouse primary keratinocytes by harvey sarcoma virus and its modulation by surrounding normal cells. *Proc. Natl. Acad. Sci. USA* **1988**, *85*, 6389–6393. [CrossRef] [PubMed]

23.   Ozdemir, B.C.; Pentcheva-Hoang, T.; Carstens, J.L.; Zheng, X.F.; Wu, C.C.; Simpson, T.R.; Laklai, H.; Sugimoto, H.; Kahlert, C.; Novitskiy, S.V.; et al. Depletion of carcinoma-associated fibroblasts and fibrosis induces immunosuppression and accelerates pancreas cancer with reduced survival. *Cancer Cell* **2014**, *25*, 719–734. [CrossRef] [PubMed]

24.   Cornil, I.; Theodorescu, D.; Man, S.; Herlyn, M.; Jambrosic, J.; Kerbel, R.S. Fibroblast cell-interactions with

human-melanoma cells affect tumor-cell growth as a function of tumor progression. *Proc. Natl. Acad. Sci. USA* **1991**, *88*, 6028–6032. [CrossRef] [PubMed]

25. Givel, A.M.; Kieffer, Y.; Scholer-Dahirel, A.; Sirven, P.; Cardon, M.; Pelon, F.; Magagna, I.; Gentric, G.; Costa, A.; Bonneau, C.; et al. Mir200-regulated cxcl12beta promotes fibroblast heterogeneity and immunosuppression in ovarian cancers. *Nat. Commun.* **2018**, *9*, 1056. [CrossRef] [PubMed]

26. Wei, D.; Geng, F.; Liang, S.; Zhao, H.; Liu, M.; Wang, H. Caf-derived hgf promotes cell proliferation and drug resistance by up-regulating the c-met/pi3k/akt and grp78 signalling in ovarian cancer cells. *Biosci. Rep.* **2017**, *37*, BSR20160470.

27. Cirri, P.; Chiarugi, P. Cancer associated fibroblasts: The dark side of the coin. *Am. J. Cancer Res.* **2011**, *1*, 482–497. [PubMed]

28. Henriksson, M.L.; Edin, S.; Dahlin, A.M.; Oldenborg, P.A.; Oberg, A.; Van Guelpen, B.; Rutegard, J.; Stenling, R.; Palmqvist, R. Colorectal cancer cells activate adjacent fibroblasts resulting in fgf1/fgfr3 signaling and increased invasion. *Am. J. Pathol.* **2011**, *178*, 1387–1394. [CrossRef] [PubMed]

29. Matsuo, Y.; Ochi, N.; Sawai, H.; Yasuda, A.; Takahashi, H.; Funahashi, H.; Takeyama, H.; Tong, Z.; Guha, S. Cxcl8/il-8 and cxcl12/sdf-1alpha co-operatively promote invasiveness and angiogenesis in pancreatic cancer. *Int. J. Cancer* **2009**, *124*, 853–861. [CrossRef] [PubMed]

30. Orimo, A.; Gupta, P.B.; Sgroi, D.C.; Arenzana-Seisdedos, F.; Delaunay, T.; Naeem, R.; Carey, V.J.; Richardson, A.L.; Weinberg, R.A. Stromal fibroblasts present in invasive human breast carcinomas promote tumor growth and angiogenesis through elevated sdf-1/cxcl12 secretion. *Cell* **2005**, *121*, 335–348. [CrossRef] [PubMed]

31. Lau, T.S.; Chan, L.K.; Wong, E.C.; Hui, C.W.; Sneddon, K.; Cheung, T.H.; Yim, S.F.; Lee, J.H.; Yeung, C.S.; Chung, T.K.; et al. A loop of cancer-stroma-cancer interaction promotes peritoneal metastasis of ovarian cancer via tnfalpha-tgfalpha-egfr. *Oncogene* **2017**, *36*, 3576–3587. [CrossRef] [PubMed]

32. Mitchell, M.I.; Engelbrecht, A.M. Metabolic hijacking: A survival strategy cancer cells exploit? *Crit. Rev. Oncol. Hematol.* **2017**, *109*, 1–8. [CrossRef] [PubMed]

33. Zhao, L.J.; Ji, G.L.; Le, X.B.; Wang, C.; Xu, L.; Feng, M.; Zhang, Y.G.; Yang, H.L.; Xuan, Y.; Yang, Y.F.; et al. Long noncoding rna linc00092 acts in cancer-associated fibroblasts to drive glycolysis and progression of ovarian cancer. *Cancer Res.* **2017**, *77*, 1369–1382. [CrossRef] [PubMed]

34. Hadler-Olsen, E.; Winberg, J.O.; Uhlin-Hansen, L. Matrix metalloproteinases in cancer: Their value as diagnostic and prognostic markers and therapeutic targets. *Tumor Biol.* **2013**, *34*, 2041–2051. [CrossRef] [PubMed]

35. Lederle, W.; Hartenstein, B.; Meides, A.; Kunzelmann, H.; Werb, Z.; Angel, P.; Mueller, M.M. Mmp13 as a stromal mediator in controlling persistent angiogenesis in skin carcinoma. *Carcinogenesis* **2010**, *31*, 1175–1184. [CrossRef] [PubMed]

36. Garinchesa, P.; Old, L.J.; Rettig, W.J. Cell-surface glycoprotein of reactive stromal fibroblasts as a potential antibody target in human epithelial cancers. *Proc. Natl. Acad. Sci. USA* **1990**, *87*, 7235–7239. [CrossRef]

37. Yang, W.; Han, W.; Ye, S.; Liu, D.; Wu, J.; Liu, H.; Li, C.; Chen, H. Fibroblast activation protein-alpha promotes ovarian cancer cell proliferation and invasion via extracellular and intracellular signaling mechanisms. *Exp. Mol. Pathol.* **2013**, *95*, 105–110. [CrossRef] [PubMed]

38. Mhawech-Fauceglia, P.; Yan, L.; Sharifian, M.; Ren, X.; Liu, S.; Kim, G.; Gayther, S.A.; Pejovic, T.; Lawrenson, K. Stromal expression of fibroblast activation protein alpha (fap) predicts platinum resistance and shorter recurrence in patients with epithelial ovarian cancer. *Cancer Microenviron.* **2015**, *8*, 23–31. [CrossRef] [PubMed]

39. Cai, J.; Tang, H.; Xu, L.; Wang, X.; Yang, C.; Ruan, S.; Guo, J.; Hu, S.; Wang, Z. Fibroblasts in omentum activated by tumor cells promote ovarian cancer growth, adhesion and invasiveness. *Carcinogenesis* **2012**, *33*, 20–29. [CrossRef] [PubMed]

40. Zhang, Y.; Ertl, H.C.J. Depletion of fap(+) cells reduces immunosuppressive cells and improves metabolism and functions cd8(+)t cells within tumors. *Oncotarget* **2016**, *7*, 23282–23299. [CrossRef] [PubMed]

41. Kraman, M.; Bambrough, P.J.; Arnold, J.N.; Roberts, E.W.; Magiera, L.; Jones, J.O.; Gopinathan, A.; Tuveson, D.A.; Fearon, D.T. Suppression of antitumor immunity by stromal cells expressing fibroblast activation protein-alpha. *Science* **2010**, *330*, 827–830. [CrossRef] [PubMed]

42. Cheng, J.D.; Valianou, M.; Canutescu, A.A.; Jaffe, E.K.; Lee, H.O.; Wang, H.; Lai, J.H.; Bachovchin, W.W.;

Weiner, L.M. Abrogation of fibroblast activation protein enzymatic activity attenuates tumor growth. *Mol. Cancer Ther.* **2005**, *4*, 351–360. [PubMed]

43. Kelly, T. Fibroblast activation protein-alpha and dipeptidyl peptidase iv (cd26): Cell-surface proteases that activate cell signaling and are potential targets for cancer therapy. *Drug Resist. Updat.* **2005**, *8*, 51–58. [CrossRef] [PubMed]

44. Wen, Y.; Wang, C.T.; Ma, T.T.; Li, Z.Y.; Zhou, L.N.; Mu, B.; Leng, F.; Shi, H.S.; Li, Y.O.; Wei, Y.Q. Immunotherapy targeting fibroblast activation protein inhibits tumor growth and increases survival in a murine colon cancer model. *Cancer Sci.* **2010**, *101*, 2325–2332. [CrossRef] [PubMed]

45. Fabregat, I.; Fernando, J.; Mainez, J.; Sancho, P. Tgf-beta signaling in cancer treatment. *Curr. Pharm. Des.* **2014**, *20*, 2934–2947. [CrossRef] [PubMed]

46. Akhurst, R.J. Targeting tgf-beta signaling for therapeutic gain. *Cold Spring Harb. Perspect. Biol.* **2017**, *9*, a022301. [CrossRef] [PubMed]

47. Abendstein, B.; Stadlmann, S.; Knabbe, C.; Buck, M.; Muller-Holzner, E.; Zeimet, A.G.; Marth, C.; Obrist, P.; Krugmann, J.; Offner, F.A. Regulation of transforming growth factor-beta secretion by human peritoneal mesothelial and ovarian carcinoma cells. *Cytokine* **2000**, *12*, 1115–1119. [CrossRef] [PubMed]

48. Yamamura, S.; Matsumura, N.; Mandai, M.; Huang, Z.; Oura, T.; Baba, T.; Hamanishi, J.; Yamaguchi, K.; Kang, H.S.; Okamoto, T.; et al. The activated transforming growth factor-beta signaling pathway in peritoneal metastases is a potential therapeutic target in ovarian cancer. *Int. J. Cancer* **2012**, *130*, 20–28. [CrossRef] [PubMed]

49. Maier, A.; Peille, A.L.; Vuaroqueaux, V.; Lahn, M. Anti-tumor activity of the tgf-beta receptor kinase inhibitor galunisertib (ly2157299 monohydrate) in patient-derived tumor xenografts. *Cell Oncol. (Dordr.)* **2015**, *38*, 131–144. [CrossRef] [PubMed]

50. Gao, Y.; Shan, N.; Zhao, C.; Wang, Y.; Xu, F.; Li, J.; Yu, X.; Gao, L.; Yi, Z. Ly2109761 enhances cisplatin antitumor activity in ovarian cancer cells. *Int. J. Clin. Exp. Pathol.* **2015**, *8*, 4923–4932. [PubMed]

51. Kovacs, R.J.; Maldonado, G.; Azaro, A.; Fernandez, M.S.; Romero, F.L.; Sepulveda-Sanchez, J.M.; Corretti, M.; Carducci, M.; Dolan, M.; Gueorguieva, I.; et al. Cardiac safety of tgf-beta receptor i kinase inhibitor ly2157299 monohydrate in cancer patients in a first-in-human dose study. *Cardiovasc. Toxicol.* **2015**, *15*, 309–323. [CrossRef] [PubMed]

52. Zhang, M.J.; Liu, T.B.; Xia, B.R.; Yang, C.Y.; Hou, S.Y.; Xie, W.L.; Lou, G. Platelet-derived growth factor d is a prognostic biomarker and is associated with platinum resistance in epithelial ovarian cancer. *Int. J. Gynecol. Cancer* **2018**, *28*, 323–331. [CrossRef] [PubMed]

53. Matei, D.; Chang, D.D.; Jeng, M.H. Imatinib mesylate (gleevec) inhibits ovarian cancer cell growth through a mechanism dependent on platelet-derived growth factor receptor alpha and akt inactivation. *Clin. Cancer Res.* **2004**, *10*, 681–690. [CrossRef] [PubMed]

54. Pietras, K.; Pahler, J.; Bergers, G.; Hanahan, D. Functions of paracrine pdgf signaling in the proangiogenic tumor stroma revealed by pharmacological targeting. *PLoS Med.* **2008**, *5*, e19. [CrossRef] [PubMed]

55. Haubeiss, S.; Schmid, J.O.; Murdter, T.E.; Sonnenberg, M.; Friedel, G.; van der Kuip, H.; Aulitzky, W.E. Dasatinib reverses cancer-associated fibroblasts (cafs) from primary lung carcinomas to a phenotype comparable to that of normal fibroblasts. *Mol. Cancer* **2010**, *9*, 1–8. [CrossRef] [PubMed]

56. Matei, D.; Emerson, R.E.; Schilder, J.; Menning, N.; Baldridge, L.A.; Johnson, C.S.; Breen, T.; McClean, J.; Stephens, D.; Whalen, C.; et al. Imatinib mesylate in combination with docetaxel for the treatment of patients with advanced, platinum-resistant ovarian cancer and primary peritoneal carcinomatosis: A hoosier oncology group trial. *Cancer* **2008**, *113*, 723–732. [CrossRef] [PubMed]

57. Matei, D.; Sill, M.W.; Lankes, H.A.; DeGeest, K.; Bristow, R.E.; Mutch, D.; Yamada, S.D.; Cohn, D.; Calvert, V.; Farley, J.; et al. Activity of sorafenib in recurrent ovarian cancer and primary peritoneal carcinomatosis: A gynecologic oncology group trial. *J. Clin. Oncol.* **2011**, *29*, 69–75. [CrossRef] [PubMed]

58. Otrock, Z.K.; Mahfouz, R.A.; Makarem, J.A.; Shamseddine, A.I. Understanding the biology of angiogenesis: Review of the most important molecular mechanisms. *Blood Cells Mol. Dis.* **2007**, *39*, 212–220. [CrossRef] [PubMed]

59. Folkman, J. Angiogenesis: An organizing principle for drug discovery? *Nat. Rev. Drug Discov.* **2007**, *6*, 273–286. [CrossRef] [PubMed]

60. Zetter, B.R. Angiogenesis and tumor metastasis. *Annu. Rev. Med.* **1998**, *49*, 407–424. [CrossRef] [PubMed]

61. Hollingsworth, H.C.; Kohn, E.C.; Steinberg, S.M.; Rothenberg, M.L.; Merino, M.J. Tumor angiogenesis in advanced stage ovarian carcinoma. *Am. J. Pathol.* **1995**, *147*, 33–41. [PubMed]

62. Hanahan, D.; Folkman, J. Patterns and emerging mechanisms of the angiogenic switch during tumorigenesis. *Cell* **1996**, *86*, 353–364. [CrossRef]

63. Ko, S.Y.; Naora, H. Therapeutic strategies for targeting the ovarian tumor stroma. *World J. Clin. Cases* **2014**, *2*, 194–200. [CrossRef] [PubMed]

64. Yoneda, J.; Kuniyasu, H.; Crispens, M.A.; Price, J.E.; Bucana, C.D.; Fidler, I.J. Expression of angiogenesis-related genes and progression of human ovarian carcinomas in nude mice. *J. Natl. Cancer Inst.* **1998**, *90*, 447–454. [CrossRef] [PubMed]

65. Barton, D.P.; Cai, A.; Wendt, K.; Young, M.; Gamero, A.; De Cesare, S. Angiogenic protein expression in advanced epithelial ovarian cancer. *Clin. Cancer Res.* **1997**, *3*, 1579–1586. [PubMed]

66. Kraft, A.; Weindel, K.; Ochs, A.; Marth, C.; Zmija, J.; Schumacher, P.; Unger, C.; Marme, D.; Gastl, G. Vascular endothelial growth factor in the sera and effusions of patients with malignant and nonmalignant disease. *Cancer* **1999**, *85*, 178–187. [CrossRef]

67. Mesiano, S.; Ferrara, N.; Jaffe, R.B. Role of vascular endothelial growth factor in ovarian cancer: Inhibition of ascites formation by immunoneutralization. *Am. J. Pathol.* **1998**, *153*, 1249–1256. [CrossRef]

68. Shen, G.H.; Ghazizadeh, M.; Kawanami, O.; Shimizu, H.; Jin, E.; Araki, T.; Sugisaki, Y. Prognostic significance of vascular endothelial growth factor expression in human ovarian carcinoma. *Br. J. Cancer* **2000**, *83*, 196–203. [CrossRef] [PubMed]

69. Duncan, T.J.; Al-Attar, A.; Rolland, P.; Scott, I.V.; Deen, S.; Liu, D.T.; Spendlove, I.; Durrant, L.G. Vascular endothelial growth factor expression in ovarian cancer: A model for targeted use of novel therapies? *Clin. Cancer Res.* **2008**, *14*, 3030–3035. [CrossRef] [PubMed]

70. Graybill, W.; Sood, A.K.; Monk, B.J.; Coleman, R.L. State of the science: Emerging therapeutic strategies for targeting angiogenesis in ovarian cancer. *Gynecol. Oncol.* **2015**, *138*, 223–226. [CrossRef] [PubMed]

71. Ruscito, I.; Cacsire Castillo-Tong, D.; Vergote, I.; Ignat, I.; Stanske, M.; Vanderstichele, A.; Glajzer, J.; Kulbe, H.; Trillsch, F.; Mustea, A.; et al. Characterisation of tumour microvessel density during progression of high-grade serous ovarian cancer: Clinico-pathological impact (an octips consortium study). *Br. J. Cancer* **2018**, *119*, 330–338. [CrossRef] [PubMed]

72. De Palma, M.; Biziato, D.; Petrova, T.V. Microenvironmental regulation of tumour angiogenesis. *Nat. Rev. Cancer* **2017**, *17*, 457–474. [CrossRef] [PubMed]

73. Holmes, D.I.; Zachary, I. The vascular endothelial growth factor (vegf) family: Angiogenic factors in health and disease. *Genome Biol.* **2005**, *6*, 209. [CrossRef] [PubMed]

74. Neufeld, G.; Cohen, T.; Gengrinovitch, S.; Poltorak, Z. Vascular endothelial growth factor (vegf) and its receptors. *FASEB J.* **1999**, *13*, 9–22. [CrossRef] [PubMed]

75. Gupta, K.; Kshirsagar, S.; Li, W.; Gui, L.; Ramakrishnan, S.; Gupta, P.; Law, P.Y.; Hebbel, R.P. Vegf prevents apoptosis of human microvascular endothelial cells via opposing effects on mapk/erk and sapk/jnk signaling. *Exp. Cell Res.* **1999**, *247*, 495–504. [CrossRef] [PubMed]

76. Cebe-Suarez, S.; Zehnder-Fjallman, A.; Ballmer-Hofer, K. The role of vegf receptors in angiogenesis; complex partnerships. *Cell. Mol. Life Sci.* **2006**, *63*, 601–615. [CrossRef] [PubMed]

77. Eskander, R.N.; Randall, L.M. Bevacizumab in the treatment of ovarian cancer. *Biologics* **2011**, *5*, 1–5. [PubMed]

78. Mabuchi, S.; Terai, Y.; Morishige, K.; Tanabe-Kimura, A.; Sasaki, H.; Kanemura, M.; Tsunetoh, S.; Tanaka, Y.; Sakata, M.; Burger, R.A.; et al. Maintenance treatment with bevacizumab prolongs survival in an in vivo ovarian cancer model. *Clin. Cancer Res.* **2008**, *14*, 7781–7789. [CrossRef] [PubMed]

79. Burger, R.A.; Brady, M.F.; Bookman, M.A.; Fleming, G.F.; Monk, B.J.; Huang, H.; Mannel, R.S.; Homesley, H.D.; Fowler, J.; Greer, B.E.; et al. Incorporation of bevacizumab in the primary treatment of ovarian cancer. *N. Engl. J. Med.* **2011**, *365*, 2473–2483. [CrossRef] [PubMed]

80. Coleman, R.L.; Brady, M.F.; Herzog, T.J.; Sabbatini, P.; Armstrong, D.K.; Walker, J.L.; Kim, B.G.; Fujiwara, K.; Tewari, K.S.; O'Malley, D.M.; et al. Bevacizumab and paclitaxel-carboplatin chemotherapy and secondary cytoreduction in recurrent, platinum-sensitive ovarian cancer (nrg oncology/gynecologic oncology group study gog-0213): A multicentre, open-label, randomised, phase 3 trial. *Lancet Oncol.* **2017**, *18*, 779–791. [CrossRef]

81. Burger, R.A.; Sill, M.W.; Monk, B.J.; Greer, B.E.; Sorosky, J.I. Phase II trial of bevacizumab in persistent or recurrent epithelial ovarian cancer or primary peritoneal cancer: A gynecologic oncology group study. *J. Clin. Oncol.* **2007**, *25*, 5165–5171. [CrossRef] [PubMed]

82. Perren, T.J.; Swart, A.M.; Pfisterer, J.; Ledermann, J.A.; Pujade-Lauraine, E.; Kristensen, G.; Carey, M.S.; Beale, P.; Cervantes, A.; Kurzeder, C.; et al. A phase 3 trial of bevacizumab in ovarian cancer. *N. Engl. J. Med.* **2011**, *365*, 2484–2496. [CrossRef] [PubMed]

83. Pujade-Lauraine, E.; Hilpert, F.; Weber, B.; Reuss, A.; Poveda, A.; Kristensen, G.; Sorio, R.; Vergote, I.; Witteveen, P.; Bamias, A.; et al. Bevacizumab combined with chemotherapy for platinum-resistant recurrent ovarian cancer: The aurelia open-label randomized phase iii trial. *J. Clin. Oncol.* **2014**, *32*, 1302–1308. [CrossRef] [PubMed]

84. Moroney, J.W.; Sood, A.K.; Coleman, R.L. Aflibercept in epithelial ovarian carcinoma. *Future Oncol.* **2009**, *5*, 591–600. [CrossRef] [PubMed]

85. Teng, L.S.; Jin, K.T.; He, K.F.; Zhang, J.; Wang, H.H.; Cao, J. Clinical applications of vegf-trap (aflibercept) in cancer treatment. *J. Chin. Med. Assoc.* **2010**, *73*, 449–456. [CrossRef]

86. Byrne, A.T.; Ross, L.; Holash, J.; Nakanishi, M.; Hu, L.; Hofmann, J.I.; Yancopoulos, G.D.; Jaffe, R.B. Vascular endothelial growth factor-trap decreases tumor burden, inhibits ascites, and causes dramatic vascular remodeling in an ovarian cancer model. *Clin. Cancer Res.* **2003**, *9*, 5721–5728. [PubMed]

87. Colombo, N.; Mangili, G.; Mammoliti, S.; Kalling, M.; Tholander, B.; Sternas, L.; Buzenet, G.; Chamberlain, D. A phase ii study of aflibercept in patients with advanced epithelial ovarian cancer and symptomatic malignant ascites. *Gynecol. Oncol.* **2012**, *125*, 42–47. [CrossRef] [PubMed]

88. Bergers, G.; Hanahan, D. Modes of resistance to anti-angiogenic therapy. *Nat. Rev. Cancer* **2008**, *8*, 592–603. [CrossRef] [PubMed]

89. Matulonis, U.A.; Berlin, S.; Ivy, P.; Tyburski, K.; Krasner, C.; Zarwan, C.; Berkenblit, A.; Campos, S.; Horowitz, N.; Cannistra, S.A.; et al. Cediranib, an oral inhibitor of vascular endothelial growth factor receptor kinases, is an active drug in recurrent epithelial ovarian, fallopian tube, and peritoneal cancer. *J. Clin. Oncol.* **2009**, *27*, 5601–5606. [CrossRef] [PubMed]

90. Hirte, H.; Lheureux, S.; Fleming, G.F.; Sugimoto, A.; Morgan, R.; Biagi, J.; Wang, L.; McGill, S.; Ivy, S.P.; Oza, A.M. A phase 2 study of cediranib in recurrent or persistent ovarian, peritoneal or fallopian tube cancer: A trial of the princess margaret, chicago and california phase ii consortia. *Gynecol. Oncol.* **2015**, *138*, 55–61. [CrossRef] [PubMed]

91. Ledermann, J.A.; Hackshaw, A.; Kaye, S.; Jayson, G.; Gabra, H.; McNeish, I.; Earl, H.; Perren, T.; Gore, M.; Persic, M.; et al. Randomized phase ii placebo-controlled trial of maintenance therapy using the oral triple angiokinase inhibitor bibf 1120 after chemotherapy for relapsed ovarian cancer. *J. Clin. Oncol.* **2011**, *29*, 3798–3804. [CrossRef] [PubMed]

92. Du Bois, A.; Kristensen, G.; Ray-Coquard, I.; Reuss, A.; Pignata, S.; Colombo, N.; Denison, U.; Vergote, I.; del Campo, J.M.; Ottevanger, P.; et al. Standard first-line chemotherapy with or without nintedanib for advanced ovarian cancer (ago-ovar 12): A randomised, double-blind, placebo-controlled phase 3 trial. *Lancet Oncol.* **2016**, *17*, 78–89. [CrossRef]

93. Pignata, S.; Lorusso, D.; Scambia, G.; Sambataro, D.; Tamberi, S.; Cinieri, S.; Mosconi, A.M.; Orditura, M.; Bartolini, S.; Arcangeli, V.; et al. Mito-11: A randomized multicenter phase ii trial testing the addition of pazopanib to weekly paclitaxel in platinum-resistant or -refractory advanced ovarian cancer (aoc). *J. Clin. Oncol.* **2014**, *32*.

94. Sawada, K.; Mitra, A.K.; Radjabi, A.R.; Bhaskar, V.; Kistner, E.O.; Tretiakova, M.; Jagadeeswaran, S.; Montag, A.; Becker, A.; Kenny, H.A.; et al. Loss of e-cadherin promotes ovarian cancer metastasis via alpha 5-integrin, which is a therapeutic target. *Cancer Res.* **2008**, *68*, 2329–2339. [CrossRef] [PubMed]

95. Iwanicki, M.P.; Davidowitz, R.A.; Ng, M.R.; Besser, A.; Muranen, T.; Merritt, M.; Danuser, G.; Ince, T.A.; Brugge, J.S. Ovarian cancer spheroids use myosin-generated force to clear the mesothelium. *Cancer Discov.* **2011**, *1*, 144–157. [CrossRef] [PubMed]

96. Davidowitz, R.A.; Selfors, L.M.; Iwanicki, M.P.; Elias, K.M.; Karst, A.; Piao, H.; Ince, T.A.; Drage, M.G.; Dering, J.; Konecny, G.E.; et al. Mesenchymal gene program-expressing ovarian cancer spheroids exhibit enhanced mesothelial clearance. *J. Clin. Investig.* **2014**, *124*, 2611–2625. [CrossRef] [PubMed]

97. Lessan, K.; Aguiar, D.J.; Oegema, T.; Siebenson, L.; Skubitz, A.P. Cd44 and beta1 integrin mediate ovarian carcinoma cell adhesion to peritoneal mesothelial cells. *Am. J. Pathol.* **1999**, *154*, 1525–1537. [CrossRef]

98. Kenny, H.A.; Chiang, C.Y.; White, E.A.; Schryver, E.M.; Habis, M.; Romero, I.L.; Ladanyi, A.; Penicka, C.V.; George, J.; Matlin, K.; et al. Mesothelial cells promote early ovarian cancer metastasis through fibronectin secretion. *J. Clin. Investig.* **2014**, *124*, 4614–4628. [CrossRef] [PubMed]

99. Janiak, A.; Zemskov, E.A.; Belkin, A.M. Cell surface transglutaminase promotes rhoa activation via integrin clustering and suppression of the src-p190rhogap signaling pathway. *Mol. Biol. Cell* **2006**, *17*, 1606–1619. [CrossRef] [PubMed]

100. Satpathy, M.; Cao, L.; Pincheira, R.; Emerson, R.; Bigsby, R.; Nakshatri, H.; Matei, D. Enhanced peritoneal ovarian tumor dissemination by tissue transglutaminase. *Cancer Res.* **2007**, *67*, 7194–7202. [CrossRef] [PubMed]

101. Shao, M.; Cao, L.; Shen, C.; Satpathy, M.; Chelladurai, B.; Bigsby, R.M.; Nakshatri, H.; Matei, D. Epithelial-to-mesenchymal transition and ovarian tumor progression induced by tissue transglutaminase. *Cancer Res.* **2009**, *69*, 9192–9201. [CrossRef] [PubMed]

102. Condello, S.; Cao, L.; Matei, D. Tissue transglutaminase regulates beta-catenin signaling through a c-src-dependent mechanism. *FASEB J.* **2013**, *27*, 3100–3112. [CrossRef] [PubMed]

103. Condello, S.; Sima, L.; Ivan, C.; Cardenas, H.; Schiltz, G.; Mishra, R.K.; Matei, D. Tissue tranglutaminase regulates interactions between ovarian cancer stem cells and the tumor niche. *Cancer Res.* **2018**, *78*, 2990–3001. [CrossRef] [PubMed]

104. Strobel, T.; Cannistra, S.A. Beta1-integrins partly mediate binding of ovarian cancer cells to peritoneal mesothelium in vitro. *Gynecol. Oncol.* **1999**, *73*, 362–367. [CrossRef] [PubMed]

105. Cannistra, S.A.; Kansas, G.S.; Niloff, J.; DeFranzo, B.; Kim, Y.; Ottensmeier, C. Binding of ovarian cancer cells to peritoneal mesothelium in vitro is partly mediated by cd44h. *Cancer Res.* **1993**, *53*, 3830–3838. [PubMed]

106. Strobel, T.; Swanson, L.; Cannistra, S.A. In vivo inhibition of cd44 limits intra-abdominal spread of a human ovarian cancer xenograft in nude mice: A novel role for cd44 in the process of peritoneal implantation. *Cancer Res.* **1997**, *57*, 1228–1232. [PubMed]

107. Slack-Davis, J.K.; Atkins, K.A.; Harrer, C.; Hershey, E.D.; Conaway, M. Vascular cell adhesion molecule-1 is a regulator of ovarian cancer peritoneal metastasis. *Cancer Res.* **2009**, *69*, 1469–1476. [CrossRef] [PubMed]

108. Mitra, A.K.; Sawada, K.; Tiwari, P.; Mui, K.; Gwin, K.; Lengyel, E. Ligand-independent activation of c-met by fibronectin and alpha(5)beta(1)-integrin regulates ovarian cancer invasion and metastasis. *Oncogene* **2011**, *30*, 1566–1576. [CrossRef] [PubMed]

109. Raab-Westphal, S.; Marshall, J.F.; Goodman, S.L. Integrins as therapeutic targets: Successes and cancers. *Cancers (Basel)* **2017**, *9*, 110. [CrossRef] [PubMed]

110. Bell-McGuinn, K.M.; Matthews, C.M.; Ho, S.N.; Barve, M.; Gilbert, L.; Penson, R.T.; Lengyel, E.; Palaparthy, R.; Gilder, K.; Vassos, A.; et al. A phase ii, single-arm study of the anti-alpha5beta1 integrin antibody volociximab as monotherapy in patients with platinum-resistant advanced epithelial ovarian or primary peritoneal cancer. *Gynecol. Oncol.* **2011**, *121*, 273–279. [CrossRef] [PubMed]

111. Trikha, M.; Zhou, Z.; Nemeth, J.A.; Chen, Q.; Sharp, C.; Emmell, E.; Giles-Komar, J.; Nakada, M.T. Cnto 95, a fully human monoclonal antibody that inhibits alphav integrins, has antitumor and antiangiogenic activity in vivo. *Int. J. Cancer* **2004**, *110*, 326–335. [CrossRef] [PubMed]

112. Chen, Q.; Manning, C.D.; Millar, H.; McCabe, F.L.; Ferrante, C.; Sharp, C.; Shahied-Arruda, L.; Doshi, P.; Nakada, M.T.; Anderson, G.M. Cnto 95, a fully human anti alphav integrin antibody, inhibits cell signaling, migration, invasion, and spontaneous metastasis of human breast cancer cells. *Clin. Exp. Metastasis* **2008**, *25*, 139–148. [CrossRef] [PubMed]

113. Mullamitha, S.A.; Ton, N.C.; Parker, G.J.; Jackson, A.; Julyan, P.J.; Roberts, C.; Buonaccorsi, G.A.; Watson, Y.; Davies, K.; Cheung, S.; et al. Phase i evaluation of a fully human anti-alphav integrin monoclonal antibody (cnto 95) in patients with advanced solid tumors. *Clin. Cancer Res.* **2007**, *13*, 2128–2135. [CrossRef] [PubMed]

114. Hersey, P.; Sosman, J.; O'Day, S.; Richards, J.; Bedikian, A.; Gonzalez, R.; Sharfman, W.; Weber, R.; Logan, T.; Buzoianu, M.; et al. A randomized phase 2 study of etaracizumab, a monoclonal antibody against integrin alpha(v)beta(3), + or - dacarbazine in patients with stage iv metastatic melanoma. *Cancer* **2010**, *116*, 1526–1534. [CrossRef] [PubMed]

115. Dolgos, H.; Freisleben, A.; Wimmer, E.; Scheible, H.; Kratzer, F.; Yamagata, T.; Gallemann, D.; Fluck, M. In vitro and in vivo drug disposition of cilengitide in animals and human. *Pharmacol. Res. Perspect.* **2016**, *4*, e00217. [CrossRef] [PubMed]

116. Soffietti, R.; Trevisan, E.; Ruda, R. What have we learned from trials on antiangiogenic agents in glioblastoma? *Expert Rev. Neurother.* **2014**, *14*, 1–3. [CrossRef] [PubMed]

117. Kaur, S.; Kenny, H.A.; Jagadeeswaran, S.; Zillhardt, M.R.; Montag, A.G.; Kistner, E.; Yamada, S.D.; Mitra, A.K.; Lengyel, E. {beta}3-integrin expression on tumor cells inhibits tumor progression, reduces metastasis, and is associated with a favorable prognosis in patients with ovarian cancer. *Am. J. Pathol.* **2009**, *175*, 2184–2196. [CrossRef] [PubMed]

118. Kenny, H.A.; Lengyel, E. Mmp-2 functions as an early response protein in ovarian cancer metastasis. *Cell Cycle* **2009**, *8*, 683–688. [CrossRef] [PubMed]

119. Schlaepfer, D.D.; Jones, K.C.; Hunter, T. Multiple grb2-mediated integrin-stimulated signaling pathways to erk2/mitogen-activated protein kinase: Summation of both c-src- and focal adhesion kinase-initiated tyrosine phosphorylation events. *Mol. Cell Biol.* **1998**, *18*, 2571–2585. [CrossRef] [PubMed]

120. Renshaw, M.W.; Price, L.S.; Schwartz, M.A. Focal adhesion kinase mediates the integrin signaling requirement for growth factor activation of map kinase. *J. Cell Biol.* **1999**, *147*, 611–618. [CrossRef] [PubMed]

121. Ward, K.K.; Tancioni, I.; Lawson, C.; Miller, N.L.; Jean, C.; Chen, X.L.; Uryu, S.; Kim, J.; Tarin, D.; Stupack, D.G.; et al. Inhibition of focal adhesion kinase (fak) activity prevents anchorage-independent ovarian carcinoma cell growth and tumor progression. *Clin. Exp. Metastasis* **2013**, *30*, 579–594. [CrossRef] [PubMed]

122. Matei, D.; Graeber, T.G.; Baldwin, R.L.; Karlan, B.Y.; Rao, J.; Chang, D.D. Gene expression in epithelial ovarian carcinoma. *Oncogene* **2002**, *21*, 6289–6298. [CrossRef] [PubMed]

123. Yakubov, B.; Chelladurai, B.; Schmitt, J.; Emerson, R.; Turchi, J.J.; Matei, D. Extracellular tissue transglutaminase activates noncanonical nf-kappab signaling and promotes metastasis in ovarian cancer. *Neoplasia* **2013**, *15*, 609–619. [CrossRef] [PubMed]

124. Satpathy, M.; Shao, M.; Emerson, R.; Donner, D.B.; Matei, D. Tissue transglutaminase regulates matrix metalloproteinase-2 in ovarian cancer by modulating camp-response element-binding protein activity. *J. Biol. Chem.* **2009**, *284*, 15390–15399. [CrossRef] [PubMed]

125. Khanna, M.; Chelladurai, B.; Gavini, A.; Li, L.; Shao, M.; Courtney, D.; Turchi, J.J.; Matei, D.; Meroueh, S. Targeting ovarian tumor cell adhesion mediated by tissue transglutaminase. *Mol. Cancer Ther.* **2011**, *10*, 626–636. [CrossRef] [PubMed]

126. Yakubov, B.; Chen, L.; Belkin, A.M.; Zhang, S.; Chelladurai, B.; Zhang, Z.Y.; Matei, D. Small molecule inhibitors target the tissue transglutaminase and fibronectin interaction. *PLoS ONE* **2014**, *9*, e89285. [CrossRef] [PubMed]

127. Burkholder, B.; Huang, R.Y.; Burgess, R.; Luo, S.; Jones, V.S.; Zhang, W.; Lv, Z.Q.; Gao, C.Y.; Wang, B.L.; Zhang, Y.M.; et al. Tumor-induced perturbations of cytokines and immune cell networks. *Biochim. Biophys. Acta.* **2014**, *1845*, 182–201. [CrossRef] [PubMed]

128. Zhang, L.; Conejo-Garcia, J.R.; Katsaros, D.; Gimotty, P.A.; Massobrio, M.; Regnani, G.; Makrigiannakis, A.; Gray, H.; Schlienger, K.; Liebman, M.N.; et al. Intratumoral t cells, recurrence, and survival in epithelial ovarian cancer. *Ne. Engl. J. Med.* **2003**, *348*, 203–213. [CrossRef] [PubMed]

129. Clarke, B.; Tinker, A.V.; Lee, C.H.; Subramanian, S.; van de Rijn, M.; Turbin, D.; Kalloger, S.; Han, G.; Ceballos, K.; Cadungog, M.G.; et al. Intraepithelial t cells and prognosis in ovarian carcinoma: Novel associations with stage, tumor type, and brca1 loss. *Mod. Pathol.* **2009**, *22*, 393–402. [CrossRef] [PubMed]

130. Sato, E.; Olson, S.H.; Ahn, J.; Bundy, B.; Nishikawa, H.; Qian, F.; Jungbluth, A.A.; Frosina, D.; Gnjatic, S.; Ambrosone, C.; et al. Intraepithelial cd8+ tumor-infiltrating lymphocytes and a high cd8+/regulatory t cell ratio are associated with favorable prognosis in ovarian cancer. *Proc. Natl. Acad. Sci. USA* **2005**, *102*, 18538–18543. [CrossRef] [PubMed]

131. Santoiemma, P.P.; Reyes, C.; Wang, L.P.; McLane, M.W.; Feldman, M.D.; Tanyi, J.L.; Powell, D.J., Jr. Systematic evaluation of multiple immune markers reveals prognostic factors in ovarian cancer. *Gynecol. Oncol.* **2016**, *143*, 120–127. [CrossRef] [PubMed]

132. Ye, Q.; Song, D.G.; Poussin, M.; Yamamoto, T.; Best, A.; Li, C.; Coukos, G.; Powell, D.J., Jr. Cd137 accurately identifies and enriches for naturally occurring tumor-reactive t cells in tumor. *Clin. Cancer Res.* **2014**, *20*, 44–55. [CrossRef] [PubMed]

133. Jimenez-Sanchez, A.; Memon, D.; Pourpe, S.; Veeraraghavan, H.; Li, Y.; Vargas, H.A.; Gill, M.B.; Park, K.J.; Zivanovic, O.; Konner, J.; et al. Heterogeneous tumor-immune microenvironments among differentially growing metastases in an ovarian cancer patient. *Cell* **2017**, *170*, 927–938. [CrossRef] [PubMed]

134. Bosmuller, H.C.; Wagner, P.; Peper, J.K.; Schuster, H.; Pham, D.L.; Greif, K.; Beschorner, C.; Rammensee, H.G.; Stevanovic, S.; Fend, F.; et al. Combined immunoscore of cd103 and cd3 identifies long-term survivors in high-grade serous ovarian cancer. *Int. J. Gynecol. Cancer* **2016**, *26*, 671–679. [CrossRef] [PubMed]

135. Garon, E.B.; Rizvi, N.A.; Hui, R.; Leighl, N.; Balmanoukian, A.S.; Eder, J.P.; Patnaik, A.; Aggarwal, C.; Gubens, M.; Horn, L.; et al. Pembrolizumab for the treatment of non-small-cell lung cancer. *N. Engl. J. Med.* **2015**, *372*, 2018–2028. [CrossRef] [PubMed]

136. Robert, C.; Schachter, J.; Long, G.V.; Arance, A.; Grob, J.J.; Mortier, L.; Daud, A.; Carlino, M.S.; McNeil, C.; Lotem, M.; et al. Pembrolizumab versus ipilimumab in advanced melanoma. *N. Engl. J. Med.* **2015**, *372*, 2521–2532. [CrossRef] [PubMed]

137. Ikarashi, H.; Fujita, K.; Takakuwa, K.; Kodama, S.; Tokunaga, A.; Takahashi, T.; Tanaka, K. Immunomodulation in patients with epithelial ovarian cancer after adoptive transfer of tumor-infiltrating lymphocytes. *Cancer Res.* **1994**, *54*, 190–196. [PubMed]

138. Kandalaft, L.E.; Chiang, C.L.; Tanyi, J.; Motz, G.; Balint, K.; Mick, R.; Coukos, G. A phase i vaccine trial using dendritic cells pulsed with autologous oxidized lysate for recurrent ovarian cancer. *J. Transl. Med.* **2013**, *11*, 149. [CrossRef] [PubMed]

139. Tumeh, P.C.; Harview, C.L.; Yearley, J.H.; Shintaku, I.P.; Taylor, E.J.; Robert, L.; Chmielowski, B.; Spasic, M.; Henry, G.; Ciobanu, V.; et al. Pd-1 blockade induces responses by inhibiting adaptive immune resistance. *Nature* **2014**, *515*, 568–571. [CrossRef] [PubMed]

140. Brahmer, J.R.; Tykodi, S.S.; Chow, L.Q.; Hwu, W.J.; Topalian, S.L.; Hwu, P.; Drake, C.G.; Camacho, L.H.; Kauh, J.; Odunsi, K.; et al. Safety and activity of anti-pd-l1 antibody in patients with advanced cancer. *N. Engl. J. Med.* **2012**, *366*, 2455–2465. [CrossRef] [PubMed]

141. Gettinger, S.N.; Horn, L.; Gandhi, L.; Spigel, D.R.; Antonia, S.J.; Rizvi, N.A.; Powderly, J.D.; Heist, R.S.; Carvajal, R.D.; Jackman, D.M.; et al. Overall survival and long-term safety of nivolumab (anti-programmed death 1 antibody, bms-936558, ono-4538) in patients with previously treated advanced non-small-cell lung cancer. *J. Clin. Oncol.* **2015**, *33*, 2004–2012. [CrossRef] [PubMed]

142. Mahoney, K.M.; Freeman, G.J.; McDermott, D.F. The next immune-checkpoint inhibitors: Pd-1/pd-l1 blockade in melanoma. *Clin. Ther.* **2015**, *37*, 764–782. [CrossRef] [PubMed]

143. Hamanishi, J.; Mandai, M.; Iwasaki, M.; Okazaki, T.; Tanaka, Y.; Yamaguchi, K.; Higuchi, T.; Yagi, H.; Takakura, K.; Minato, N.; et al. Programmed cell death 1 ligand 1 and tumor-infiltrating cd8+ t lymphocytes are prognostic factors of human ovarian cancer. *Proc. Natl. Acad. Sci. USA* **2007**, *104*, 3360–3365. [CrossRef] [PubMed]

144. Krempski, J.; Karyampudi, L.; Behrens, M.D.; Erskine, C.L.; Hartmann, L.; Dong, H.; Goode, E.L.; Kalli, K.R.; Knutson, K.L. Tumor-infiltrating programmed death receptor-1+ dendritic cells mediate immune suppression in ovarian cancer. *J. Immunol.* **2011**, *186*, 6905–6913. [CrossRef] [PubMed]

145. Darb-Esfahani, S.; Kunze, C.A.; Kulbe, H.; Sehouli, J.; Wienert, S.; Lindner, J.; Budczies, J.; Bockmayr, M.; Dietel, M.; Denkert, C.; et al. Prognostic impact of programmed cell death-1 (pd-1) and pd-ligand 1 (pd-l1) expression in cancer cells and tumor-infiltrating lymphocytes in ovarian high grade serous carcinoma. *Oncotarget* **2016**, *7*, 1486–1499. [CrossRef] [PubMed]

146. Webb, J.R.; Milne, K.; Kroeger, D.R.; Nelson, B.H. Pd-l1 expression is associated with tumor-infiltrating t cells and favorable prognosis in high-grade serous ovarian cancer. *Gynecol. Oncol.* **2016**, *141*, 293–302. [CrossRef] [PubMed]

147. Duraiswamy, J.; Freeman, G.J.; Coukos, G. Therapeutic pd-1 pathway blockade augments with other modalities of immunotherapy t-cell function to prevent immune decline in ovarian cancer. *Cancer Res.* **2013**, *73*, 6900–6912. [CrossRef] [PubMed]

148. Varga, A.; Pihapaul, S.A.; Ott, P.A.; Mehnert, J.M.; Bertonrigaud, D.; Johnson, E.A.; Cheng, J.D.; Yuan, S.; Rubin, E.H.; Matei, D.E. Antitumor activity and safety of pembrolizumab in patients (pts) with pd-l1 positive advanced ovarian cancer: Interim results from a phase ib study. *J. Clin. Oncol.* **2015**, *33*, 5510. [CrossRef]

149. Disis, M.L.; Patel, M.R.; Pant, S.; Infante, J.R.; Lockhart, A.C.; Kelly, K.; Beck, J.T.; Gordon, M.S.; Weiss, G.J.; Ejadi, S.; et al. Avelumab (msb0010718c), an anti-pd-l1 antibody, in patients with previously treated, recurrent or refractory ovarian cancer: A phase ib, open-label expansion trial. *J. Clin. Oncol.* **2015**, *33*, 5509. [CrossRef]

150. Lau, E. Mismatch repair deficiency predicts benefit of anti-pd-1 therapy. *Lancet Oncol.* **2015**, *16*, e319. [CrossRef]

151. Le, D.T.; Uram, J.N.; Wang, H.; Bartlett, B.R.; Kemberling, H.; Eyring, A.D.; Skora, A.D.; Luber, B.S.; Azad, N.S.; Laheru, D.; et al. Pd-1 blockade in tumors with mismatch-repair deficiency. *N. Engl. J. Med.* **2015**, *372*, 2509–2520. [CrossRef] [PubMed]

152. Strickland, K.C.; Howitt, B.E.; Shukla, S.A.; Rodig, S.; Ritterhouse, L.L.; Liu, J.F.; Garber, J.E.; Chowdhury, D.; Wu, C.J.; D'Andrea, A.D.; et al. Association and prognostic significance of brca1/2-mutation status with neoantigen load, number of tumor-infiltrating lymphocytes and expression of pd-1/pd-l1 in high grade serous ovarian cancer. *Oncotarget* **2016**, *7*, 13587–13598. [CrossRef] [PubMed]

153. Noy, R.; Pollard, J.W. Tumor-associated macrophages: From mechanisms to therapy. *Immunity* **2014**, *41*, 49–61. [CrossRef] [PubMed]

154. Rabinovich, G.A.; Gabrilovich, D.; Sotomayor, E.M. Immunosuppressive strategies that are mediated by tumor cells. *Annu. Rev. Immunol.* **2007**, *25*, 267–296. [CrossRef] [PubMed]

155. Bronte, V.; Serafini, P.; Apolloni, E.; Zanovello, P. Tumor-induced immune dysfunctions caused by myeloid suppressor cells. *J. Immunother.* **2001**, *24*, 431–446. [CrossRef] [PubMed]

156. Almand, B.; Clark, J.I.; Nikitina, E.; van Beynen, J.; English, N.R.; Knight, S.C.; Carbone, D.P.; Gabrilovich, D.I. Increased production of immature myeloid cells in cancer patients: A mechanism of immunosuppression in cancer. *J. Immunol.* **2001**, *166*, 678–689. [CrossRef] [PubMed]

157. Youn, J.I.; Nagaraj, S.; Collazo, M.; Gabrilovich, D.I. Subsets of myeloid-derived suppressor cells in tumor-bearing mice. *J. Immunol.* **2008**, *181*, 5791–5802. [CrossRef] [PubMed]

158. Zhang, M.; He, Y.; Sun, X.; Li, Q.; Wang, W.; Zhao, A.; Di, W. A high m1/m2 ratio of tumor-associated macrophages is associated with extended survival in ovarian cancer patients. *J. Ovarian Res.* **2014**, *7*, 19. [CrossRef] [PubMed]

159. Pollard, J.W. Tumour-educated macrophages promote tumour progression and metastasis. *Nat. Rev. Cancer* **2004**, *4*, 71–78. [CrossRef] [PubMed]

160. Wang, X.; Deavers, M.; Patenia, R.; Bassett, R.L., Jr.; Mueller, P.; Ma, Q.; Wang, E.; Freedman, R.S. Monocyte/macrophage and t-cell infiltrates in peritoneum of patients with ovarian cancer or benign pelvic disease. *J. Transl. Med.* **2006**, *4*, 30. [CrossRef] [PubMed]

161. Yin, M.; Li, X.; Tan, S.; Zhou, H.J.; Ji, W.; Bellone, S.; Xu, X.; Zhang, H.; Santin, A.D.; Lou, G.; et al. Tumor-associated macrophages drive spheroid formation during early transcoelomic metastasis of ovarian cancer. *J. Clin. Investig.* **2016**, *126*, 4157–4173. [CrossRef] [PubMed]

162. Hagemann, T.; Wilson, J.; Kulbe, H.; Li, N.F.; Leinster, D.A.; Charles, K.; Klemm, F.; Pukrop, T.; Binder, C.; Balkwill, F.R. Macrophages induce invasiveness of epithelial cancer cells via nf-kappa b and jnk. *J. Immunol.* **2005**, *175*, 1197–1205. [CrossRef] [PubMed]

163. Ko, S.Y.; Ladanyi, A.; Lengyel, E.; Naora, H. Expression of the homeobox gene hoxa9 in ovarian cancer induces peritoneal macrophages to acquire an m2 tumor-promoting phenotype. *Am. J. Pathol.* **2014**, *184*, 271–281. [CrossRef] [PubMed]

164. Cui, T.X.; Kryczek, I.; Zhao, L.; Zhao, E.; Kuick, R.; Roh, M.H.; Vatan, L.; Szeliga, W.; Mao, Y.; Thomas, D.G.; et al. Myeloid-derived suppressor cells enhance stemness of cancer cells by inducing microrna101 and suppressing the corepressor ctbp2. *Immunity* **2013**, *39*, 611–621. [CrossRef] [PubMed]

165. Horikawa, N.; Abiko, K.; Matsumura, N.; Hamanishi, J.; Baba, T.; Yamaguchi, K.; Yoshioka, Y.; Koshiyama, M.; Konishi, I. Expression of vascular endothelial growth factor in ovarian cancer inhibits tumor immunity through the accumulation of myeloid-derived suppressor cells. *Clin. Cancer Res.* **2017**, *23*, 587–599. [CrossRef] [PubMed]

166. Taki, M.; Abiko, K.; Baba, T.; Hamanishi, J.; Yamaguchi, K.; Murakami, R.; Yamanoi, K.; Horikawa, N.; Hosoe, Y.; Nakamura, E.; et al. Snail promotes ovarian cancer progression by recruiting myeloid-derived suppressor cells via cxcr2 ligand upregulation. *Nat. Commun.* **2018**, *9*, 1685. [CrossRef] [PubMed]

167. De Sanctis, F.; Bronte, V.; Ugel, S. Tumor-induced myeloid-derived suppressor cells. *Microbiol. Spectr.* **2016**, *4*. [CrossRef] [PubMed]

168. Engblom, C.; Pfirschke, C.; Pittet, M.J. The role of myeloid cells in cancer therapies. *Nat. Rev. Cancer* **2016**, *16*, 447–462. [CrossRef] [PubMed]

169. Pulaski, H.L.; Spahlinger, G.; Silva, I.A.; McLean, K.; Kueck, A.S.; Reynolds, R.K.; Coukos, G.; Conejo-Garcia, J.R.; Buckanovich, R.J. Identifying alemtuzumab as an anti-myeloid cell antiangiogenic therapy for the treatment of ovarian cancer. *J. Transl. Med.* **2009**, *7*, 49. [CrossRef] [PubMed]

170. Penn, C.A.; Yang, K.; Zong, H.; Lim, J.Y.; Cole, A.; Yang, D.; Baker, J.; Goonewardena, S.N.; Buckanovich, R.J. Therapeutic impact of nanoparticle therapy targeting tumor-associated macrophages. *Mol. Cancer Ther.* **2018**, *17*, 96–106. [CrossRef] [PubMed]

171. Zhu, H.; Bengsch, F.; Svoronos, N.; Rutkowski, M.R.; Bitler, B.G.; Allegrezza, M.J.; Yokoyama, Y.; Kossenkov, A.V.; Bradner, J.E.; Conejo-Garcia, J.R.; et al. Bet bromodomain inhibition promotes anti-tumor immunity by suppressing pd-l1 expression. *Cell Rep.* **2016**, *16*, 2829–2837. [CrossRef] [PubMed]

172. Stone, M.L.; Chiappinelli, K.B.; Li, H.; Murphy, L.M.; Travers, M.E.; Topper, M.J.; Mathios, D.; Lim, M.; Shih, I.M.; Wang, T.L.; et al. Epigenetic therapy activates type i interferon signaling in murine ovarian cancer to reduce immunosuppression and tumor burden. *Proc. Natl. Acad. Sci. USA* **2017**, *114*, E10981–E10990. [CrossRef] [PubMed]

173. Burges, A.; Wimberger, P.; Kumper, C.; Gorbounova, V.; Sommer, H.; Schmalfeldt, B.; Pfisterer, J.; Lichinitser, M.; Makhson, A.; Moiseyenko, V.; et al. Effective relief of malignant ascites in patients with advanced ovarian cancer by a trifunctional anti-epcam x anti-cd3 antibody: A phase i/ii study. *Clin. Cancer Res.* **2007**, *13*, 3899–3905. [CrossRef] [PubMed]

Permissions

List of Contributors

Monika Sobočan
Department of Pharmacology, Faculty of Medicine, University of Maribor, 2000 Maribor, Slovenia
Divison of Gynecology and Perinatology, University Medical Centre Maribor, 2000 Maribor, Slovenia
Department of Obstetrics and Gynecology, Faculty of Medicine, University of Maribor, 2000 Maribor, Slovenia

Jure Knez and Iztok Takač
Divison of Gynecology and Perinatology, University Medical Centre Maribor, 2000 Maribor, Slovenia
Department of Obstetrics and Gynecology, Faculty of Medicine, University of Maribor, 2000 Maribor, Slovenia

Suzana Bračič
Department of Pathology, Hospital Graz II, West, 8020 Graz, Austria
Department of Pathology, Faculty of Medicine, University of Maribor, 2000 Maribor, Slovenia

Johannes Haybaeck
Department of Pathology, Medical Faculty Otto-von-Guericke University Magdeburg, 39120 Magdeburg, Germany
Department of Pathology, Neuropathology and Molecular Pathology, Medical University of Innsbruck, 6020 Innsbruck, Austria
Diagnostic and Research Institute of Pathology, Medical University of Graz, 8036 Graz, Austria

Claudia B. Colon-Echevarria, Tatiana Ortiz, Lizette Maldonado, Melanie J. Hidalgo-Vargas, Alexandra N. Aquino-Acevedo and Roberto Herrera-Noriega
Department of Basic Sciences, Pharmacology Division, School of Medicine, Ponce Health Sciences University, Ponce, PR 00716, USA

Jaileene Pérez-Morales
Department of Cancer Epidemiology, H. Lee Mott Cancer Center and Research Institute, Tampa, FL 33612, USA

Margarita Bonilla-Claudio
Division of Cancer Biology, Ponce Research Institute, Ponce, PR 00716, USA

Eida M. Castro
Clinical Psychology Program, School of Behavior and Brain Sciences, Ponce Health Sciences University, Ponce, PR 00716, USA

Mental Health Division, Ponce Research Institute, Ponce, PR 00716, USA

Guillermo N. Armaiz-Pena
Department of Basic Sciences, Pharmacology Division, School of Medicine, Ponce Health Sciences University, Ponce, PR 00716, USA
Division of Cancer Biology, Ponce Research Institute, Ponce, PR 00716, USA
Division of Women's Health, Ponce Research Institute, Ponce, PR 00716, USA

Galaxia M. Rodriguez, Kristianne J. C. Galpin, Curtis W. McCloskey and Barbara C. Vanderhyden
Cancer Therapeutics Program, Ottawa Hospital Research Institute, 501 Smyth Road, Ottawa, ON K1H 8L6, Canada
Department of Cellular and Molecular Medicine, University of Ottawa, 451 Smyth Road, Ottawa, ON K1H 8M5, Canada

Sudha S. Savant
Medical Sciences, Indiana University School of Medicine, Bloomington, IN 47405, USA

Shruthi Sriramkumar
Cell, Molecular and Cancer Biology Graduate Program, Indiana University, Bloomington, IN 47405, USA

Heather M. O'Hagan
Indiana University Melvin and Bren Simon Cancer Center, Indianapolis, IN 46202, USA

Laurie G. Hudson
Department of Pharmaceutical Sciences, University of New Mexico Health Sciences Center, Albuquerque, NM 87131, USA
Comprehensive Cancer Center, University of New Mexico Health Sciences Center, Albuquerque, NM 87131, USA

Jennifer M. Gillette, Melanie R. Rivera and Angela Wandinger-Ness
Comprehensive Cancer Center, University of New Mexico Health Sciences Center, Albuquerque, NM 87131, USA
Department of Pathology, University of New Mexico Health Sciences Center, Albuquerque, NM 87131, USA

Huining Kang
Comprehensive Cancer Center, University of New Mexico Health Sciences Center, Albuquerque, NM 87131, USA
Department of Medicine, University of New Mexico Health Sciences Center, Albuquerque, NM 87131, USA

Jillian R. Hufgard Wendel, Xiyin Wang and Shannon M. Hawkins
Department of Obstetrics and Gynecology, Indiana University School of Medicine, Indianapolis, IN 46202, USA

Tyvette S. Hilliard
Department of Chemistry and Biochemistry, Harper Cancer Research Institute, University of Notre Dame, Notre Dame, IN 46617, USA

Lynn Roy
Harper Cancer Research Institute, South Bend, IN 46617, USA
Department of Biochemistry and Molecular Biology, Indiana University School of Medicine-South Bend, South Bend, IN 46617, USA

Karen D. Cowden Dahl
Harper Cancer Research Institute, South Bend, IN 46617, USA
Department of Biochemistry and Molecular Biology, Indiana University School of Medicine-South Bend, South Bend, IN 46617, USA

Department of Chemistry and Biochemistry, University of Notre Dame, Notre Dame, IN 46617, USA
Indiana University Melvin and Bren Simon Cancer Center, Indianapolis, IN 46202, USA

Subramanyam Dasari and Yiming Fang
Medical Sciences Program, Indiana University School of Medicine, Bloomington, IN 47401, USA

Anirban K. Mitra
Medical Sciences Program, Indiana University School of Medicine, Bloomington, IN 47401, USA
Indiana University Melvin and Bren Simon Cancer Center, Indianapolis, IN 46202, USA
Department of Medical and Molecular Genetics, Indiana University School of Medicine, Indianapolis, IN 46202, USA

Nkechiyere G. Nwani and Livia E. Sima
Department of Obstetrics and Gynecology, Northwestern University, Chicago, IL 60611, USA

Wilberto Nieves-Neira and Daniela Matei
Department of Obstetrics and Gynecology, Northwestern University, Chicago, IL 60611, USA
Robert H. Lurie Comprehensive Cancer Center, Chicago, IL 60611, USA

Index

A

Albumin, 33
Antiapoptotic Protein, 78
Antitumoral Response, 36, 41, 44
Autophosphorylation, 7, 9

B

Basement Membrane, 75, 77, 151, 186, 191-192
Bevacizumab, 39, 80, 91-92, 207, 209, 218-219
Bisphosphonate, 20, 28

C

Carcinogenesis, 3, 5-8, 10, 12, 15, 17, 81-82, 85, 114, 137, 142, 145, 155, 159, 177-178, 184, 194, 199, 201, 215-216
Cell Activating Factor, 31
Cell Proliferation, 2, 5, 8-9, 12, 15-17, 20, 28, 33, 43, 45-46, 49, 56, 62, 64, 72, 84, 86-87, 92, 96, 99, 104, 112, 123, 126, 144, 151, 158-159, 167, 173, 175, 192-193, 203-207, 211, 213, 216
Chronic Inflammation, 64-65, 67-70, 82, 124, 193
Cilengitide, 211, 220
Cisplatin, 17, 62, 74, 78-80, 88-89, 91, 97-98, 108, 119, 135, 147, 168, 170-171, 175-176, 181-182, 184, 199, 206, 217
Collagen, 78, 107, 151, 156, 203
Colony Stimulating Factor, 43
Cyclooxygenase, 43, 56-57, 66, 83, 87, 89, 92, 107, 125, 194

D

Deep Infiltrating Endometriosis, 121, 125
Dendritic Cell, 40, 54, 56, 63, 202
Diaminobenzidine, 30-31

E

Endometrial Cancer, 1-3, 6, 9, 13-17, 68, 82-83
Epinephrine, 20, 28, 31
Epithelial Cell, 19, 21, 31, 135, 144-147, 192, 214
Epithelial Hyperplasia, 131
Estrogen Receptor, 2, 14, 123-124, 130, 135, 141-142
Eukaryotic Initiation Factors, 10
Everdimus, 171, 176
Exosome, 49

F

Fibronectin, 76, 78, 99, 106-107, 109, 151, 157, 160, 193, 198, 204-205, 209-210, 220-221

G

Gene Ontology, 23, 31
Granulocyte Macrophage, 43, 65
Gynecological Cancer, 1, 3, 5, 8-9, 13-14

H

Hyaluronic Acid, 167

I

Immunohistochemistry, 6, 30-32, 122, 130, 168, 170
Interleukin, 9, 13, 19, 31, 33, 43, 50, 62, 65, 81-86, 88, 90-91, 109, 124-125, 140, 193, 197, 203, 207, 215

L

Laminin, 76, 78, 151, 205
Lysophosphatidic, 81, 86-87, 89-90, 97, 157, 182, 205, 215

M

Macrophage, 9, 19-20, 23, 25-26, 28-29, 31-34, 37, 43, 65, 71, 81-83, 88, 90, 123-124, 141, 160, 194, 213
Mammalian Target of Rapamycin, 7, 140
Migration Inhibitory Factor, 19, 31, 33, 71, 86
Myeloma Cells, 78, 91

N

Natural Killer Cell, 60, 157
Neoantigen, 36, 38-42, 51, 53, 58, 212, 223
Neutrophil-activating Peptide, 19, 31
Neutrophils, 65-66, 69, 75, 194, 201, 215

O

Overall Survival, 1, 26, 30-31, 42-44, 47-48, 80, 97, 104-105, 107-108, 117-118, 162, 171, 173-174, 206-207, 209, 211, 213, 222

P

Paclitaxel, 33, 54, 61-62, 74, 78-80, 88, 91-92, 159, 165, 168, 170-172, 175, 179, 181, 200, 202, 207, 209, 218-219
Pathophysiology, 5, 13, 82, 87, 141, 157
Peritoneum, 66-67, 75-76, 108-109, 118, 124, 142, 149-151, 157, 178, 188, 203, 211
Phosphoinositide, 5, 7, 89
Phosphorylation, 5, 8-9, 13, 15-16, 34, 68, 71-74, 77, 80, 98, 107, 113, 140, 171, 174-175, 182, 195, 205, 210-211, 221
Plasminogen Activator, 10, 66, 77, 206
Platelet-derived Growth Factor, 19-20, 28, 31, 33-34, 186-188, 204, 217
Polycystic Ovarian Syndrome, 67, 69, 82

Pro-inflammatory Cytokine, 19-20, 28, 80

Prognostic Factor, 62, 90, 107, 117, 119, 137, 159

Progression-free Survival, 26, 30-31, 37, 42, 48, 60, 168, 171, 173-174, 207, 209

Prostaglandins, 64, 66, 69, 72, 74

Prostate Cancer, 5, 12, 34, 79-80, 97, 108, 116, 118, 188, 198

Protein-protein Interaction, 29, 32, 116, 211

Pyruvate Dehydrogenase Kinase, 7

R

Reactive Oxygen Species, 48, 64, 69, 84, 87, 90-91, 115, 186, 191, 205

Retrograde Menstruation, 67, 69, 122, 130, 140

S

Spheroid Formation, 167, 171-172, 175

Stem Cell Maintenance, 167, 169, 175-176, 202

T

Temsirolimus, 2-3

Threonine Kinase, 5, 12, 77, 121

Tissue Homeostasis, 64-65, 192, 205

Transferrin Receptor, 19, 32

Transgenic Mouse Model, 171, 187, 206

Tumor Initiation, 62, 69, 71, 79, 81, 131, 166-167, 169, 202, 205

Tumor Necrosis Factor, 32, 43, 65, 82-83, 85, 88, 91, 99, 124-125, 142, 203

Tumor-infiltrating Lymphocytes, 53, 56-57, 60, 221

Tyrosine Kinase Receptor, 167

V

Vascular Endothelial Growth Factor, 5-9, 19, 32-33, 43, 58, 61, 71, 86, 88-89, 96, 112, 122, 188, 204-205, 207, 218-219

Z

Zoledronic Acid, 19-20, 25, 29, 31-32, 34